T0174635

The Digital Divide

This book provides an in-depth comparative analysis of inequality and the stratification of the digital sphere.

Grounded in classical sociological theories of inequality, as well as empirical evidence, this book defines "the digital divide" as the unequal access and utility of internet communications technologies and explores how it has the potential to replicate existing social inequalities, as well as create new forms of stratification. *The Digital Divide* examines how various demographic and socio-economic factors including income, education, age and gender, as well as infrastructure, products and services affect how the internet is used and accessed. Comprised of six parts, the first section examines theories of the digital divide, and then looks in turn at:

- Highly developed nations and regions (including the USA, the EU and Japan);
- Emerging large powers (Brazil, Russia, India, China);
- Eastern European countries (Estonia, Romania, Serbia);
- Arab and Middle Eastern nations (Egypt, Iran, Israel);
- Under-studied areas (East and Central Asia, Latin America, and sub-Saharan Africa).

Providing an interwoven analysis of the international inequalities in internet usage and access, this important work offers a comprehensive approach to studying the digital divide around the globe. It is an important resource for academics and students in sociology, social policy, communication studies, media studies and all those interested in the questions and issues around social inequality.

Massimo Ragnedda teaches Mass Communications at Northumbria University, UK. Previously he was an affiliated visitor at the Department of Sociology, University of Cambridge, UK and in 2011 he was Academic Visiting at the Oxford Internet Institute, University of Oxford, UK.

Glenn W. Muschert is Associate Professor in the Sociology, Criminology, and Social Justice Studies Programs at Miami University, USA.

Routledge Advances in Sociology

For a full list of titles in this series please visit: www.routledge.com/books/series/SE0511

Play, Creativity, and Social Movements
If I can't dance, it's not my revolution
Benjamin Shepard

Undocumented Workers' Transitions
Legal status, migration, and work in Europe
Sonia McKay, Eugenia Markova and Anna Paraskevopoulou

The Marketing of War in the Age of Neo-Militarism
Edited by Kostas Gouliamos and Christos Kassimeris

Neoliberalism and the Global Restructuring of Knowledge and Education
Steven C. Ward

Social Theory in Contemporary Asia
Ann Brooks

Foundations of Critical Media and Information Studies
Christian Fuchs

A Companion to Life Course Studies
The social and historical context of the British birth cohort studies
Michael Wadsworth and John Bynner

Understanding Russianness
Risto Alapuro, Arto Mustajoki and Pekka Pesonen

Understanding Religious Ritual
Theoretical approaches and innovations
John Hoffmann

Online Gaming in Context
The social and cultural significance of online games
Garry Crawford, Victoria K. Gosling and Ben Light

Contested Citizenship in East Asia
Developmental politics, national unity, and globalization
Kyung-Sup Chang and Bryan S. Turner

Agency without Actors?
New approaches to collective action
Edited by Jan-Hendrik Passoth, Birgit Peuker and Michael Schillmeier

The Neighborhood in the Internet
Design research projects in community informatics
John M. Carroll

Managing Overflow in Affluent Societies
Edited by Barbara Czarniawska and Orvar Löfgren

Refugee Women
Beyond gender versus culture
Leah Bassel

Socioeconomic Outcomes of the Global Financial Crisis
Theoretical discussion and empirical case studies
Edited by Ulrike Schuerkens

The Digital Divide

The internet and social inequality in international perspective

Edited by
Massimo Ragnedda and
Glenn W. Muschert

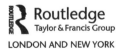

Routledge
Taylor & Francis Group

LONDON AND NEW YORK

First published 2013
by Routledge
2 Park Square, Milton Park, Abingdon, Oxon, OX14 4RN

Simultaneously published in the USA and Canada
by Routledge
711 Third Avenue, New York, NY 10017

Routledge is an imprint of the Taylor & Francis Group, an informa business

British Library Cataloguing in Publication Data
A catalogue record for this book is available from the British Library

Library of Congress Cataloging in Publication Data
The digital divide : the Internet and social inequality in
international perspective / edited by Massimo Ragnedda and
Glenn W. Muschert.
pages cm. -- (Routledge advances in sociology ; 73)
1. Digital divide. 2. Information society. 3. Equality. I. Ragnedda,
Massimo, 1976- II. Muschert, Glenn W.
HM851.D52444 2013
302.23'1--dc23
2012046956

ISBN: 978-0-415-52544-2 (hbk)
ISBN: 978-0-203-06976-9 (ebk)

Typeset in Baskerville
by Saxon Graphics Ltd, Derby

Contents

Author biographies   viii
Preface   xviii

Introduction   1
MASSIMO RAGNEDDA AND GLENN W. MUSCHERT

SECTION 1
Theories of the digital divide   15

1 The reproduction and reconfiguration of inequality:
Differentiation and class, status and power in the
dynamics of digital divides   17
BRIDGETTE WESSELS

2 A theory of the digital divide   29
JAN A.G.M. VAN DIJK

SECTION 2
Highly developed nations and regions   53

3 The digital divide in Europe   55
NICOLE ZILLIEN AND MIRKO MARR

4 The Internet and social inequalities in the U.S.   67
JAMES WITTE, MARISSA KISS AND RANDY LYNN

5 Missing in the midst of abundance: The case of
broadband adoption in Japan   85
MITO AKIYOSHI, MOTOHIRO TSUCHIYA AND TAKAKO SANO

SECTION 3
Rapidly developing large nations – the BRIC nations   105

6   The digital divide in Brazil: Conceptual, research and
    policy challenges   107
    BERNARDO SORJ

7   Digitizing Russia: The uneven pace of progress toward
    ICT equality   118
    INNA F. DEVIATKO

8   The digital divide in India: Inferences from the
    information and communication technology
    workforce   134
    P. VIGNESWARA ILAVARASAN

9   The digital divide in China, Hong Kong and Taiwan:
    The barriers of first order and second order digital
    divide   147
    SHU-FEN TSENG AND YU-CHING YOU

SECTION 4
Eastern Europe   165

10 The Internet and digital divide in South Eastern
    Europe: Connectivity does not end the digital divide,
    skills do   167
    DANICA RADOVANOVIĆ

11 Closing the gap, are we there yet?: Reflections on the
    persistence of second-level digital divide among
    adolescents in Central and Eastern Europe   179
    MONICA BARBOVSCHI AND BIANCA BALEA

12 Behind the slogan of "e-State": Digital stratification
    in Estonia   193
    VERONIKA KALMUS, KAIRI TALVES AND
    PILLE PRUULMANN-VENGERFELDT

SECTION 5
The Middle East region 207

13 Digitally divided we stand: The contribution of digital
media to the Arab Spring 209
DAVID M. FARIS

14 Explaining digital inequalities in Israel: Juxtaposing
the conflict and cultural perspectives 222
GUSTAVO MESCH, ILAN TALMUD AND TANYA KOLOBOV

15 An analysis of the second-level digital divide in Iran:
A case study of University of Tehran undergraduate
students 237
HAMID ABDOLLAHYAN, MEHDI SEMATI AND MOHAMMAD AHMADI

SECTION 6
Under-studied countries and regions 251

16 The digital divide in the Latin American context 253
DANIELA TRUCCO

17 The Central Asian digital divide 270
BARNEY WARF

18 The double digital divide and social inequality in Asia:
Comparative research on Internet cafes in Taiwan,
Singapore, Thailand, and the Philippines 285
TOMOHISA HIRATA

19 Dimensions of the mobile divide in Niger 297
GADO ALZOUMA

*Afterword: Internet freedom, nuanced digital divides, and
the Internet craftsman* 309
SASCHA D. MEINRATH, JAMES LOSEY AND BENJAMIN LENNETT

Index 316

Author biographies

Hamid Abdollahyan is an Associate Professor of Communication at the Department of Communication, Faculty of Social Sciences, University of Tehran, Iran. His research interests include new media and cultural differences, media and the public sphere, cultural studies and the generation gap, consumer culture and the automobile industry, research methods in communications studies, comparative dimensions of sociology, communication and history, historical sociology, social networking, human-computer interaction, the Internet world and its problematic for science. His writing includes the books *Conceptualization of reality in historical sociology: Narrating absentee-landlordism in Iran* (2004) and *Comparative Perspectives in Sociology, Anthropology and Communication* (2008). He has also published a number of articles in journals such as *Alternate Routes, Critique; Critical Middle Eastern Studies, WeltTrends, Asian Journal of Social Sciences, Journal of Media and Religion, Iranian Social Science Letter, Communication and Culture, Global Media Journal,* and in *Women's Studies*. He has done extensive research on the generation gap in Iran and his latest research reports came out in spring 2005, spring 2006 and spring 2007. He is currently working on theoretical dimensions of the Internet and pathology. He has also worked on comparative aspects of university professors' work load versus salaries.

Mohammad Ahmadi is a PhD student in the Department of Media and Communication Studies at the University of Tehran. His research interests include areas of digital literacy, digital divide and new media. He has published articles in these fields in scholarly journals such as *Amity Journal of Media and Communication Studies*.

Mito Akiyoshi is a professor in the Department of Sociology at Senshu University. Professor Akiyoshi has written and lectured widely on social implications of information and communication technologies. Her publications include "The diffusion of mobile Internet in Japan" (with Hiroshi Ono, *Information Society* 24(5)) and "Les Japonais en ligne: Le prisme des générations et des classes sociales" (*Hermès* 55).

Gado Alzouma is Associate Professor of Anthropology at the American University of Nigeria (AUN), Yola. He did his undergraduate and graduate studies in France (Bordeaux and Strasbourg). He also is the holder of a PhD in Anthropology from Southern Illinois University, Carbondale, USA. Before joining AUN, he was Assistant Professor at the Department of Sociology, Abdou Moumouni University, Niamey, Niger. His research and publications focus on information and communication technologies for development. He is the author of several papers in refereed journals. *Contact:* American University of Nigeria, Lamido Zubairu Way, Yola By-Pass, Yola, Adamawa, Nigeria Email: Alzouma@aaun.edu.ng

Bianca Balea (PhD) got her doctoral degree in November 2012 with a thesis on "Digital inequalities among children" at the Faculty of Sociology and Social Work, Babeş-Bolyai University, Cluj-Napoca, Romania. Since September 2011 she has been a member of the EU Kids Online project with the Romanian team. Her current research interests are new media and society, social and digital inequalities, and children's use of new digital technologies.

Monica Barbovschi is a postdoctoral fellow at the Institute for Research of Children, Youth and Family (Masaryk University, Brno, Czech Republic) and an associated researcher at the Institute of Sociology, Romanian Academy. Her research interests are at the intersection between sociology of childhood and children's rights, and are currently materialised into projects related to children's Internet and mobile Internet use. She is the contact person for Romania in the EU Kids Online Project (EC Safer Internet Programme).

Inna F. Deviatko is Professor of Sociology at the National Research University Higher School of Economics where she is Head of the Department of Analysis of Social Institutions. She has also been the editor-in-chief of *Sociology: Methodology, Methods, Mathematical Modeling*, an academic peer-reviewed journal since 2010. Her current research interests include classical and contemporary sociological theory and sociological methodology (including online research methods). Her main books are *Diagnostic procedure in sociology: An essay on history and theory* (1993); *Models of explanation and logic of sociological research* (1996); *Sociological theories of agency and practical rationality* (2003); and *Methods of sociological research*, 6th Edition (2010).

David M. Faris is Assistant Professor of Political Science and Director of International Studies at Roosevelt University. He is the author of *Dissent and revolution in a digital age: Social media, blogging and activism in Egypt* (IB Tauris and Co., 2012). His work has appeared in *Arab Media & Society*, *Middle East Policy*, *Politique Etrangere*, as well as in *The Routledge Participatory Cultures Handbook*. Faris also serves as Strategy Group

Advisor for the Meta-Activism Project (MAP), which seeks to build foundational knowledge about digital activism. He has also written for the *Christian Science Monitor,* NPR.org, *The Daily News Egypt, The Philadelphia City Paper,* and *Insights on Law and Society.*

Tomohisa Hirata is a postdoctoral fellow of JSPS in Kyoto University. He is a member of the External Committee of the Society of Socio-Informatics and was previously a member of the Research Committee of the Japan Society for Socio-Information Studies. His recent research is to clarify the relation between Internet uses in Asian countries and their cultural backgrounds by focusing on Internet cafes from the perspectives of theoretical sociology, anthropology, and human geography.

P. Vigneswara Ilavarasan (PhD-IIT Kanpur) is Associate Professor at the Department of Management Studies, Indian Institute of Technology, Delhi. He teaches and researches social aspects of production and consumption of information and communication technologies in India. Research areas include labor process in software work, small software firms and inter-firm linkages, labor segmentation in the ICT workforce, research and development centers of ICT multinationals in India, use of ICTs by urban micro-entrepreneurs, ICT clusters and electronic governance. His works have appeared in the leading international and national journals. He is the recipient of the Prof. M. N. Srinivas Memorial Prize, 2009 of the Indian Sociological Society and the Abdul Al Sagar Outstanding Young Faculty Fellowship at the Indian Institute of Technology Delhi, New Delhi. Further details are at: http://www.tinyurl.com/vigneswara

Veronika Kalmus is Professor of Media Studies at the Institute of Journalism and Communication, University of Tartu. Her research interests are socialization and inter-generational relationships in the emerging information society, and value change in transition culture. She leads the research project Generations and Inter-Generational Relations in the Emerging Information Society and participates in several national and international projects, including EU Kids Online. She has published extensively in international journals, for instance, *Childhood, Children & Society, Cyberpsychology, Discourse & Society, East European Politics and Societies, Journal of Baltic Studies, Journal of Children and Media, Journal of Computer-Mediated Communication* and *Young.*

Marissa Kiss is a research analyst at National Opinion Research Center (NORC) at the University of Chicago. Kiss has over five years of experience performing data collection management tasks and delivery activities including training materials development, field interviewer training, instrument testing, data coding and analysis, and data delivery for various large scale, multi-level research projects. Ms. Kiss recently completed writing her master's thesis on social inequalities in Internet use at George Mason University.

Tanya Kolobov is a PhD student in the Department of Sociology at the University of Haifa (Israel). Her research interests are medical sociology, inequalities in access to health and medical information and the effects of information and communication technologies on changes in patients' and physicians' interactions.

Benjamin Lennett, Policy Director for the Open Technology Institute at the New America Foundation, contributes to the program's efforts to develop and advocate policy proposals aimed at achieving universal and affordable broadband access through policy research, writing, and outreach. Prior to joining New America, Mr. Lennett served as Associate Communications and Development Manager for the Media Access Project, where he managed outreach and fundraising efforts. Mr. Lennett holds a Bachelor's Degree in Political Science from the University of Florida. He is also a graduate of American University's School of Public Affairs, where he received a Master's Degree in Public Policy, with a concentration in economic and regulatory policy.

James Losey is a fellow with the Open Technology Institute at the New America Foundation. He focuses on communications and digital divide issues in the United States and Europe. Mr. Losey has published articles and chapters with *Advances in Computing, Ars Technica, CommLaw Conspectus, IEEE Internet Computing, IEEE Spectrum,* and *Slate.* Prior to joining New America, Mr. Losey worked with Citizens for Responsibility and Ethics in Washington and interned in the Office of Congressman Donald J. Cazayoux (D-LA). Before coming to Washington, D.C., Mr. Losey was a sound engineer and youth mentor at Verge Concerts. Mr. Losey graduated from the University of California, Berkeley with a BA in interdisciplinary studies with a research focus on the relationship between power and the media. His undergraduate thesis discussed the dilemma created by the different definitions of truth used in political and press fields.

Randy Lynn is a PhD candidate in the Department of Sociology and Anthropology at George Mason University. Mr. Lynn has an MA in Sociology from the University of Missouri-St. Louis, and is currently a Presidential Scholar research assistant at the George Mason University Center for Social Science Research. His research examines the intersections of youth, education, digital technologies, and social networks.

Mirko Marr is Head of Market and Media Research at Publicitas, a leading sales house for print and digital media in Switzerland, and board member of IAB-Switzerland. He earned his PhD in communications from the University of Zurich with his dissertation on the consequences of the digital divide. His current research is focused on convergent media use and its implications for the media and advertising industry as well as for the methodology of audience research.

Sascha Meinrath is Vice President of the New America Foundation and Director of the Open Technology Institute. In 2012 he was named one of the top 100 in *Newsweek*'s Digital Power Index and he has been described as a "community Internet pioneer" and an "entrepreneurial visionary." He is a well-known expert on community wireless networks, municipal broadband, and telecommunications policy. In 2009 he was named one of *Ars Technica*'s Tech Policy "people to watch" and is also the 2009 recipient of the Public Knowledge IP3 Award for excellence in public interest advocacy. Sascha founded the Commotion Wireless Project (a.k.a., the "Internet-in-a-suitcase") and, along with Vint Cerf, is the co-founder of Measurement Lab (M-Lab), a distributed server platform for researchers around the world to deploy Internet measurement tools, advance network research, and empower the public with useful information about their broadband connections. He coordinates the Open Source Wireless Coalition, a global partnership of wireless integrators, researchers, implementers and companies dedicated to the development of open source, interoperable, low-cost wireless technologies. Sascha has worked with Free Press, the Cooperative Association for Internet Data Analysis (CAIDA), the Acorn Active Media Foundation, the Ethos Group, and the CUWiN Foundation. He blogs regularly at www.saschameinrath.com

Gustavo S. Mesch is a professor at the Department of Sociology, University of Haifa (Israel). His research interests are Internet and social media effects on society, the diffusion of information and communication technologies and youth media use. He served as the Chair of the Communication and Information Technologies Section of the American Sociological Association and is currently a member of the Board of Directors of the Israel Internet Association.

Glenn W. Muschert is Associate Professor in the Sociology, Criminology, and Social Justice Studies Programs at Miami University. He received his PhD in Sociology from the University of Colorado at Boulder in 2002, and has been in his current position since 2003. Glenn's areas of scholarly interest lie in the sociological study of crime and social problems, including the mass media framing of high profile crimes, school shootings, missing persons, and social control through surveillance technologies. He has published various materials in the fields of sociology, criminology, and media studies.

Pille Pruulmann-Vengerfeldt is Associate Professor at the Institute of Journalism and Communication, University of Tartu. She also works in the Estonian National Museum. Her research interests focus on Internet user typologies and user-friendly online spaces as possible venues for participation. Her practical interests are mostly focused on public engagement and user participation in public institutions and politics. She is the leader of the research project Developing Museum Communication in the 21st Century Information Environment and is participating in several national and international projects. She has recently published in *Journal of Baltic Studies*, *Journal of Computer-Mediated Communication* and *Journal of Children and Media*.

Danica Radovanović is a digital media specialist, and internet researcher at the Belgrade Center for Digital Humanities. She will have defended her dissertation on social media dynamics and communication practices within internet communities at the University of Belgrade in 2013. She was a Chevening PhD scholar (2009/2010) at the Oxford Internet Institute, University of Oxford. Danica worked for the United Nations (FAO) as an information management specialist on an international project on technology, science and education. She has published extensively in the fields of internet studies, social media, digital divide, and new communication practices in academic journals, and in print and online media: Index on Censorship, Global Voices Online, Scientific American, Australian Science. Danica blogs at: http://www.danicar.org/ and tweets @DanicaR.

Massimo Ragnedda, teaches mass communications at Northumbria University (UK). In the academic year 2006/2007 he was an affiliated visitor at the Department of Sociology, University of Cambridge (UK) and in 2011 he was Academic Visiting Scholar at the Oxford Internet Institute (University of Oxford, UK). He has a strong interest in developments in new media and theories of media, communication and culture. His recent research interests include digital divide and social media research; and focusing on the stratification in the access and use of the Internet. In particular he is interested in the new digital exclusion in a society of information, where having or not having access to information and the new public sphere may create new forms of digital inequalities. He is the author of five books and several articles in Italian, English and Spanish.

Takako Sano is Senior Researcher of the Institute for Information and Communications Policy, Ministry of Internal Affairs and Communications. She graduated from the Graduate School of Saitama University for Policy Sciences in 1993. She has been working at the Ministry of Internal Affairs and Communications since 1988, including a stint at the Institute for Posts and Telecommunication Policy Study.

Mehdi Semati is Professor of Communication at Northern Illinois University. His writings on international communication, cultural politics of globalization, Muslims and the Middle East in Western popular and political imagination, and Iranian media and culture have appeared in various scholarly journals. His books include *Media, culture, and society in Iran: living with globalization and the Islamic state* (Routledge, 2007), *New frontiers in international communication theory* (Rowman and Littlefield, 2004), and *Studies in terrorism: Media scholarship and enigma of terror* (Southbound, 2003). His Persian writings include *The age of CNN and Hollywood: National interests, transnational communication* (Nashr-e Nay, 2006).

Bernardo Sorj, (www.bernardosorj.com), is Director of the Edelstein Center for Social Research. He was Visiting Professor in several universities in Europe, United States and Latin America and is a retired professor of sociology from the Federal University of Rio de Janeiro. He is Director of Plataforma Democrática (www.plataformademocratica. org) and coordinator of the *Scielo Social Sciences English Edition* (http:// socialsciences.scielo.org/scielo.php/lng_es). He is the author of 27 books and more than a hundred articles published in several languages related to the impact of new technologies, the international system, contemporary social theory, and Latin American development. His recent books on the information society include *Brazil@digitaldivide: Confronting inequality in the information society* (UNESCO, 2003), *Internet y pobreza* (UNESCO/ Ediciones Trilce, 2005), and *Information societies and digital divides: An introduction* (Polimetrica, 2008).

Ilan Talmud is an associate professor at the Department of Sociology and Anthropology, University of Haifa (Israel). His research interests include economic sociology, network models of social structure, Internet research, youth online, technology and social structure, and the social organization of venture capital.

Kairi Talves is a researcher at the Institute of Sociology and Social Policy, University of Tartu. Currently she is working on her PhD thesis in sociology, focusing on the influence of flexible labor practices on work-life balance, proceeding from the conflict paradigm. Her main fields of research are related to gender studies, more specifically to labor force involvement, work-life balance and gender stratification of societies. She has participated in several international research projects tackling gender inequalities. She has published a number of research papers in international and national academic journals and chapters in edited volumes.

Daniela Trucco is a sociologist from the Pontificia Universidad Católica de Chile with a Master's Degree in Public Policy and Business Administration from the University of Maryland, U.S.A. Her professional experience has concentrated on research and social policy advisory, particularly in the education field. Currently, she is a social affairs officer, from the Social Development Division in UN-ECLAC, where she actively participates in the project Alliance for the Information Society (@LIS2) financed by the European Union, focusing on the research area of ICT and education.

Shu-Fen Tseng is Associate Professor in the Graduate Program of Social Informatics at Yuan Ze University, Taiwan. She earned her PhD in Sociology from the University of Illinois, Chicago. Her research interests include social informatics, digital divide and social media research. Her current research focuses on the use of social media and its implication for reputation management and social capital.

Motohiro Tsuchiya is Professor of the Graduate School of Media and Governance and Deputy Director of the Global Security Research Institute (G-SEC) at Keio University in Japan. Prior to joining the Keio faculty, he was Associate Professor at the Center for Global Communications (GLOCOM), International University of Japan. He researched in Washington, DC, as a visiting scholar at the Center for International Development and Conflict Management (CIDCM), University of Maryland, and at the Cyberspace Policy Institute (CPI), George Washington University. From March 2008 to March 2009 he was a visiting scholar at the MIT (Massachusetts Institute of Technology) Center for International Studies. He is interested in the impact of the information revolution on international relations; regulations regarding telecommunications and the Internet; and global governance and information technologies. He is also a member of the Information Security Policy Council of the Japanese government. He authored *Information and global governance* (Tokyo: Keio University Press, 2001, in Japanese), *Net Politics* (Tokyo: Iwanami Publishing, 2003, in Japanese), *Network power* (Tokyo: NTT Publishing, 2007, in Japanese), *Intelligence and national security* (Tokyo: Keio University Press, 2007, in Japanese), *Network hegemony* (Tokyo: NTT Publishing, 2011, in Japanese), *Cyber terrorism* (Tokyo: Bungei Shunju, 2012, in Japanese), and co-authored *Cybersecurity: Public sector threats and responses* (Boca Raton, FL, US: CRC Press, 2012) and 20 other books. He earned his BA in political science, an MA in international relations, and a PhD in Media and Governance from Keio University.

Jan A.G.M. van Dijk is Professor of Communication Science and the Sociology of the Information Society at the University of Twente, the Netherlands. Van Dijk has been investigating the social aspects of information and communication technology since 1984. His key publication is *De netwerkmaatschappij* (first edition 1991), in English: *The network society* in three editions (1999, 2006 and 2012). Other books in English are *Digital democracy* (2000), *Information and communication technology in organizations* (2005) and *The deepening divide: Inequality in the* *information society* (2005), all Sage Publications. Van Dijk is an advisor to, among others, the European Commission. Personal website: http://www.gw.utwente.nl/vandijk

Barney Warf is Professor of Geography at the University of Kansas. His research interests are diverse, but focus largely on the geographies of services, telecommunications, the Internet, and time-space compression as viewed through the conceptual lenses of social theory and political economy. He is the author of several books and more than a hundred journal articles.

Bridgette Wessels is Director of the Centre of Interdisciplinary Research in Socio-Digital Worlds and is Senior Lecturer in Sociology at the University of Sheffield. She has conducted funded research that addresses digital technology in public services, everyday life, public spheres, new media, and identity. She was an expert on the EU Fifth Framework IST programme, OST/DTI and the Royal Society cybertrust programmes and is an expert for the EU on the social web and communication in Europe. Her current projects are: Mainstreaming Telehealth (ESRC and TSB); Participating in Search Design: A Study of George Thomason's Newsbooks (AHRC); Augmenting Participation in the Arts (DCMS and KT). Her books include *Inside the digital revolution: Policing and changing communication with the public* (Ashgate, 2007); *Information and joining up services: The case of an information guide for parents of disabled children* (Policy Press, 2002); *Understanding the Internet: A socio-cultural perspective* (Palgrave, 2010), and *The cultural dynamics of the innovation of new media: The case of telematics* (VDM Verlag). She has published on digital services in journals such as *New Media and Society*, *The Information Society*, and the *Journal of Computer Supported Communication*.

James Witte is a professor of sociology and Director of the George Mason University Center for Social Science Research (CSSR). Witte is a past chair of the Communications and Information Technology section of the American Sociological Association (CITASA). Witte is the author of two books, *The Internet and social inequalities* (Routledge, 2010) and *Labor force integration and marital choice* (Westview, 1992). In 2009, Witte was the guest editor for a special edition of *Sociological methods and research* on web based survey research. Professor Witte holds a PhD in Sociology from Harvard University. He was previously on the faculty of Northwestern University and received postdoctoral training in demography from the University of North Carolina at Chapel Hill.

Yu-Ching You is a PhD candidate in sociology at National Taiwan University. Her research interests include non-standard employment, social inequality and mobility. Her current research is focused on digital inequality and exclusion, and the relationship between the Internet and social inequality.

Nicole Zillien (PhD) is Assistant Professor in the Department of Sociology at the University of Trier, Germany. Her current research interests include media sociology, society and technology, the digital divide, social inequalities, science communication and health-related Internet use. Her publications have appeared in numerous books and peer-reviewed journals. She has currently published a book on information justice (together with André Schüller-Zwierlein) and is writing a textbook on knowledge gap research (forthcoming 2014).

Preface

This book is about connecting the fascinating and rapidly-evolving body of multidisciplinary work in Internet studies and the network society with the comparatively long-established body of work in the sociology of stratification. In particular, the goal of the book is to connect studies of digital divides (that is, unequal access to and usage of the digital sphere) with sociological traditions for understanding social stratification (including inequalities in wealth, moral authority, social class, prestige, cultural capital, and political influence). Certainly, numerous sociologists have an on-going contribution to the study of digital divides (indeed, many of them appear in this volume), and we certainly respect the work of the seminal academic figures in the field of digital divides. However, what such studies at times seemed to lack was a theoretical perspective which was strongly tied to classical (and resulting) traditions in the sociology of stratification.

The book emerged from a scholarly discussion between the editors (sociologists who study, among other things, mass media, and social stratification), as to the relative under-emphasis of classical theoretical perspectives among digital divide studies. Of course, many such studies come from scholars outside sociology, in fields such as informatics, mass communications, and information technology; however, it is our sense that sociologists have something uniquely important to contribute to studies of inequality in the network society. Given the foundational role of theories of stratification in the development of sociology from the nineteenth century onward, we were sure that sociology should contribute a strong voice to on-going debates about how digital divides were articulated, and in some cases attenuated or exacerbated, worldwide.

Around the same time that we (the editors) were wondering at the relative underrepresentation of sociologists in this debate concerning the emergent form(s) of inequality in the digital sphere, there appeared a text which applied the classical schools of sociology (Durkheimian, Marxist, and Weberian) to digital inequality in the United States: James Witte and Susan Mannon's (2010) *The Internet and social inequalities*. Indeed, the Witte and Mannon volume served as an approximate point of departure for the volume, as the reading of their volume helped to solidify our sense that the theoretical and empirical approaches of classical sociology had much to say in regards to inequality in the digital sphere. While Witte and Mannon (2010) examined the relevance of this approach to studying digital divides in the United States, another contribution of the volume was that it laid a rough theoretical and empirical groundwork for the application of the approach to other countries or regions of the world. This volume is the outgrowth of our attempt to see an international and comparative examination of digital divides in a variety of settings across the world.

Each of the contributors to this volume was asked to consider Witte and Mannon's (2010) book as a point of departure, and then to add their own interpretations and perspectives to the discussion of digital divides observed within a specific national or regional context. There were very few stipulations placed upon the contributors, as these would not have led to fruitful scholarly exploration and discourse. Thus, contributors were free to select empirical data and one or more theoretical tradition within sociology around which they would center their discussion. The only stipulations we set were that each chapter needed a conceptual connection to a classical tradition of stratification in sociology, and that each chapter should be at least in some way grounded to empirical evidence. Such a loose set of stipulations meant that contributors were free to decide their own conceptual and empirical/analytical strategies, and allowed contributors to be creative and free in their contributions. However, what was gained in the setting of general parameters for contribution is that each of the chapters in this volume honors two crucial aspects of sociology: first, that the discipline is based on the foundational work of its early theorists, and second, that sociology is an empirical discipline. What was also gained was the ability to infer comparisons among the nations and regions studied in the various chapters, as such comparisons can emerge along both the theoretical lines and the empirical approaches employed in the various chapters.

This volume, the outcome of our endeavor, reflects a sociological approach in its analysis of the international connection between the related issues of the social inequalities, and the social consequences of the new digital discrimination in use of new communications technologies. Our volume contributes to the literature by collecting contributions from many different areas of the world and by publishing them in one location. Seeing country/region studies side by side will allow readers to understand the similarities and differences in the digital divide phenomena observed in the three categories of national settings, viewed via a unified lens. In connecting information about these different social and economic areas of the world, previously poorly connected (yet intimately related) aspects of the digital divide can become clear. Our volume integrates the constructionist work on digital divide, policy analysis of new digital discrimination policies, and finally offers an implied forward-looking (and perhaps proscriptive) view of how social scientists and policy analysts can effectively understand and respond to varying forms of new digital inequalities. With expert contributors from a variety of areas of the world and social science disciplines, this book turns a critical eye to the current state of the digital divide and new social inequality practices (and policies), while exploring the lessons learned from successes and failures in international and comparative perspectives. We anticipate that the comparative examination of these dynamics will be helpful to clarify the mechanisms and consequences of the digital divide in a variety of settings.

Introduction

Massimo Ragnedda
Northumbria University

Glenn W. Muschert
Miami University

Defined as stratification in the access and use of the Internet, the so-called digital divide is inevitably tied with the concept of social inequalities (van Dijk, 2005), a classic sociological concept. Strangely, the discipline of sociology has been slow to contribute to the debate on the Internet and social inequalities. This is surprising, because sociology has a long and fruitful tradition of studies in aspects of social inequalities, and because sociology has contributed to the debates about stratification more than any other discipline. Indeed, even if social stratification is a crucial part of all human organization ever observed, it was in the writings of the "fathers of sociology" such as Marx, Weber, and Durkheim, that the study of this topic became more systematic, articulated using concepts that remain with us to this day. It is inevitable therefore, from a sociological point of view, to study the digital divide using these conceptual and analytical tools. Despite this, the phenomenon of the digital divide (a fundamental aspect of social inequity in the information age) has received less sociological attention than it should (though this is changing – see, for example, DiMaggio *et al.*, 2001; Witte and Mannon, 2010; Stern, 2010), at least using the traditions within sociology.

In this volume, the analysis of the digital divide is driven by the sociological perspective(s) and is intended to understand the nature of social inequalities and the new digital discrimination/virtual inequality (Mossberger *et al.*, 2003). However, the sociological dimensions of the digital divide are also explored in comparative perspective, as the reader encounters studies focusing on stratification in the digital sphere, as explored in a variety of national and cultural settings. We are interested in the social consequences of Internet use (Katz and Rice, 2002) and how people's online activities are influenced by socioeconomic background (Zillien and Hargittai, 2009), but also in a comparative global context.

The digital divide is a complex and dynamic phenomenon (van Dijk and Hacker, 2003) and in its simplistic sense, conceptualized as a form of stratification exhibiting itself in unequal access and use of the Internet. This concept is typically measured via access to the Internet (versus non-access), number of sites at which the Internet is accessed, users' skill at using the Internet, amount of time spent online, and the variety of activities carried out digitally. In its many forms, the digital divide has more commonly been conceptualized (and measured) as the differences between those who have access to the web versus those who do not. Clearly, academic research should go beyond just studying access (Castells, 2001; Stanley, 2003) because such a binary classification limits digital divide research (Hargittai, 2002). Certainly those who are completely excluded are at one extreme end of the digital divide, however even among those with web access, there are nuances to the digital divide, ones which add finer gradients to the discussion. Today the biggest concern is not always concerning access, but the divide among information "haves" and "have-nots", resulting from the ways in which people use the Internet (Dobson and Willinsky, 2009; Eshet and Aviram, 2006; Eshet-Alkalai and Chajut, 2009; Hargittai, 2005, 2009; Jenkins *et al.*, 2006; Livingstone and Helsper, 2010; Perez-Tornero, 2004). In other words, differences in digital proficiencies create new inequalities (Gui and Argentin, 2011) and are the main focus of studies of the so-called second-level digital divide (Hargittai, 2002; van Deursen and van Dijk, 2010).

One core theme in the book is to explain how online activities vary according to crucial sociological dimensions, including gender (Bimber, 2000; DiMaggio *et al.*, 2001; Clark and Gorski, 2002a; Cooper and Weaver, 2003; Losh, 2003; Ono and Zavodny, 2003; Cooper, 2006), age/generation (Loges and Jung, 2001; Soker, 2005; Palfrey and Gasser, 2008; Hargittai, 2010), education (Clark and Gorski,, 2001; Attewell, 2001; Clark and Gorski, 2002b), income and social class/caste (Bucy, 2000; Zillien and Hargittai, 2009), country (Chen, 2004; Chinn and Fairlie, 2007), employment, and race/ethnicity (Hoffman and Novak, 2001; Fairlie, 2003; Fairlie, 2004); and, further, to explain the practical consequences of these differences, in terms of social status, power or profit. Where else to find an arsenal of academic concepts to address such dimensions of the digital divide than in sociology? Indeed, a sociological perspective is needed and our goal has been to tie the study of digital divides to the concepts of social inequality and stratification as understood within classical theories of sociology. Stratification studies proceed from a multiplicity of approaches including perspectives of class inequality (Scott, 2000) or other forms of material inequality (Crompton, 1998). For social scientists who study digital divides, it is vital to reframe the crucial concepts as social stratification. In light of social changes and emergent social movements (Therborn, 2000), it can be informative to reframe contemporary studies of the digital sphere within classical perspectives of social stratification, as studied by Marx, Weber and Durkheim.

The Marxist-derived or conflict perspective focuses on the economic aspects of social stratification, and clearly this perspective (and its derivatives) has been most strongly represented in the field of digital divide studies. Classically, Marx describes the ownership of property as the basis of class divisions, and the social stratification as inevitably tied with economic class (1976). The scholars influenced by the Marxist approach to social stratification tend to emphasize the sphere of production in which the ruling class (or bourgeoisie) derives its power from its ownership and control of the forces of production. According to some authors, the Marxist approach is still important in the digital age, particularly after the world economic crisis (Žižek, 2010). Various scholars weigh in on the connection: Graham talks about a digital dark age in which the knowledge economy is seen as alienation (2001). Lauer (2008) argues about the process of alienation in the information economy, while Rey (2012) explains how the social media users are subject to levels of exploitation relatively consistent with industrial capitalism, which is a new iteration of alienation. Similarly, Fuchs in various studies has argued that online advertising is a mechanism by which corporations largely take advantage of Web 2.0 users (Fuchs, 2009, 2010, 2011). Vincent Mosco argued that a Marxist theory of communications should "demonstrate how communication and culture are material practices, how labor and language are mutually constituted, and how communication and information are dialectical instances of the same social activity, the social construction of meaning" (2009, 44). Furthermore a special issue of *tripleC – Open Access Journal for a Global Sustainable Information Society* edited by Fuchs and Mosco (2012) on "Marx is back: The importance of Marxist theory and research for critical communication studies today" shows the enduring importance of a Marxist approach for critical communication studies. This approach is crucial in order to understand the formation of dominant groups in the communications sector and the capital accumulation dynamics that reproduce social inequalities. The digital divide could be seen, in this perspective, as a way in which the social inequalities are (re)produced (not to mention consumed) in the digital age using the new technologies of communication.

The Weberian perspective offers the basis for integrating what have been considered, up to now, divergent approaches to stratification studies (Scott, 1996). Social stratification in a Weberian approach comprises three independent factors, each one with its own hierarchy and therefore role in constituting social ranking: economic class, social status (prestige), and political power (party) (Weber, 1947). The main element of his model of social structure is the power, and this is articulated differently than in Marx's work, as class is based on the economic order, which rather than being the totality of social life, is one aspect of life, albeit an important one. The interaction among the three aspects of stratification constitutes the way in which social hierarchies come about. Each of these elements relates to the digital divide, because access to new technologies of communication, digital skills/literacy, and capacity to create income throughout the new technologies all contribute to increased political power, social prestige, and economic influence. The digital divide, according to this approach, creates social inequalities in a new media society, because it influences social status by giving increased prestige to those in positions to use new technologies of communication, mastering new specializations/skills, and increasing the ability of digital literati to create new opportunities to realize their goals in social, political, or economic spheres. In a number of studies in this volume, we observe that the Internet is a powerful tool for indicating and maintaining social status, and such conclusions can be immediately reflective of the Weberian tradition. For example, a clear link emerges between education (a marker of prestige and economic influence) and the ability to transform knowledge (via digital fluency) into social, economic, or political influence.

Finally, the Durkheimian perspective focuses on the importance of the division of labor as the social mechanism that reproduces particular types of social bonds while suppressing others. Specifically Durkheim (1984) conceived two distinct types of inequalities: external inequality (imposed on the individual by the social circumstances of birth) and internal inequality (inequalities based on achieved status or individual talent). Both of those inequalities recur in different ways in the digital age. Durkheim also wrote about the external regulation of social behaviors, via external forces of social control, and the individual's internal integration of a society's norms and values. Thus, social solidarity reflected in the collective social consciousness was a crucial element for any society, one that echoes the underlying moral order which undergirds social coherence. Of course, education was a crucial aspect of the (re)production of the moral order in any society (Durkheim, 1956, 1961), and indeed we find in our studies that the use of information and communication technologies (ICTs) in education is a focus in many settings around the world. The role of digital divides in new forms of education (including lifelong learning) cannot be underestimated, and clearly, these connect readily with the Durkheimian tradition.

Each of the contributing authors have been invited to discuss the phenomenon of the digital divide as related to their chosen countries (or regions) of expertise, using one or more of these sociological perspectives to illustrate the dimensions of social inequalities in digital spheres. Certainly, sociologists are adept at examining inequalities as they exist in the world at large, yet there is much to be learned about how such inequalities exist in the digital world. For example, do the traditional inequalities simply replicate themselves in the digital sphere, or does the digital divide operate under its own dynamics? Similarly, it is unclear whether the digital divide simply exacerbates traditional inequalities, or whether it also includes counter-trends that might mitigate traditional inequalities, even while forming new forms of stratification. Finally, it is unclear whether inequalities in the digital world translate culturally, or whether they manifest themselves in culturally-specific ways. Such comparative perspectives have also been underemphasized in the scholarly discourse about the digital divide, and this under-emphasis leads to gaps in our understanding of the digital divide, as social inequalities may vary widely from country to country. This volume is a first step at addressing this gap.

Organization of the book

In *The Internet and social inequalities*, Witte and Mannon (2010) present a theoretical perspective for understanding the digital divide, and the contributors to this volume have used Witte and Mannon's theoretical and empirical approaches as points of departure for their own examinations of the digital divide in their respective settings. From this unified perspective, the book proceeds with an introductory section, a theoretical section to provide the conceptual framework for the volume, and five region-focused sections: the first including case studies examining the digital divide in highly modernized countries (the EU, the USA, and Japan), the second in rapidly emerging world powers (Brazil, Russia, India, and China), the third Eastern European countries (Romania, Estonia, and Serbia), the fourth examining Middle Eastern countries (Israel, Egypt, and Iran), and the fifth focusing on less developed countries, especially areas that have received little study thus far (Latin America, the Former Soviet Republics of Central Asia, countries in East Asia, and Niger).

Theoretical section

The first part of this book provides a theoretical starting point for the volume, by exploring the digital divide as academic concepts within stratified societies. In the first chapter, entitled "The reproduction and reconfiguration of inequality: Differentiation and class, status and power in the dynamics of digital divides," Bridgette Wessels integrates the study of digital divides with the sociology of stratification from the founding fathers of sociology, who in the nineteenth and early twentieth centuries grappled with the revolutionary changes of industrialization. Although in different ways, she argues that class, status and power are key factors in people's ability to be included in a networked society.

In the second chapter, entitled "A theory of the digital divide," Jan van Dijk describes the way in which four types of access to digital media are distributed among people with different social positions and/or personal characteristics. Here, the digital divide is analyzed in the context of the network society in which structural inequality is potentially growing between the information elite, a participating majority, and those who are excluded, as these three segments of society have differential opportunities for connecting to the network.

Section 2: Highly developed nations and regions

The second section concentrates on digital divides in highly developed nations and regions, specifically the EU, the US, and Japan. In the opening chapter of Section 2, entitled "The digital divide in Europe," Nicole Zillien and Mirko Marr base their analysis on the countries of the European Union (with particular focus on Germany) showing how high status users succeed in utilizing the Internet to increase existing resources supporting the notion that the digital divide is an important new dimension of social inequality.

In the fourth chapter, entitled "The Internet and social inequalities in the U.S.," James Witte, Marissa Kiss, and Randy Lynn consider whether the gaps in Internet use according to income and education have persisted, increased, or decreased as widely-used Internet applications and devices have become ubiquitous. In the concluding chapter of Section 2, "Missing in the midst of abundance: The case of broadband adoption in Japan," Mito Akiyoshi, Motohiro Tsuchiya and Takako Sano discuss empirically and theoretically the digital divide as it exhibits itself in Japan, using high quality data made available by the Ministry of International Affairs and Communications. It specifically focuses on the issues concerning broadband and mobile Internet access and user and examines what demographic and social-economic factors suppress the adoption of broadband technologies.

Section 3: Rapidly developing large nations – the BRIC nations

In this section, the digital divide is analyzed in the rapidly emerging large nations, the so-called BRIC (Brazil, Russia, India and China) nations. In particular, in the first chapter of this section, entitled "The digital divide in Brazil: Conceptual, research and policy challenges," Bernardo Sorj examines how the various levels of access to products, services, and benefits of new ICTs affect different segments of the Brazilian population. This case exemplifies the general argument that, from a policy perspective, the struggle for digital inclusion is a struggle against time. In the second chapter of this section, "Digitizing Russia: The uneven pace of progress toward ICT equality," Inna F. Deviatko addresses major dimensions of Internet-related inequalities in contemporary Russia, including relevant regional, urban/rural, income, gender, education and age-related predictive variables commonly used in order to operationalize differences in socioeconomic positions of individuals and families and, correspondingly, in their access to Internet. The analysis is based on multiple data sources – from 2007–2010 Russian Federal State Statistics Service Household Budget Survey data to Public Opinion Research Foundation (FOM) Internet Use Survey (2002–2011) data, and other opinion and market research data on Internet coverage.

In the eighth chapter, "The digital divide in India: Inferences from the information and communication technology workforce," P. Vigneswara Ilavarasan uses indicators delineated by the International Telecommunications Union (ITU) on core ICT indicators (2010) and by the Organization for Economic Co-operation and Development (OECD) (2011) to measure digital inequalities. The chapter also compares this with the status in 1991 when the national economy was opened for liberalization, providing possible reasons for a shrinking divide in the last two decades. Finally, in the last chapter of this section, Shu-Fen Tseng and Yu-Ching You examine the first and second order digital divides in newly industrialized countries (NICs) such as Hong Kong and Taiwan, and the rapidly developing economy of China. These are compared and tested for the normalization/ stratification hypothesis of Internet penetration. In their chapter entitled "The digital divide in China, Hong Kong and Taiwan: The barriers of first order and second order digital divide," the continuous expansion of ICTs is addressed, and this analysis reveals new disparities, specifically in the second order digital divide – inequality in ICT usage.

Section 4: Eastern Europe

In this section, the analyses of the digital divide are oriented to understand how and if the digital divide is reinforcing or reducing the social inequalities in the former Communist areas, with coverage of Serbia, Romania, Hungary, Poland, Bulgaria, and Estonia. This section opens with a chapter entitled "The Internet and digital divide in South Eastern Europe: Connectivity does not end the digital divide, skills do" in which Danica Radovanović explores the social inequalities not only in the context of technological infrastructure, but examines issues such as literacies (information, digital, media, and network), online social networks, knowledge gaps, and collaborative/non-collaborative practices. The fundamental concept of social stratification is examined from socio-technological and educational perspectives.

Next, Monica Barbovschi and Bianca Balea, present a chapter built on the data from the EU Kids Online II project. This chapter, entitled "Closing the gap, are we there yet? Reflections on the persistence of second-level digital divide among adolescents in Central and Eastern Europe," investigates the differences in digital competencies along the lines of socio-economical dimensions in four countries in the Central and Eastern European region: Romania, Hungary, Bulgaria and Poland. The authors utilize a conflict perspective which emphasizes how Internet use, understood as a package of knowledge and skills, plays an important role in maintaining inequalities.

In the final chapter of this section, entitled "Behind the slogan of 'e-State': Digital stratification in Estonia," Veronika Kalmus, Kairi Talves and Pille Pruulmann-Vengerfeldt demonstrate the shift in the literature to exploring "digital inclusion" and "digital stratification," where qualitative parameters of inclusion/exclusion and ICT use matter. The authors use empirical data from several nationwide quantitative studies carried out in Estonia – a "new" EU member state whose success in information society development is internationally recognized.

Section 5: The Middle East region

In this section the authors examine the digital divide in the Middle East region. We have invited scholars from Egypt, Israel, and Iran with the aim of covering these three important countries: the first chapter was written after the revolt that culminated with the resignation of Hosni Mubarak, the second chapter analyses the digital divide in Israel, and finally the digital divide is examined in the demographically young (about 70 percent of Iran's population is under the age of 30) and large (with a population of 70 million) country of Iran.

In the first chapter of this section, entitled "Digitally divided we stand: The contribution of digital media to the Arab Spring," David M. Faris presents new data which suggests access to the Internet is still dependent on income and country across the entirety of the Arab world. This inequality undermines the egalitarian potential of online public spheres, while simultaneously empowering a set of actors who are best positioned to take advantage of their privileged access. In Egypt, a group of young, tech-savvy urban elites used the power of digital activism to harness long-simmering resentment against Egyptian state practices. This online movement culminated in the resignation of Hosni Mubarak and the movement of the country toward more democratic and pluralist rule. Faris explains how digital inequalities both at the level of access and at the level of substantive input structured the Egyptian digital activist movement, empowered some Egyptians, and marginalized the voices of other important actors like organized labor.

In the second chapter of this section, "Explaining digital inequalities in Israel: Juxtaposing the conflict and cultural perspectives," Gustavo Mesch, Ilan Talmud and Tanya Kolobov analyze the rapid expansion of Internet adoption and its use, often associated with the formation of social networks, the accumulation of social capital, and increasing wages. Thus, a lack of Internet access seems to reflect other social inequalities, leading to inequality amplification. The authors investigated gaps over time in access and use of the Internet in Israel, moving from the central assumption that in deeply divided societies where there is a partial, but significant, overlap between ethnicity and the occupational structure, disadvantaged minorities lack digital access, as they are concentrated in occupations that are not exposed to computers and the Internet.

In the final chapter of this section, Hamid Abdollahyan, Mehdi Semati and Mohammad Ahmadi examine dimensions of digital divide in Iran with an emphasis on secondary digital divide. This chapter, entitled "An analysis of the second-level digital divide in Iran: A case study of University of Tehran undergraduate students," is structured around two major parts. First, the authors review and analyze data about second-level digital divide in Iran and they discuss the historical turn in digital divide studies that has been diverted from studying technology haves and have-nots towards studying a skilled-based divide among different groups. Then, the authors elaborate their digital literacy survey among undergraduate students at the University of Tehran, offering an argument as to why they believe second-level digital divide is an issue in Iran.

Section 6: Under-studied countries and regions

For the final section of the volume, we have invited scholars to cover some of the under-represented and under-studied areas of the world. Naturally it is difficult to cover all parts of the world, but we have tried to offer an international perspective giving space also to the digital divide in Latin America, in the Former Soviet Republics in Central Asia, in East Asia, and finally in Sub-Saharan Africa. The section opens with a chapter that explores the process by which ICTs are integrated and used in Latin America, with an approach that views ICTs as instruments for addressing the development needs of the region, paying attention to the risks inherent in the process. Daniela Trucco Horwitz, in her chapter "The digital divide in the Latin American context," states that this is one of the most unequal regions of the world and the mass dissemination of ICT could be generating new and rapidly growing forms of stratification. In Latin America, there are different types and levels of digital divides that operate simultaneously. The access gap, which is still substantial, is compounded by a second gap of use and appropriation. The analysis uses empirical data collected through international household surveys and through international educational assessment tests.

The chapter about the digital divide in the Former Soviet Republics of Central Asia is written by Barney Warf and is entitled "The Central Asian digital divide." It traces the changing geographies of internet access in the region in light of the legacy of Soviet policies, the uneven introduction of fiber optic cables, the rapid growth of netizens, unequal patterns of prices, mobile technologies, the heavy bias in favor of urban areas, and government attempts to censor internet content.

The third chapter of this section, entitled "The double digital divide and social inequality in Asia: Comparative research on Internet cafes in Taiwan, Singapore, Thailand, and the Philippines," examines the digital divide in the East Asian context. Tomohisa Hirata, using statistical data provided by the ITU, states that there is a significant difference in the proportion of households with the Internet in Asia. In this chapter, this phenomenon in Asia is designated as "the double digital divide," which indicates both the digital divide within each Asian country and that across the whole of Asia. The author discusses it from the perspective of the cultural theory in Weberian socio-economics, drawing on extensive ethnographic fieldwork and interviews conducted at Internet cafes which provide relatively poor people with the Internet and personal computers in Asian countries.

In the final chapter of this section, and indeed of the volume as a whole, Gado Alzouma fills a void in the literature caused by the fact that African countries are most commonly studied in relation to more developed countries, rather than as sites of study themselves. Indeed, only a few of the studies have so far analyzed how the use of technology relates to economic standing, prestige acquisition and power relations, the three dimensions of inequality and social stratification identified by Weber. For this reason in this chapter, entitled "Dimensions of the mobile divide in Niger," the author explores the unequal adoption, appropriation and use of computers in the country. Alzouma shows how access to computers, computer ownership, and Internet use are stratified across the West African country. The paper is based on a Weberian perspective and uses Bourdieu's field theory, analyzing data drawn from fieldwork and semi-structured interviews carried out in the capital city, Niamey. Interview data are supplemented using various sources such as statistics from the ITU, from the Government of Niger and from various studies and surveys concerning access to ICTs in Niger.

Finally, in addition to these nineteen chapters, Sascha Meinrath, James Losey, and Ben Lennett, (director and fellows with the Open Technology Institute at the New America Foundation), contribute a brief Afterword entitled "Internet freedom, nuanced digital divides, and the Internet craftsman." They start by reminding us that "the international consensus that communications is a fundamental human right is emerging as we begin to understand the key role that the Internet plays in numerous spheres of social life." However, rather than focus on the benefits of broadband and Internet connectivity, the authors center their discussion on two significant dilemmas that have received less attention from policy makers and commentators. First, the challenges faced by the unconnected and, second, that all connectivity is not created equal. Indeed, the authors argue that "in the Internet age, which technologies and devices you use to connect increasingly determines your online opportunities." These different opportunities are at the bases of the new digital and social inequalities in the Internet age.

Overall, the nineteen chapters in this book provide an interwoven analysis of the digital divide in relation with the social stratification. Although some authors move in independent directions (whether methodologically or theoretically), there are many areas of overlap, providing room for distinctions and/or connections across countries, cultures, and regions. The authors highlight the processes that bring social inequalities to knowledge societies, and they offer a way forward toward a comprehensive approach to the digital divide around the world. Ultimately, they remind us how the foundations laid by the founding fathers of sociology are extremely important as starting points to understand how the Internet is disseminated and used and that they are still relevant, even if not exhaustive, to understanding the current critical issue of stratification in the digital sphere.

References

Attewell, P. (2001). The first and second digital divides. *Sociology of Education,* 74 (3), 252–259.

Bimber, B. (2000). Measuring the gender gap on the Internet. *Social Science Quarterly,* 81, 868–876.

Bucy, E.P. (2000). Social access to the Internet. *Harvard International Journal of Press/Politics,* 5 (1), 50–61.

Castells, M. (2001). *The Internet galaxy: Reflections on the Internet, business and society.* Oxford, UK: Oxford University Press.

Chen, W. (2004). The global digital divide within and between countries. *IT & Society,* 1(7), 39–45.

Chinn, M.D. and Fairlie, R.W. (2007). The determinants of the global digital divide: A cross-country analysis of computer and Internet penetration. *Oxford Economic Papers,* 59(1), 16–44.

Clark, C. and Gorski, P. (2001). Multicultural education and the digital divide: Focus on race, language, socioeconomic class, sex, and disability. *Multicultural Perspectives,* 3(3), 39–44.

Clark, C. and Gorski, P., (2002a). Multicultural education and the digital divide: Focus on gender. *Multicultural Perspectives,* 4(1), 30–40.

Clark, C. and Gorski, P. (2002b). Multicultural education and the digital divide: Focus on socioeconomic class background. *Multicultural Perspectives,* 4(3), 25–36.

Cooper, J. (2006). The digital divide: The special case of gender. *Journal of Computer Assisted Learning,* 22(5), 320–334.

Cooper, J. and Weaver, K.D. (2003). *Gender and computers: Understanding the digital divide.* Mahwah, NJ, US.: Erlbaum Associates.

Crompton, R. (1998). *Class and stratification,* 2nd Edition. Cambridge, MA, US: Polity Press.

DiMaggio, P., Hargittai, E., Neuman, W.R. and Robinson, J. (2001). The social implications of the Internet. *Annual Review of Sociology* 27, 307–336.

Dobson, T.M. and Willinsky, J. (2009). Digital literacy. In D.R. Olson and N. Torrance (eds). *The Cambridge handbook of literacy* (286–312) Cambridge, UK: Cambridge University Press.

Durkheim, E. (1956). *Education and sociology.* Glencoe, IL, US: The Free Press.

Durkheim, E. (1961). *Moral education.* New York: The Free Press of Glencoe.

Durkheim, E. (1984). *The division of labour in society.* London: Macmillan.

Eshet, Y. and Aviram, R. (2006). Towards a theory of digital literacy: Three scenarios for the next steps, *European Journal of Open Distance E-Learning.*

Accessed 12 July 2012 from: http://www.eurodl.org/index.php?p=archivesandy
ear=2006andhalfyear=1andarticle=223

Eshet-Alkalai, Y. and Chajut, E. (2009). Changes over time in digital literacy. *Cyberpsychology & Behavior,* 12(6).

Fairlie, R.W. (2003). Is there a digital divide? Ethnic and racial differences in access to technology and possible explanations. Final report to the University of California, Latino Policy Institute and California Policy Research Center. Accessed 15 September 2012 from: http://www.cjtc.ucsc.edu/docs/r_techreport5.pdf

Fairlie, R.W. (2004). Race and the digital divide. *Contributions in Economic Analysis & Policy,* 3(1), Article 15.

Fuchs, C. (2009). Information and communication technologies and society: A contribution to the critique of the political economy of the Internet. *European Journal of Communication,* 24(1), 69–87.

Fuchs, C. (2010). Class and knowledge labour in informational capitalism and on the Internet. *The Information Society,* 26(3), 179–196.

Fuchs, C. (2011). *Foundations of critical media and information studies.* New York: Routledge.

Fuchs, C. and Mosco, V. (eds). (2012). Marx is back – the importance of Marxist theory and research for critical communication studies today. *tripleC – Open Access Journal for a Global Sustainable Information Society,* 10(2), 127–632.

Graham, Philip W. (2001). The digital dark ages: The knowledge economy as alienation. In H. Brown, G. Lovink, H. Merrick, N. Rossiter, D. Teh and M. Willson (eds). *The fibreculture reader: Politics of a digital present.* Melbourne, Australia: Fibreculture Publications.

Gui, M. and Argentin, G. (2011). Digital skills of the Internet natives: Differences of digital literacy in a random sample of northern Italian high school students. *New Media & Society,* 2(17): 1–18.

Hargittai, E. (2002). Second-level digital divide: Differences in people's online skills. *First Monday,* 7(4). Accessed 20 September 2012 from: http://firstmonday.org/issues/issue7_4/hargittai/index.html.

Hargittai, E. (2005). Survey measures of web-oriented digital literacy. *Social Science Computer Review,* 23(3), 371–379.

Hargittai, E. (2009). An update on survey measures of web-oriented digital literacy. *Social Science Computer Review,* 27(1), 130–137.

Hargittai, E. (2010). Digital na(t)ives? Variation in Internet skills and uses among members of the "Net Generation." *Sociological Inquiry,* 80(1), 92–113.

Hoffman, D.L and Novak, T.P. (2001). The evolution of the digital divide: Examining the relationship of race to Internet access and usage over time. In M. Benjamin (ed.), *The digital divide: Facing a crisis or creating a myth?* Cambridge, MA, US: MIT Press, 47–97.

ITU. (2010). *Core ICT indicators, 2010.* Geneva: International Telecommunication Union.

Jenkins, H., Clinton, K., Purushotma, R., Robinson, A.J. and Weigel, M. (2006). Confronting the challenges of participatory culture: Media education for the 21st century, an occasional paper written for the MacArthur Foundation. Accessed 15 July 2012 from: http://digitallearning.macfound.org/atf/cf/%7B7E45C7E0-A3E0-4B89-AC9C-E807E1B0AE4E%7D/JENKINS_WHITE_PAPER.PDF

Katz, J.E. and Rice, R.E. (2002). *Social consequences of Internet use: Access, involvement and interaction.* Cambridge, MA, US: MIT Press.

Lauer, J. (2008). Alienation in the information economy: Toward a Marxist critique of consumer surveillance. In *Participation and media production*, N. Carpentier and B. De Cleen (eds), Newcastle, UK: Cambridge Scholars, 41–53.

Livingstone, S. and Helsper, E. (2010), Balancing opportunities and risks in teenagers' use of the Internet: the role of online skills and the Internet self-efficacy, *New Media & Society*, 12(2), 309–329.

Loges, W.E. and Jung, J-Y. (2001). Exploring the digital divide, Internet connectedness and age. *Communication Research*, 28(4), 536–562.

Losh, S.C. (2003). Gender and educational digital chasms in computer and Internet access and use over time: 1983–2000. *IT & Society*, 1(4), 73–86.

Marx, K. (1976) *Capital: A critique of political economy.* Harmondsworth, UK: Penguin.

Mosco, V. (2009). *The political economy of communication*, 2nd Edition. London: Sage.

Mossberger, K., Tolbert, C. J. and Stansbury, M. (2003). *Virtual inequality: Beyond the digital divide.* Washington, DC: Georgetown University Press.

Ono, H. and Zavodny, M. (2003). Gender and the Internet. *Social Science Quarterly*, 84, 111–121.

Palfrey, J. and Gasser, U. (2008). *Born digital: Understanding the first generation of digital natives.* New York: Basic Books.

Perez-Tornero, J. M. (2004). A new model for promoting digital literacy. Accessed 20 August 2012 from: http://ec.europa.eu/education/archive/elearning/doc/workshops/Digital_literacy/position_papers/perez_tornero_jose.pdf Rey, P. J. (2012). Alienation, Exploitation, and Social Media. *American Behavioral Scientist* 56(4), 399–420

Scott J. (1996). *Stratification and power: Structures of class, status and command.* Cambridge, MA, US: Polity Press.

Scott, J. (2000). Class and stratification. In G. Payne (ed.). *Social divisions.* London: Macmillan.

Soker, Z. (2005). Age, gender, ethnicity and the digital divide: University students' use of web based instruction. *Electronic Journal of Sociology.* Accessed 20 September 2012 from: http://www.sociology.org/content/2005/tier1/soker.html

Stanley, L. D. (2003). Beyond access: Psychosocial barriers to computer literacy. *Information Society*, 19(5), 407–416.

Stern, M.J. (2010). Inequality in the Internet age. *Sociological Inquiry*, 80(1), 28–33.

Therborn, G. (2000). At the birth of second century sociology: Times of reflexivity, spaces of identity and nodes of knowledge. *British Journal of Sociology*, 51(1), 37–59.

van Deursen, A.J.A.M. and van Dijk, J.A.G.M. (2010). The Internet skills and the digital divide. *New Media & Society*, 11(11), 1–19.

van Dijk, J. (2005). *The deepening divide: Inequality in the information society.* Thousand Oaks, CA, US: Sage.

van Dijk, J. and Hacker, K. (2003). The digital divide as a complex and dynamic phenomenon. *Information Society*, 19(4), 315–327.

Weber, M. (1947). *The theory of social and economic organization.* New York: Free Press.

Witte, J.C. and Mannon, S.E. (2010). *The Internet and social inequalities.* New York: Routledge.

Zillien, N. and Hargittai, E. (2009). Digital distinction: Status-specific types of Internet usage. *Social Science Quarterly,* 90, 274–291.

Žižek, S. (2010). *Living in the end times.* London: Verso.

Section 1

Theories of the digital divide

1 The reproduction and reconfiguration of inequality

Differentiation and class, status and power in the dynamics of digital divides

Bridgette Wessels
University of Sheffield

Introduction

The development and expanding use of digital technology within economic, political, social and cultural life on a global scale is raising concerns about the emergence of new inequalities and the reproduction of existing inequalities (Wyatt *et al.*, 2000). These developments are part of rapid social change, which is ushering in an information and networked society (Castells, 1996, 2001; Webster, 2004). Some commentators argue that the global informational capitalism underpinning an information and networked society is generating increasingly fragmented and unequal societies (Robins and Webster, 1999; Fuchs, 2008). This chapter draws on the work of the founding fathers of sociology to address inequality in a global information society. To trace this link, the chapter introduces the idea of a digital divide before considering the way technology is situated in socio-cultural change and inequality. It then discusses digital divides in global informational capitalism and the formation of new inequalities. This is followed by the conclusion.

Digital technology, social relations, and the digital divide

For many people across the world the pervasiveness of digital technology – whether experienced as a presence or an absence – is significant. A distinctive aspect to digital technology is that it is both an artifact and a communication medium, which Silverstone and Hirsch (1994) call "double articulation." This is important in terms of assessing inequality in a digitally enabled network society: it is not only the networked structuring of the technology and the ability to access and use it that are contributing factors in inequality but it also provides access to information and the public sphere, which is a key resource in an information society. In overall terms the significance of the technology lies in the way in which it is embedded within the relations of production; in information flows; and in the way it underpins participation. The utilization of technology within the economic, political, and socio-cultural processes of society shape inequality.

One can start to assess the significance of exclusion from social networks based on digital technology when one sees that it is the use of technology within social relations that produces inequality. One can see that inclusion into digitally enabled networks is significant in terms of the opportunities people have to engage in economic life and to participate in political, social, and cultural life. The embedding of digital technology in social, economic, democratic process and cultural forms is materializing and is experienced unevenly and differently by people across the globe. The differential development and use of digital technology within contexts of global inequality is creating a dynamic that is generating new forms of poverty and exclusion as well as reproducing existing inequalities and social divisions.

The current inequalities and divisions within information and networked society are often thought about in terms of a digital divide (Norris, 2000). The idea of a digital divide is a useful starting point in exploring the dynamics of inequality within a global information culture (Lash, 1999). Castells (2001) argues that the digital divide goes beyond those who have access to the Internet and those who do not have access. He writes that differing levels of access to, and usage of, digital services "adds a fundamental cleavage to existing sources of inequality and social exclusion in a complex interaction" (Castells, 2001, p. 247). The dimensions of digital divide can be understood as the dynamic of inclusion and exclusion that articulates the levels of digital and other resources that people have available to them within the social divisions of society. This means that people have unequal levels of opportunity to develop digital skills, to participate in democratic process, and enter the labor market (Garnham, 2005). The digital divide involves social, democratic and global divides (Norris, 2000), and is multi-dimensional (Wessels, 2010).

Some of the dimensions of the digital divide are as follows. First, ethnicity, age, gender, levels of education and socio-economic background and status are influential in the dynamics of the digital divide (Wessels, 2010). Second, there is a technological divide amongst world regions with different levels of infrastructure that prevent some regions linking into a global economy. Third, as Zillien and Marr (in Chapter 3 of this volume) point out, there is widening knowledge gap for those with low access, low skills, and little cultural capital to use digital resources. These dimensions configure in different ways across the globe. In the US the ethnic divide is still significant amongst digital inequalities (Wessels, 2010; Witte, Kiss and Lynn, Chapter 4 of this volume). The contributors of this volume show that the digital divide in developing countries is uneven with some cities and regions developing rapidly whilst others are disconnected. There are specific development needs of particular countries and if access and support is not provided inequalities will deepen, as seen for example in the Latin American context (Horwitz, Chapter 16 of this volume). Status and cultural factors interact with the take up of digital services, which fosters inequalities seen for example in Sub-Saharan Africa (Alzouma, Chapter 19 of this volume) and in Japan (Akiyoshi, Chapter 5 of this volume). Faris (Chapter 13 of this volume) outlines the dynamics of a democratic divide in accessing an online public sphere. The dynamics of these aspects are fostering greater inequality globally as the gap between the wealthy and poor widens around the digital divide (Castells, 2001).

The theoretical insights of Marx, Durkheim, and Weber about inequality are based on greater differentiation in a capitalist economy and its resulting organization of class, power and status in society. These themes can be traced into the current situation of a global networked society, its reconfiguration of class and its inequalities at local, national and global levels (Castells, 2001; Webster, 2004). Inequalities coalesce around the way technology is embedded within social relations.

Situating technology within the dynamics of socio-cultural change and inequality

The social shaping approaches to technology address the way in which technology is embedded in social relations. It argues that technology is shaped by social factors such as economic concerns and gender relations (MacKenzie and Wajcman, 1985). The way in which technology becomes meaningful within social relations is through the culture in which is it produced and consumed. Pfaffenberger (1988), for instance, argues that:

> Technology expresses an embedded social vision, and it engages us in what Marx would call a form of life, including political, social and symbolic aspects of social life. It has a legal dimension, it has a history, it entails a set of social relationships and it has meaning (1988, p. 244).

Robins and Webster (1999) follow a similar type of analysis in which they see digital technology as: "articulating the social relations of the societies in which they are mobilized …. [that includes] power relations" (p. 2). These types of conceptualizations encompass the social relations of digital technology, which address the social, political, and cultural dynamics of inequality and the digital divide.

Durkheim (1984), Marx (1976), and Weber (1922) raise the issue of inequality, and ask:

- Why does the pursuit of wealth seem to generate poverty on an unprecedented scale?
- Why do the principles of liberty and equality appear to go hand in hand with monstrous new forms of oppression? (Abrams, 1982, p. 4).

These classical sociologists address these questions in different ways. Weber (1922) emphasizes the development of bureaucracy, which is related to the increase in scale of organizations and to the division of labor. He sees distinctions between people based on class, status and power. Weber identifies rationalization as a fine calculation of means to ends rather than the value of ends, which celebrates efficiency in a dominant cult of technique. The combination of divisions based on class and status combines with rationalization to create an iron cage that locks people into specific positions and restricted life-worlds. Each of these positions influences the power individuals have to shape their life chances.

Marx (1976; Marx and Engels, 1968) addresses the division of labor and alienation within the capitalist mode of production when he identifies alienation in the labor process and in the productive activity of the worker. Alienation expresses the fact that the organization of productive relationships constitutes a class system resting on the exploitative dominance of one class by another, and the division of labor identifies occupational specialization as the source of fragmentation of work into routine and undemanding tasks (Giddens, 1979). For Marx the hallmark of capitalism is the emergence of a class of producers who own nothing but their own labor-power that they are forced to sell in return for wages paid by the owners of the means of production. The work of Marx (and Engels) highlights the relationships of inequality in a market economy and in political arrangements associated with capitalism (Abrams, 1982).

Durkheim (1984) argues that structural differentiation fosters individualism as he observes that labor is becoming more divided and specialized. The division of labor results from the struggle of individuals to flourish in the face of the increasing volume and density of the population and pressures on resources (Abrams, 1982). For Durkheim differentiation creates inequalities that are part of a larger, more complex social system. Within this system, institutions are important in supporting social cohesion. Thus education is important in supporting organic solidarity and in supporting individuals to develop specialisms so that each could integrate into the labor market. The education system is also significant in sustaining a sense of conscience collective – a collective sense of values and morals – that underpins social order.

Marx (1976), Weber (1922), and Durkheim (1984) identify the emergence of inequalities through increased differentiation in market based economies. These inequalities are about material resources, about personal fulfillment and enchantment, and about senses of belonging to a community or collective. These issues are traced into global capitalism in the following section.

Situating the dynamics of digital divides in global informational capitalism

The innovation of digital technology alongside globalization, neo-liberalism, and consumerism is generating social transformation and is ushering in what some commentators call an "information society" (Webster, 2004) or a "networked society" (Castells, 2001). In changes to a network and information society there is continuity in that the economy is still based on capitalism (Robins and Webster, 1999). The use of digital technology in economic activity is situated within global capitalism that is based on a networked organization of production processes and patterns of consumption (Fuchs, 2008).

This networked organization of social and economic life is facilitated by a digital infrastructure for an e-economy and information society (Castells, 2001). For economies to be competitive in a global market, they need to be connected to the digital infrastructure and they require a labor force that has the education and skills to work in an e-economy. From the point of view of ordinary people their life chances are linked to having the capability to work in the e-economy to ensure employment. The acquisition of the appropriate education and skills to enable people to engage in economic life is differentiated amongst class, cultural capital and status, gender, ethnicity, digital literacy and opportunities across the life course at the local, regional, and national level. Furthermore as digital technology is embedded in political communication, individuals need access and skills to engage in the democratic process (Wessels, 2010). Access to social and cultural networks is highly differentiated along class, status, and ethnic lines in terms of cultural capital, which relates to inequality in participation (Kolko, Nakamura and Rodman, 2000). Age and gender cuts across all of these divisions and undermines older people and women's ability to engage and participate (Cockburn, 1983; Hacker, 1990).

The e-economy facilitates the agile development of global value chains of production and consumption. Global corporations are able to produce, distribute, and market products and services efficiently and cheaply by taking advantage of national and regional low labor costs and just-in-time production processes. A consequence of this type of networked process is that it dis-empowers nation states and weakens national economies (Castells, 2001; Freeman, 2000). This interacts with the provision of welfare, both for Western advanced economies and for developing countries.

In various corporate settlements after the Second World War, governments in European nation states created types of welfare systems that could mitigate to some degree the inequalities inherent in a capitalist economy by providing basic support for those living in poverty and those unemployed; by providing greater equality of opportunity through education; and providing a universal health care system free at the point of delivery (Steinert and Pilgram, 2007). Although these settlements varied between nation states, nation states took some responsibility in addressing disadvantage (Roche, 1992). However, with the development of globalization nation states have less power and resource to draw on to fund national welfare support. This has disempowered nation states and is resulting in the retrenchment of state-provided welfare.

Developing countries, each locked into their specific historical trajectory, are experiencing new senses of disempowerment. These countries have been disempowered from colonial and imperial rule onwards. When seeking and being granted self-determination in terms of gaining nation state status, these countries were, and still are, locked into dependencies with the more advanced economies and global multinational companies (Frank, 1969). Very often, these dependencies create the development of underdevelopment, which reinforces poverty and limits the available resource for such countries to develop. These dynamics are still at work and they have an added dimension in that the speed of development and change when harnessed to digital technology is fast and flexible, which makes it difficult for developing countries to catch up (Castells, 2001).

The development of networked production processes on a global scale means that multi-nationals can exploit low labor costs in developing countries often by using their own infrastructures, which means that these countries are locked into dependencies. Another aspect of this is that if countries and regions are not connected to a high quality digital infrastructure and do not have a skilled labor force, they are locked out of the global economy and therefore slip more into poverty. Both of these dynamics point to the way in which neo-liberal globalization and an e-enabled economy either exploit poorer countries or disconnect them. This when taken with the overall rural exodus to urban areas is creating absolute poverty for many people in developing regions, with women and children often bearing the extreme ravages of such poverty (Castells, 2001; Goddard and Richardson, 1996).

One of the defining features of global capitalism with its digital infrastructure is that of the networked organization of social life. In terms of production, the organizational form that underpins is the "network" (Castells, 2001). The network is becoming pervasive across all of social life extending beyond the process of production into the organization of welfare, social movements and into everyday life. Change to institutional arrangements in society based on the network interacts with change in the lives of individuals, as seen in the development of networked individualism (Wellman and Haythornthwaite, 2002). Networked individualism points to the way in which individuals create their own networks of communication and contacts – some being strong ties others being weak ties – whereby they manage their social lives. The transition to networked individualism is characterized as being one that moves from "groups" with "each in their place" to "networks" involving the "mobility of people and goods." The rise of networks is in the context of a market capitalist economy with its inherent inequities.

There is continuity with the key themes that Marx, Durkheim, and Weber identified. This is seen in the way in which production networks are structuring work in terms of a flexible highly competitive labor market, whereby politics and cultural life is organized via flows of information within networks shaped by status, class and power; and the differentiation of social life is ongoing and is accelerated with heightened senses of individualism. Alongside these trends the state and the corporate sector are using more and more techniques of surveillance to control populations via rationalization. These trends – as continuations – of processes from market based industrialization into market based networked information society create the new conditions of inequality.

The formation of new conditions of inequality

Given the networked context of inequality, an expansion of the definition of digital divides is one that addresses the multi-dimensional aspect of inequality in a digital age. The multi-dimensional approach includes the dynamics of socio-economic position, geographic location, ethnicity and language, as well as educational capacities and digital literacy. These dynamics are further complicated at the global level, where lower Internet penetration in developing countries (although this can be uneven within these countries), combined with the rapid change of the Internet-based technological paradigm, requires that the less-developed countries have to outperform advanced economies just to stay where they are, thus fostering and reproducing global inequalities (Castells, 2001). Under the current social and institutional conditions of transnational-networked capitalism there is uneven development that is putting many at risk of poverty and social exclusion (Wessels, 2010).

The dynamics of inclusion and exclusion require consideration of the restructuring of the capitalist economy, its networked logic underpinned by digital technology and trends towards post-Fordist welfare. The dynamics of transnational informational capitalism within an ethos of neo-liberalism is interacting with social and economic life at the local, regional, national and global level (Room, 1995). Situations of exclusion are experienced at the local level, which link to regional and national economic conditions and policy, whilst also relating to trends in the global economy (Steinert and Pilgram, 2007; Young, 2000). A phenomenology of exclusion points to different dimensions, such as political exclusion (via citizenship), economic exclusion (through lack of means), social exclusion (through isolation), and cultural exclusion (through deficits in education). Steinert's (2007) definition captures the dynamics of exclusion, arguing that social exclusion is a:

...dynamic and multi-dimensional process ... as the continuous and gradual exclusion from full participation in the social, including material as well as symbolic, resources produced, supplied and exploited in a society for making a living, organizing a life and taking part in the development of a (hopefully better) future (p. 5).

The dynamics of exclusion are embedded in post–Fordist relations of production and the processes of globalization (Bauman, 1998; Hutton and Giddens, 2001). There is a lack of employment security, with actors having to be flexible to survive in the labor market (Sennett, 2001). There is need for labor with skills to work as symbolic analysts (Robins and Webster, 1999) and as knowledge workers with appropriate skills and education to use digital technology to turn information into knowledge, and knowledge into action (Castells, 2001; Dutton, 2001). There are others who are on the "outside" of these developments, who do not have the necessary skills and resources, including geographical mobility to compete successfully in the market (Bauman, 1998). Very often, these dynamics produce geographical spaces of exclusion in the form of ghettos, run-down estates, with few local services and a general lack of opportunity (Madanipour, 1998).

When post-Fordist trends in welfare are combined with lightly regulated market economies, this triggers remote forms of control that reinforce social exclusion, managed, in part, through various technologies of surveillance. Digital technology is part of these dynamics in two main ways. First, its networking logic makes it a perfect tool for post-Fordist and global production processes. Second, its use within bureaucracies and by the state means it can be used to as a tool of surveillance over the populace. Baggulay (1994) draws these aspects together to state that advanced nations are grouped by the ways their traditional social welfare policies are constructed and how these influence employment and social structure. He draws on Esping Andersen's (1992) term "regime" to illustrate that the relation between the state and the economy is systematically woven from a complex of legal and organizational features. The way in which situations of exclusion emerge and are managed is, therefore, a result of the ways in which the economy and the state interact to produce either opportunities for participation in open societies or it may foster increasing levels of surveillance in society.

Theories of the way power operates in society vary (Westwood, 2002) from ideas regarding oppression (Freire, 1972), hegemony (Gramsci, 1992), and technologies of power and discipline (Foucault, 1977). However, with regard to digital technology, there are two main dimensions of power and exclusion. First, access to digital technology as it materializes in the relations of production provides the economic opportunity to participate in the labor market and economy and thus for individuals to have some power over their life chances. Second, digital technology gives states and commercial organizations the potential to control individuals through the information they can electronically gather about them. Any lack of transparency in the workings of the state and the commercial sector is a form of power that can either be used to incorporate or exclude. In this context individuals need access to the data held on them and the skills, education and power to protect their rights and identity (with the state having the responsibility to ensure freedoms are maintained through proper legislation).

The levels of access and the quality of resources are key aspects in enabling individuals and groups to participate in the life of society (Pelikan *et al.*, 2007). The question therefore involves ensuring that individuals and groups have access to the relevant resources to enable them to participate. When digital technology is seen as resource then it can be seen as part of a virtuous circle, where those with access to (fast) Internet (Fox, 2005), good education and socio-economic background are in good positions to take advantage of economic development. Those on the other hand who lack access to any of these resources are at a disadvantage and at risk of exclusion. The allocation of resources is related to positions of power, with those with the least resources having less power in determining their futures, securities, and freedoms to participate. Given the ways in which digital technology is becoming embedded in the relations of production, in working life, in public policy and in everyday life, it becomes a resource for participation – social, economic, political, and cultural. However, this does not reduce exclusion merely to access to digital technology, rather digital-related resources become one aspect embedded within the multi-dimensionality of exclusion and the digital divide.

Conclusion

The key themes that Marx, Weber, and Durkheim identified about inequality are still relevant in the contemporary, digitally enabled, networked society. The relevance of market positions, rationalization, and differentiation are still key in the development of capitalism in a global informational form. In many ways these factors have become heightened because the digital infrastructure of global capitalism is enabling faster and more agile production processes that push for a more individualistic and flexible approach to the labor market. The need to control populations remotely is pushing ever more rationalization through increased surveillance techniques and the pervasive networked organization of social life is undermining strong social ties and senses of community. When these trends are combined with a retrenchment of welfare in the West and an ever-growing gap between developed and developing counties then the risk of exclusion is high, creating greater inequality.

Digital technology is a key resource for accessing resources and for participating in social life. It works in two related ways: one, as a structuring network for generating production and participation as an infrastructure in global capitalism; and two, as a resource for individuals that enable them to compete to enter the labor market; to engage in politics, culture and education and to participate in social life. It is only one resource amongst others and it cannot be utilized without other resources such as education, language and writing skills, and good socio-economic conditions. The general circumstance of an individual's life is a prerequisite to be able to utilize the potential of digital technology. Therefore, people's living conditions such as housing, health, and access to local resources such as good food, water, transport and public utilities and hygiene are the backdrop for making full use of the Internet. Nonetheless, given that digital services are the vehicle for production and participation the need to be connected is real and significant: being disconnected from digital services pushes people into exclusion and poverty.

These risks interact with existing social divisions such as socio-economic status, class background, gender, age, ethnicity, levels of education, geographical location and cultural capital. These configure in a highly individualized market based society with weak ties and connections. The general condition of a digital divide is one of insecurity and uncertainty for many people. Given the complexity of differentiation in a society organized through networks, the digital divide needs to be considered in terms of the dynamics of inclusion and exclusion in global informational capitalism. The multi-dimensional character of exclusion points to the way barriers to participation configure through the lack of different sets of resources. One dimension of exclusion is people's access and ability to use digital technology to support life chances and to facilitate participation in social life. Digital technology is a key resource for people in a networked society because it provides information and resources, and access to online public spheres. However, the use of digital services coalesces around social divisions, and in situations with low resources, which adds a fundamental cleavage to existing inequalities. Social inequality and disadvantage is being reproduced and reconfigured within the networked society, specifically as digital divides. The insights of the founding fathers about inequality are pertinent in assessing the dynamics of the digital divide because inequality is being reproduced in digital networks through differentiation, rationalization, and individualism.

References

Abrams, P. (1982). *Historical sociology*. Ithaca, NY, US: Cornell University Press.
Baggulay, P. (1994). Prisoners of the Beveridge Dream? The political mobilisation of the poor against contemporary welfare regimes. In R. Burrows and B. Loader (eds.) *Towards a post-Fordist welfare state?* London: Routledge.

Bauman, Z. (1998). *Globalization: The human consequences,* Cambridge, UK: Polity Press.

Castells, M. (1996). *The rise of the network society,* Oxford, UK: Blackwell.

Castells, M. (2001). *The Internet galaxy: Reflections on the Internet, business and society.* Oxford, UK: Oxford University Press.

Cockburn, C. (1983). *Brothers: Male dominance and technological change.* London: Pluto.

Dutton, D. (2001). *Society on the line: Information politics in the digital age.* Oxford, UK: Oxford University Press.

Durkheim, E. (1984). *The division of labor in society.* London, Basingstoke, UK: Macmillan.

Esping Andersen, G. (1992). *The three worlds of welfare capitalism.* Cambridge, UK: Polity Press.

Foucault, M. (1977). *Discipline and punish: The birth of the prison.* London: Allen Lane.

Fox, S. (2005). *Digital divisions: There are clear differences among those with broadband connections, dial-up connections, and no connections at all to the Internet/* Pew Internet & American Life Project.

Frank, G. (1969). *Latin America: Underdevelopment or revolution: Essays on the development of underdevelopment and immediate enemy.* New York: Monthly Review.

Freeman, C. (2000). Social inequality, technology and economic growth. In S. Wyatt, F. Henwood, N. Miller and P. Senker (eds.) *Technology and in/equality: Questioning the information society.* London: Routledge, pp. 149–171.

Freire, P. (1972). *Pedagogy of the oppressed.* London: Sheed and Ward.

Fuchs, C. (2008). *Internet and society: Social theory in the information age.* New York: Routledge.

Garnham, N. (2005). *Political economy of the information society.* London: Taylor and Francis.

Giddens, A. (1979). *Capitalism and modern social theory: An analysis of the writings of Marx, Durkheim and Max Weber.* Cambridge, UK: Cambridge University Press.

Goddard, J. and Richardson, R. (1996). Why geography will still matter: What jobs go where? In L. Dutton and M. Peltu (eds.) *Information and Communication Technologies: Visions and Realities.* Oxford. UK: Oxford University Press.

Gramsci, A. (1992). *Prison notebooks.* New York: Columbia University Press.

Hacker, S. (1990). *Doing it the hard way: Investigations of gender and technology.* Winchester, MA, US: Unwin Hyman.

Hutton, W. and Giddens, A. (2001). *On the edge: Living with global capitalism.* London: Vintage.

Kolko, B., Nakamura, L. and Rodman, G. (eds.) (2000). *Race in cyberspace.* London: Routledge.

Lash, S. (1999). *Another modernity: A different rationality.* Oxford, UK: Blackwell Publisher.

MacKenzie, D. and Wajcman, J. (eds.) (1985). *The social shaping of technology.* Maidenhead, UK: Open University Press.

Madanipour, A. (1998). *Social exclusion in European cities.* London: Jessica Kingsley.

Marx, K. and Engels, F. (1968). *Selected Works,* Vols. 1–2. London: Lawrence and Wishart.

Marx, K. (1976). *Capital: A critique of political economy.* Harmondsworth, UK: Penguin.

Norris, P. (2000). *Digital divide: Civic engagement, information poverty, and the Internet worldwide.* Cambridge, UK: Cambridge University Press.

Pelikan, C., Pilgram, A., Steinert, H. and Vobruba, G. (2007). Welfare policies as resource management. In H. Steinert and A. Pilgram (eds.) *Welfare from below: Struggles against social exclusion in Europe: Towards a dynamic understanding of participation.* Aldershot, UK: Ashgate.

Pfaffenberger, B. (1988). Fetishized objects and humanised nature: Toward an anthropology of technology. *Man* 23, pp. 236–252.

Robins, K. and Webster, F. (1999). *Times of the technoculture: From the information society to virtual life.* London: Routledge.

Roche, M. (1992). *Rethinking citizenship, welfare, ideology and change in modern society.* Cambridge, UK: Polity Press.

Room, G. (1995). *Beyond the threshold: The measurement and analysis of social exclusion.* Bristol, UK: Policy Press.

Sennett, R. (2001). Street and office: Two sources of identity. In W. Hutton and A. Giddens (eds.) *On the Edge: Living with Global Capitalism.* London: Vintage.

Silverstone, R. and Hirsch, E. (1994). *Consuming technologies: Media and information in domestic spaces.* London: Routledge.

Steinert, H. and Pilgram, A. (2007). *Welfare policy from below: Struggles against social exclusion in Europe.* Aldershot, UK: Ashgate.

Steinert, H. (2007). Introduction: the cultures of welfare and exclusion. In Steinert, H. and Pilgram, A. (eds.) *Welfare policy from below: Struggles against social exclusion in Europe.* Aldershot, UK: Ashgate.

Weber, M. (1922). *Economy and society: An outline of interpretive sociology.* New York: Bedminster Press.

Webster, F. (ed.). (2004). *The information society reader.* London: Routledge.

Wellman, B. and Haythornthwaite, C. (eds.). (2002). *The Internet in everyday life.* Malden, UK: Blackwell Publishing.

Westwood, S. (2002). *Power and the social,* London: Routledge.

Wessels, B. (2010). *Understanding the Internet: A socio-cultural perspective,* Basingstoke, UK: Palgrave.

Wyatt, S., Henwood, F., Miller, N. and Senker, P. (eds.). (2000). *Technology and in/equality: Questioning the information society.* London: Routledge.

Young, J. (2000). *The exclusive society.* London: Sage.

2 A theory of the digital divide[1]

Jan A.G.M. van Dijk
University of Twente

A relational view of inequality

Contemporary research of the digital divide and digital skills is marked by a descriptive nature (van Dijk, 2006a). Inequalities are described using simple demographics of individuals who have more or less access to computers and the Internet and a different level of digital skills. The explanation of these differences has received far less attention. One of the reasons for this state of affairs is the predominance of individualistic notions of inequality. Like most social, scientific and economic investigations, digital divide research works based on so-called methodological individualism (Wellman and Berkowitz, 1988). Differential access to information and computer technologies (ICTs) is related to individuals and their characteristics: level of income and education, employment, age, sex, and ethnicity, to mention the most important ones. This is the usual approach in survey research, which measures the properties and attitudes of individual respondents. Making multivariate analyses of several individual properties and aggregating them to produce properties of collectivities, one hopes to find background explanations.

This kind of research might produce useful data, but it does not automatically result in explanations, as it is not guided by theory or by hypotheses derived from theory. They remain on a descriptive level of reasoning. One is not able to explain, for example, what it is about age and gender that produces the differences observed. Another disadvantage of the individualistic approach to inequality is the social and political effect of simply blaming inequality of access on attributes of individuals such as a lack of motivation or the urge to spend money on things other than digital technology and the correction of inadequate digital skills.

An alternative notion of inequality uses a relational or network approach (Wellman and Berkowitz, 1988). Here the prime units of analysis are not individuals but the positions of individuals and the relationships between them. Inequality is not primarily a matter of individual attributes but of categorical differences between groups of people. This is the point of departure of the groundbreaking work *Durable Inequality* by the American sociologist Charles Tilly (1999). "The central argument runs like this: Large, significant inequalities in advantages among human beings correspond mainly to categorical differences such as black/white, male/female, citizen/ foreigner, or Muslim/Jew rather than to individual differences in attributes, propensities, or performances" (p. 7). The point of departure of this notion of inequality is that neither the essences of individuals nor the essences of particular collectives or systems (e.g., capitalism, patriarchy) but rather the bonds, relationships, interactions, and transactions between people. "I claim that an account of how transactions clump into social ties, social ties concatenate into networks, and existing networks constrain solutions of organizational problems clarifies the creation, maintenance and change of categorical inequality" (p. 21).

On the issues of the digital divide and digital skills the most important categorical distinctions are employers and (un)employed, management and employees, people with high and low levels of education, males and females, the old and the young, parents and children, whites and blacks, citizens and migrants. At the macro level of countries, we can observe the categorical inequality of developed and developing countries, sometimes indicated as countries from the North and countries from the South of the globe. In every case, the first of these pairs is the dominant category in almost every part of the world, the white-black distinction excluded. With two exceptions (the aged and parents), this also goes for digital access and skills, as we will see in the remainder of this chapter.

A first instance of the insight offered by the relational view is an explanation of the differential appropriation of technology. Access to new technological means is a part of this. The dominant category is the first to adopt the new technology. It uses this advantage to increase power in its relationship with the subordinate category. I will give a preliminary example of the type of explanation the relational view is able to produce here. Gender differences in the appropriation of technology start very early in life. Little boys are the first to pick up technical toys and devices, passing the little girls, most often their sisters and small female neighbors or friends. These girls leave the operation to the boys, perhaps at first because the girls are less secure in handling them. Here a long process of continual reinforcement starts in which the girls "never" learn to operate the devices and the boys improve. This progresses into adulthood, where males are able to appropriate the great majority of technical and strategically important jobs and, in practice, keep females out of these jobs, whether they are conscious of this fact or not. This kind of explanation will unearth more of the actual mechanisms creating inequality than will an explanation in terms of individual attributes (females being less technical or less motivated, etc.).

A second advantage of the relational view of inequality is the capacity to make better distinctions between types of inequality. Individualistic notions of inequality produce an endless number of differences that can be observed between individuals, with no particular priority among them. Instead, distinctions have to be made between types of difference and attention has to be called to the structural aspects of society who refer to the relatively permanent and systemic nature of the differentiation called inequality. In Tilly's definition, inequality is the unequal distribution of resources in society as a result of the competition of categorical pairs, which produces systems of social closure, exploitation, and control (Tilly, 1999, pp. 7–9). Although this competition and the resulting distributions are changing continually, the categorical pairs reproduce themselves through mechanisms of social closure, exploitation, and control. In this way, inequality becomes a systematic or structural characteristic of societies. Using Tilly's terminology, it is "durable" as soon as it depends heavily on the institutionalization of categorical pairs in social, economic and cultural systems such as capitalism, bureaucracy and patriarchy (p. 8).

A third advantage of the relational view is that it is not necessary to give priority to any of the pairs in advance. Their relative importance is a matter of empirical observation, producing different results for every society. Moreover, the pairs overlap with individuals. Take, for instance, a relatively poor, young, single, female, Jamaican teacher living in the United Kingdom. Her inclusion in the categories of educational workers, young people, and inhabitants of a developed country would put her on the "right" side of the digital divide, as we will observe in the next four chapters. However, being a female with relatively low income, perhaps living alone without a partner or children to share a computer or Internet connection, and being part of an ethnic minority means that she would most likely be on the "wrong" side of the divide. This example shows the complexity of this type of inequality. In this chapter we will argue that labor market position, educational position, age, and sex, or gender, are the most important categorical inequalities determining the present digital divide.

A final benefit of the relational view of equality is that it directs our attention to relative inequality between people and their positions and resources. All too often, the metaphor of the digital divide suggests a yawning gap and the absolute exclusion of certain people. Earlier, I claimed that the simple picture of a two-tiered information society might better be replaced by the image of a continuum or a spectrum of positions across the population that is stretched when inequality increases (van Dijk, 1999). The absolute exclusion of access to digital media remains important, even in the developed countries, but the emphasis is shifting to the relative differences between people who already have access in a certain way or to a particular extent. These differences are relative inequalities of skills and usage. They are becoming even more important in the information society and the network society. In my opinion, individualistic notions of inequality are inadequate if one is to understand these relatively new kinds of inequality as they are increasingly linked to relationships, social networks and being first in the appropriation of information ("information is power").

Resources and appropriation theory

In my book, *The Deepening Divide* (van Dijk, 2005), I have developed a theory based upon this relational view of inequality. I call it a resources and appropriation theory of the diffusion, acceptance and adoption of new technologies. The following four are the core concepts of this theory:

1 a number of personal and positional categorical inequalities in society;
2 the distribution of resources relevant to this type of inequality;
3 a number of kinds of access to ICTs;
4 a number of fields of participation in society.

Items 1 and 2 are held to be the causes, and 3 is the phenomenon to be explained, together with 4, the potential consequence of the whole process. Being part of a process, 4 feeds back upon 1 and 2, as more or less participation in several fields of society will change the relationships of categorical inequalities and the distribution of resources in society. Finally, a fifth state of affairs determining the type of inequality to be explained has to be added as a side factor: the special characteristics of information and communication technology. In this way, a dynamic model can be drawn that forms the representation of this theory, as illustrated in Figure 2.1.

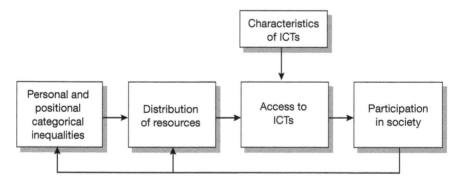

Figure 2.1 A causal model of resources and appropriation theory

The core argument can be summarized in the following statements:

1 Categorical inequalities in society produce an unequal distribution of resources.
2 An unequal distribution of resources causes unequal access to digital technologies.
3 Unequal access to digital technologies also depends on the characteristics of these technologies.
4 Unequal access to digital technologies brings about unequal participation in society.
5 Unequal participation in society reinforces categorical inequalities and unequal distributions of resources.

The following *personal categorical inequalities* can be frequently observed in digital divide research:

- age (young/old)
- gender (male/female)
- race/ethnicity (majority/minority)
- intelligence (high/low)
- personality (extravert/introvert; self-confident/not self-confident)
- health (abled/disabled).

The same goes for the following *positional categorical inequalities*:

- labor position (entrepreneurs/workers; management/employees; employed/unemployed)
- education (high/low)
- household (family/single person)
- nation (developed/developing).

In most empirical observations, the first of these relational categories has more access than does the second.

   The following *resources* frequently figure in digital divide research, sometimes under other labels such as economic, social, and cultural capital:

- temporal (having time to use digital media)
- material (possession and income)
- mental (technical ability; motivation)
- social (having a social network to assist in using digital media)
- cultural (status and preference for being in the world of digital media).

The core part of the model is a number of *kinds of access* in succession. Here the multi-faced concept of access is refined and conceived as the total process of appropriation of a new technology. This is partly responsible for the theory's name of Resources and Appropriation Theory. To appropriate a new technology one should first be motivated to use it. When sufficient motivation is developed one should be able to acquire physical access to a computer, the Internet or another digital medium. Additionally, one needs the material resources to keep using the technology that consists of peripheral equipment, software, ink, paper, subscriptions and so on. Having physical and material access does not automatically lead to appropriation of the technology as one first has to develop several skills to use the medium concerned. The more these skills are developed the more appropriate use can be made of the technology in several applications. The concept of usage can be measured, among others by the observation of the frequency of usage and the number and diversity of applications. This process is depicted in Figure 2.2, which is the framework for the relative long exposition of the following section.

The *characteristics of ICT* as a technology are sideward factors in Figure 2.1. When a technology is experienced to be complex, expensive, multi-faced (multimedia) and leading to problems of accessibility and usability this will increase access problems in general. Computer devices simply are not equal to, for example, television sets. In the first decades of the existence of ICT the characteristics mentioned were widespread in the supply of this technology. In the most recent decade considerable progress has been made in making the hardware and software concerned more accessible and usable for larger parts of the population. Understandably, this has reduced the gaps of digital skills and usage.

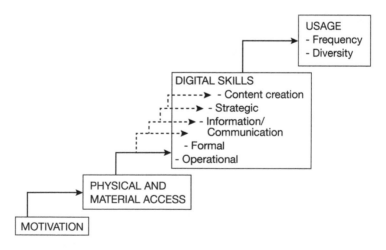

Figure 2.2 Four successive kinds of access in the appropriation of digital technology

The final factor in Figure 2.1 is the stake of the digital divide. The consequences of unequal access of all kinds are more or less participation in several fields of society: economic (such as jobs), social (e.g. social contacts), political (voting and other kinds of political participation), cultural (participating in cyber-culture), spatial (being able to lead a mobile life) and institutional (such as realizing citizenship rights).

The following section presents the main results to date of empirical research following the four kinds of access distinguished. Most results presented are from the Netherlands where the author of this chapter was able to test his theory in a large number of surveys and skill performance tests. Most likely the state of affairs in Germany will be not much different from the Netherlands. The only two differences between the countries are that the Netherlands has a bit higher Internet access rate than Germany (91 percent of Internet household access as compared to 82 percent in 2010, according to Eurostat) and a larger proportion of users with a low educational background. The popularization of the Internet has advanced a bit more in the Netherlands than in Germany.

Research on motivation, physical access, skills and usage

Motivation

Prior to physical access comes the wish to have a computer and to be connected to the Internet. Many of those who remain at the "wrong" side of the digital divide have motivational problems. It appears that there are not only "have nots," but also "want nots" considering digital technology. With the advent of a new technology, acceptance problems in terms of motivation always are highest. In the 1980s and 1990s many people gave answers in survey questions that they did not need a computer or Internet connection. When the technology has largely diffused in society the motivation to obtain a computer and reach Internet access increases fast. In countries with a high diffusion of ICTs even people that are far above age 80 are motivated to get access, if only to communicate with their grandchildren. In the year 2011 it was observed that 95 percent of the Dutch population was motivated to have access to the Internet (van Deursen and van Dijk, 2011). In the age of Internet hype and afterwards when diffusion rose fast, research for the motivation to have access has been relatively ignored. At the turn of the century German and American surveys (ARD/ZDF, 1999a; NTIA, 2000) showed that the main reasons for the refusal were:

- no need or significant usage opportunities;
- no time or desire;
- rejection of the medium (the Internet and computer games as "dangerous" media);

- lack of money;
- lack of skills.

In several European and American surveys reported between 1999 and 2003 it was revealed that half of the unconnected to the Internet at that time explicitly responded that they would refuse to get connected, for the list of reasons just mentioned (e.g., ARD/ZDF, 1999b) and a Pew Internet and American Life survey (Lenhart *et al.*, 2003).

These observations lead us to one of the most confusing myths produced by popular ideas about the digital divide: that people are either in or out, included or excluded. The last referenced survey revealed that the Internet population in fact is ever shifting (Lenhart *et al.*, 2003). First, there are so-called intermittent users: people who go offline for extended periods for some reason. A second often unnoticed group is the drop-outs that more or less permanently lost connection to the Internet. Their number was 10 percent of the American population in 2002 (Lenhart *et al.*, 2003). The next group is the "net-evaders" that simply refuse to use the Internet and it does not matter whether they have the resources or not (among them older managers charging their secretaries to use e-mail and search the Internet and persons being proud of not using that "filthy medium" or operating computers as that is deemed to be "women's work" by some macho-male workers). However, the number of intermittent users, drop-outs and net-evaders is decreasing as the technology becomes a necessary tool for daily life. In the year 2011 the proportion of drop-outs in the Dutch population fell to 9 percent among a total of complete non-users also comprising 9 percent. The most important reasons for complete non-use and for drop-out from earlier use are lack of interest (47 percent), feeling too old to use it (26 percent), not needing it (22 percent), and having insufficient skills to use it (15 percent) (van Deursen and van Dijk, 2011). However, the most important result of this 2011 survey was that only 7.3 percent of non-users in the Netherlands were prepared to potentially use the Internet in the future. So, in this country the hard core of refusing non-users has already been reached.

The ever-shifting Internet population focuses our attention on a second, perhaps even more important myth produced by the misleading dichotomy of the digital divide. This is the assumption that those who have a computer or Internet connection are actually using it. Many presumed users use the computer or the Internet only once a week or a couple of times a month, a few people even never use them. Measuring computer and Internet access in survey questions often conflates possession or connection with use or usage time. Time diary studies and the like show much larger differences or divides between categories of people as will be argued in the subsection on usage below.

The factors explaining motivational access are both of a social or cultural and a mental or psychological nature. A primary social explanation is that "the Internet does not have appeal for low-income and low-educated people" (Katz and Rice, 2002, p. 93). To dig deeper into the reasons for this lack of interest it seems appropriate to complete the large-scale surveys with qualitative studies in local communities and cultural groups. This was done for instance by Laura Stanley in a San Diego study in poor Latino and African American working class neighborhoods (Stanley, 2001) and by the University of Texas in poor communities of Austin (Rojas *et al.*, 2004). They discovered the importance of traditional masculine cultures (rejecting computer work that is not "cool" and "something girls do") and of particular minority and working class lifestyles.

However, most pronounced are mental and psychological explanations. Here the phenomena of computer anxiety and technophobia come forwards. Computer anxiety is a feeling of discomfort, stress, or fear experienced when confronting computers (Brosnan, 1998; Chua, Chen and Wong, 1999; Rockwell and Singleton, 2002). Technophobia is a fear of technology in general and distrust in its beneficial effects. According to a representative UCLA survey of 2003, more than 30 percent of new American Internet users reported that they were moderately to highly technophobic and the same applied to 10 percent of experienced Internet users (UCLA, 2003, p. 25). Computer anxiety and technophobia are still major barriers to computer and Internet access in many countries, especially among seniors, people with a low educational level and a part of the female population. These phenomena are decreasing, but do not completely disappear with a further diffusion of computers and Internet access in society.

The continuation of anxiety is partly explained by personality characteristics. The Big Five personality dimensions (agreeableness, conscientiousness, neuroticism, extraversion, and openness) are known to be related to computer use, attitude and stress (Hudiburg, 1999). For example, neuroticism aggravates problems experienced in approaching and using computers and extraversion alleviates them. See Hudiburg (1999) and Finn and Korukonda (2004) for the personality dimensions related to computer use.

Physical and material access

The overwhelming majority of digital divide investigations are dedicated to the observation of divides of physical access to personal computers and the Internet among demographical categories that are obvious in this respect: income, education, age, sex, and ethnicity. The first nation-wide surveys in the developed countries at the end of the 1990s and the turn of the century all showed growing gaps of access between people with high and low income or education and majority ethnicities as compared to minority ethnicities. However, the gender physical access divide has closed in those years, complete closure for this gap only happened in the Northern American and North-Western European countries. Considering age, the relationship is curved: physical access peaks in the age group of 25 to 40 and sharply declines afterwards. Clearly, the youngest generation and women benefit from the household possession of computers, as households are the most familiar survey unit of measurement. From the years 2000–2002 onwards the physical access divides in the northern European, American and Eastern-Asian developed countries started to decline as the categories with high income and education reached partial saturation and people with lower income and education started to catch up (NTIA, 2002; Horrigan and Rainie, 2002; Eurobarometer 56–63, 2001–2010). However, in the developing countries the physical access divide kept widening and is still widening (United Nations Statistics Division, 2004; van Dijk, 2005).

Probably, the path of the physical access divide follows the familiar S-curve of the adoption of innovations. However, the path is much more complex and differentiated among groups of the population than the S-curve projects and there are serious problems with mainstream diffusion theory considering computer and Internet technology (see van Dijk, 2005, p. 62–65). One of these problems is treated by Norris (2001) who makes a distinction between normalization and stratification models of diffusion. In the normalization model it is presupposed that the differences between groups only increase in the early stages of adoption and that differences disappear with saturation in the last stages. In the stratification model it is assumed that first, there is a different point of departure of the access curve for the higher and the lower social strata and second, a different point of arrival: for some strata it might never reach 90 to 100 percent.

The two models lead to quite different projections of the evolution of the digital divide. (See Figure 2.2 above.) This figure compares the curve of adoption of the highest and lowest social strata in terms of physical access. In all countries, there is higher access for people with high education and income and a low age and there is lower access for people with low education and income and a high age. It shows how they come together after reaching a particular tipping point and in this way gradually close the physical access divide. The model projects (almost) complete future closure when a normalization model applies and the continuation of a (smaller) gap when the stratification model applies. In the Netherlands and other rich countries it seems that the normalization model applies (van Deursen and van Dijk, 2011); in poorer countries the stratification model gives a better reflection of the current and the probable coming situation. The developed countries on average crossed the tipping point between the years of 2000 and 2005. The developing countries have not yet reached this state (see the annual ITU (International Telecommunications Union) figures of the diffusion of PCs and Internet connections across countries with different level of development [United Nations Statistics

Division, 2004]). A tipping point is a concept of network theory. It refers to a sudden acceleration or slow-down in the diffusion of an innovation. Concerning the digital divide two tipping points appear. The first is the acceleration that happens when sufficient other people are connected to a network; then it makes more sense to also connect. This occurs at around 20 to 25 percent of diffusion. The higher social strata and the young are the first to experience this drive to connect. In this way the divide broadens. The second tipping point happens when a majority is connected and saturation sets in, usually at around a two-thirds access rate. On this occasion the lower social strata and the seniors are starting to catch up and the divide narrows. It is this second point that we are talking about here and that is indicated in Figure 2.3.

The background variables mentioned reveal that material and social types of inequality are prevalent in digital divide research explaining differences of physical access. The concepts of economic, social, and cultural capital are the most popular ones. Others defend a resource based approach (van Dijk *et al..* 2000; de Haan, 2003; Dutta-Bergman, 2005). The author of this chapter combines a resource based and a network approach that focuses on social positions (van Dijk, 2005). According to this theory, differences of physical access are related to a distribution of resources (temporal, mental, material, social and cultural) that in turn is explained by personal categories such as age, sex, intelligence, personality and ability and positions in society (of labor, education and household position).

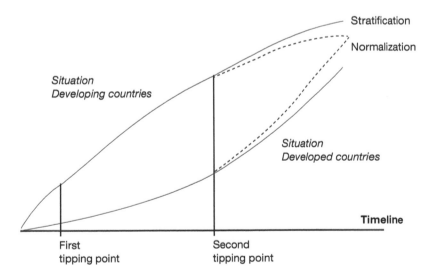

Figure 2.3 Evolution of the digital divide of physical access in time (line below: access of categories of low education, low income and higher age; line above: access of categories of high education, high income and lower age)

Unfortunately digital divide research with a focus on physical access is rather descriptive and does not relate to such theories. The most common exception is the S-curve of adoption derived from diffusion of innovations theory and partly reflected in Figure 2.3.

Next to physical access the broader concept of *material access* can be distinguished. This applies when not only the core hardware of a computer, smart phone or Internet connection is considered but also peripheral equipment, materials such as paper and ink, software and not forgetting subscriptions. They comprise a growing part of the total expenses for digital media. While hardware costs for single devices tend to decline, the number of devices purchased these days tends to rise. Evidently, sufficient income remains an important condition here. So, when the physical access gap is closing, income inequalities remain important for material access at large.

Digital skills

After having acquired the motivation to use computers and some kind of physical access to them, one has to learn to manage the hardware and software. Here the problem of a lack of skills might appear, according to the model in Figure 2.2. This problem is framed with terms such as "computer, information or multimedia literacy" and "computer skills" or "information capita." Steyaert (2000) and van Dijk (1999 2003, 2005) introduced the concept of "digital skills" as a succession of several types of skill. The most basic are "instrumental skills" (as per Steyaert) or "operational skills" (as per van Dijk), the capacities to work with hardware and software. These skills have acquired much attention in the literature and in public opinion.

The most popular view is that skills problems are solved when these skills are mastered. However, many scholars engaged with information processing in an information society have called attention to all kinds of content-related skills required to successfully use computers and the Internet. Steyaert distinguishes between "structural skills" and "strategic skills." Van Dijk (2005) proposed a comparable distinction between "information skills" and "strategic skills." Information skills are the skills to search, select, and process information in computer and network sources. They can be defined as the capacities to use computer and network sources as the means for particular goals and for the general goal of improving one's position in society.

In the last four years the author of this chapter and his Ph.D. student Alexander van Deursen have considerably refined the concept of digital/Internet skills into six types of digital/Internet skills and several kinds of measurement ranging from large-scale surveys to performance tests of Internet tasks in a media laboratory (van Deursen and van Dijk, 2010). The following medium-related and content-related Internet skills have been distinguished and (already) partly measured, as in Figure 2.4. The focus of Internet skills can easily be enlarged to encompass other digital media.

Very little scientific research has been done on the actual level of digital skills possessed by people. Unfortunately it is extremely difficult to determine the actual level because most digital skills are not the result of computer courses, but of learning through practice in particular social user environments (van Dijk, 2005). So far, there are only few estimates of skills. A number of large-scale surveys have revealed dramatic differences of skills among populations, also among populations of countries with large new media diffusion (van Dijk, 2005; Warschauer, 2003). However, these surveys measure the actual level of digital skills possessed only by questions asking respondents to estimate their own level of digital skills. This kind of measurement has obvious problems of validity (Hargittai, 2002; Merritt, Smith and Renzo, 2005; Talja, 2005).

Measurements of real performances only occur in small educational settings or as a part of computer classes. The problem of these measurements is that they are fully normative: whether the goal of a particular course has been reached. A problem for both types of measurements, surveys and course exams is that they mostly use a limited definition of digital skills that does not go beyond the operational skills listed in Figure 2.4. There is virtually no attention to the "higher" content-related skills mentioned in this figure.

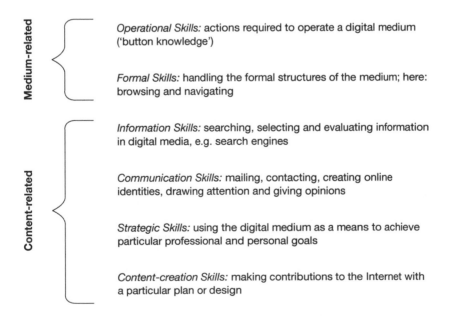

Figure 2.4 Six types of digital skills applied to Internet skills

The only way to obtain a valid and complete measurement of digital skills is to charge people with performance tests of computer and Internet tasks that they regularly meet in daily life. Performance tests have so far only been done by Hargittai (2002). She charged 54 demographically diverse American experimental subjects with five rather different Internet search tasks that belong to the information skills (as in Figure 2.4). The results revealed enormous differences of accomplishment of these tasks and the time needed for them.

The labor-intensive performance tests of van Deursen and van Dijk in a university media lab where they invited a cross-section of the Dutch population (adding up to more than 300 people) to perform nine comprehensive Internet tasks during 1.5 hours, have provided a more valid picture of the actual skills possessed by people (van Deursen, 2010). So far, operational, formal, information and strategic Internet skills have been measured (van Deursen and van Dijk, 2010). At the time of writing the communication and content-related skills are being tested.

The main conclusion of these tests is that in these tasks Dutch citizens showed a fairly high-level of operational and formal skills. On average 80 percent of the operational skill assignments and 72 percent of the formal skill assignments were successfully completed. However, the levels of information skills and strategic Internet skills attained were much lower. Information skill assignments were completed on average by 62 percent and strategic skill assignments on average by only 25 percent of those subjected to these performance tests. Unfortunately, there are no standards of comparison since comparable performance tests in other countries are non-existent.

The second main conclusion was that there were significant differences of performance between people of different ages and education. The most important factor appeared to be educational background. People with higher education perform better on all skills than people with a lower educational background. Age primarily appears to be a significant contributor to medium-related skills. Younger people perform better on these skills than older people do. However, the results regarding content-related skills prove different. In fact, age positively contributes to the level of content-related skills, meaning that older people perform better in information and strategic skills than young people on the condition that they have an adequate level of medium-related skills. However, due to the lack of medium-related Internet skills, many seniors are seriously limited in their content-related skills. This observation puts the abilities of the so-called "digital generation" in another perspective than it is known in public opinion. It also shows that the skills inequality problem will not automatically disappear in the future and that substantial education of all kinds and life experience remain vital for digital skills too. In none of the series of performance tests done so far has any gender difference been observed, despite the fact that in pre-test questionnaires males indicated that their skills were significantly better than those of females.

Usage

Evidently, the purpose of the total process of appropriation is usage, according to Figure 2.2. Having sufficient motivation, physical access and skills to apply digital media are necessary but not sufficient conditions of actual use. Usage has its own grounds or determinants. As a dependent factor it can be measured in at least four ways:

1 usage time and frequency;
2 number and diversity of usage applications;
3 broadband or narrowband use;
4 more or less active or creative use.

In the remainder of this chapter I will concentrate on the first two ways. Current computer and Internet use statistics are notoriously unreliable with their shifting and divergent operational definitions of use, most often made by market research bureaus. They only give some indication how much actual use differs from physical access. Clearly, actual use diverges far from potential use. In the U.S. more exact measures of daily, weekly or monthly Internet use are reported in the annual surveys of, for instance, the Pew Internet and American Life Project (www.pewinternet.org) and the UCLA Internet Reports (www.digitalcenter.org). In Europe the same is done by the annual Eurobarometer and Eurostat statistics. However, the most valid and reliable estimations of actual usage time are made in detailed daily time diary studies that are representative for a particular country. They sometimes produce striking results. For example the Dutch Social and Cultural Planning Agency found in a 2001 time diary study that the number of weekly hours of computer and Internet use of males at that time was double as compared to females (Steyaert and de Haan, 2001). Ten years later this gender gap of computer and Internet usage time has almost closed in the Netherlands (van Deursen and van Dijk, 2011). Anyway, this still means that when a physical access gap for a particular social category closes, this does not mean that the comparable usage gap also disappears. This goes for frequency and time of usage but also for usage applications and the other two factors mentioned above. For example, in all countries males and females still have different preferences for particular Internet applications. We will see that there is still a gender usage gap in terms of applications.

A usage factor that is likely to equalize first is usage time. In 2010, van Deursen and van Dijk observed for the first time in history that Dutch people with low education were using the Internet in their leisure time for more hours a day than people with high education, specifically 3.2 hours a day against 2.6 hours. This turned the computer and Internet usage time of the social classes in terms of education completely upside down as compared to the situation in the 1980s and 1990s when usage was completely dominated by the high educated. This was seen as a sign of the growing popularization of the Internet. This medium is merging completely with daily life and everyday activities and has become an essential facility for the large majority of people in the developed countries.

With this observation in mind it becomes relevant to look at the number and diversity of usage applications. What are the people with lower and higher education doing on the Internet? It appeared that people with low education used a smaller number of applications but for a much longer period of time. Popular applications requiring a relative long usage time for people with low education were chatting, online gaming, receiving audio-visual programs, social networking and trading places for products (e.g. eBay). Chatting and online gaming were the only Internet applications that were used significantly more by people with low education than with high education in the Netherlands.

These observations are confirmations of the thesis of the appearance of a so-called *usage gap* in terms of computer and Internet use that was suggested by van Dijk (1999, 2003, 2005), Bonfadelli (2002), Park (2002), Cho *et al.*, (2003), Zillien and Hargittai (2009) and others. The basic statement is that some sections of the population will more frequently use the *serious applications* with the highest advantageous effects on capital and resources (work, career, study, societal participation etc.), while other sections will use the *entertainment applications* with no, or very little, advantageous effects on capital and resources. This statement was first applied to people with low and high education, by van Dijk, Bonfadelli and others, in this way framing an education usage gap. This thesis is clearly related to the knowledge gap thesis of the 1970s (Tichenor *et al.*, 1970) that stated that the high educated derived more knowledge from the mass media such as television and newspapers than the low educated. Only, the usage gap is much broader and potentially more effective in terms of social inequality than the knowledge gap because the usage gap concerns differential uses and activities in all spheres of daily life, not just the perception and cognition of mass media.

An education usage gap was confirmed in an Internet usage trend survey in the Netherlands (van Dijk and van Deursen, 2012). Of the 31 Internet applications investigated (15 applications labeled "serious," 6 labeled "entertainment," and 10 "neutral," being "general every-day life applications" such as e-mail and search engine use) people with low education used significantly more entertainment than serious applications and for the high educated it was the opposite. However, age and gender usage gaps were also observed and in the year 2010 they were stronger than the education usage gap (van Deursen and van Dijk, 2013). Young people (ages 16–35) used significantly more social networking, uploading and downloading of music and video files, chatting, gaming and free surfing, but also more serious applications such as news services, discussion groups, job hunting and educational applications than people of medium and old age. None of the 31 Internet applications were used significantly more by people of medium and old age. A gender usage gap was revealed by a significant higher use of 18 of the total of 31 Internet applications by males. Females significantly more often used the applications of e-mail, social networking, online gaming and slightly more often used patient websites or self-help groups.

Surveying the growing number of usage application surveys in the world, the author of this chapter draws the conclusion that, increasingly, all familiar social and cultural differences in society are reflected in computer and Internet use. He expects that the age usage gap will be the first to become smaller, with a large number of Internet applications that previously were mainly used by young people, such as social networking, online gaming, chatting and downloading audiovisuals, spreading to other age groups.

Research of unequal access effects

Strangely enough, research of the social effects of all these inequalities of access is very scarce. Apparently, researchers take the advantages of access to computers and the Internet for granted. But actually what is the stake of these inequalities? Do people with no, or limited access of the four kinds distinguished experience real disadvantages? So far, an important argument has been that people still have the old channels at their disposal that also deliver the information and communication channels they need. For those who have no Internet, plenty of radio and television stations and newspapers are available. For those who have no access to e-commerce, the number of physical shops abounds. People who need new social contacts or a romantic encounter do not necessarily need a social-networking site or an online dating service. They still have the choice of innumerable physical meeting places. Those who want to make a reservation can still pick up the phone.

To investigate the real advantages and disadvantages of having or not having access of the four kinds portrayed above, the Internet use trend surveys of 2010 and 2011 in the Netherlands (van Deursen and van Dijk, 2010, 2011) proposed to the respondents a number of precise statements about the potential advantages of Internet use that actually are measurement items of the concept of participation in Figure 2.1. These statements and their support are in Table 2.1. This is measured via the level of support among the respondents for ten statements which indicated the advantages of Internet usage. Among the Dutch Internet users surveyed, the average respondent agreed with four of the ten statements, as illustrated in Table 2.1. However, there are big inequalities between people of different ages, educational levels and kinds of occupation. (See Figure 2.5.) In the end this is the most important figure concerning the digital divide. Here it is shown that access to computers and the Internet really matters. That those without access have a clear disadvantage and that those who only have access to traditional channels of information and communication lag behind. With the growing diffusion of these digital media in society they will probably lag further and further behind to finally become excluded from large parts of society. This is why more or less participation is the legitimate final effect of unequal access in the model of Figure 2.1.

Table 2.1 Percentage of Internet users in the Netherlands giving positive answers to potential advantages of Internet use in 2011

Statement	*Percentage Affirming*
After an online application concerning a vacancy I have obtained a job	19
Via the Internet I was able to buy a product cheaper than in a shop	80
Via the Internet I was able to sell or exchange something I otherwise would have taken as a loss	63
Via the Internet I have discovered which political party I would like to vote for	37
Via the Internet I have come across an association I became a member of (such as a sports club, a cultural association, a trade union or a political organization)	22
Via the Internet I have acquired one or more friends that I have really met later	32
Via a dating site I have made an appointment with a potential partner	14
Via the Internet I have discovered which medical illness I had	27
Via the Internet I have booked an economical holiday trip	60
Via the Internet I have achieved a discount on a product	42

Source: van Deursen and van Dijk, 2011.

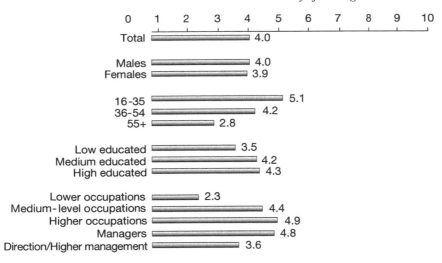

Figure 2.5 Average number of positive answers to 10 potential advantages of Internet use in the Netherlands in 2011. Source: van Deursen & van Dijk, 2011

Conclusion: Inequality in the network society

In the former section, we saw that unequal access to computers and the Internet has shifted from unequal motivation and physical access to inequalities of skills and usage. This observation is known in the literature as the so-called *Second Level Divide* (Hargittai, 2002; DiMaggio *et al.*, 2004) or the *Deepening Divide* (van Dijk, 2005). With the gradual close of the physical access divide, the digital divide problem as a whole is not solved. On the contrary, the problem gets deeper. Differences of skills and preferences for particular Internet use applications will become ever more important for society. The unequal benefits of Internet use as portrayed in Table 2.1 and Figure 2.5 are most likely caused by differences of skills, motivations and preferences of use that belong to a particular age, gender, educational level and occupation. Here it has to be admitted that seniors are at a disadvantage concerning some applications in Table 2.1 as they most likely search fewer jobs and partners online than younger people. However, this does not apply to other applications. The same survey revealed, for example, that young people also obtain much more information about their medical illness via the Internet than elderly people, who clearly need this information more (van Deursen and van Dijk, 2011).

According to a relational view of inequality differences of physical access (connectivity), skills and usage will become much more strategically important in a network society. A network society can be defined as a society that is increasingly based upon a combined infrastructure of social and media networks (van Dijk, 1999, 2006b, 2012). In this society, occupying particular positions and having relations with this position become decisive for one's place, opportunities and chances in society (van Dijk, 2005). Access to and being able to use social and media networks increasingly merge in a network society. Those who have less connection in social networks usually also have less access to and ability to use media networks such as the Internet. Inclusion and exclusion in both social and media networks combined might be a powerful creator of structural inequality in the network society. It could create the following tripartite structure.

The core of this concentric picture of a network society portrays an information elite of about 15 percent of the population in high-access developed societies that has very dense and overlapping social and media networks. They are people with high levels of income and education, they have the best jobs and societal positions and they have more than 95 percent Internet access. These elite are accustomed to living in dense social networks. They are extended with a large number of long-distance ties that are part of a very mobile lifestyle.

The majority of the population (50 to 60 percent) in these societies has fewer social and media network ties and less Internet access, skill and use. The Internet applications used are of a relatively less serious and more of an entertainment kind as in the case of the usage gap thesis discussed earlier.

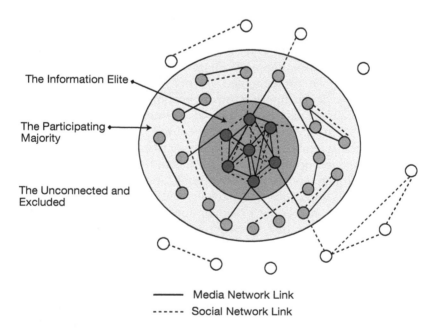

Figure 2.6 Potential tripartite structure of the network society. Source: van Dijk (1999, 2006, 2012)

Finally we have the unconnected and excluded part of society that is relatively isolated in terms of both social networks and media network connections. They comprise at least a quarter of the population of (even) developed societies. They consist of the lowest social classes, the unemployed, particular elderly people, ethnic minorities and a large group of migrants. They participate considerably less in several fields of society.

Such a dark picture of structural inequality does not have to appear. The inequalities of the digital divide and digital skills can be mitigated by deliberate policies for the labor market, for the training of employees and for educational improvements at all levels, including adult education (see van Dijk, 2005, for a complete policy program).

References

ARD/ZDF-Arbeitsgruppe Multimedia. (1999a). ARD/ZDF-online-studie 1999: Wird online alltagsmedium? [ARD/ZDF online study: Is online becoming an everyday medium?]. *Media Perspektiven* 1999(8), 388–409.

ARD/ZDF-Arbeitsgruppe Multimedia. (1999b). Nichtnutzer von online: Einstellungen und zugangsbarrieren. Ergebnisse der ARD/ZDF-offline-studie 1999 [Online nonusers: Attitudes and access barriers. Results of the ARD/ZDF offline study 1999]. *Media Perspektiven* 1999(8), 415–422.

Bonfadelli, H. (2002). The Internet and knowledge gaps: A theoretical and empirical investigation. *European Journal of Communication*, 17(1), 65–84.

Brosnan, M. J. (1998). The impact of computer anxiety and self-efficacy upon performance. *Journal of Computer Assisted Learning*, 14, 223–234.

Cho, J., de Zúñiga, H., Rojas, H. and Shah, D. (2003). Beyond access: The digital divide and Internet uses and gratifications. *IT & Society*, 1(4), 46–72.

Chua, S. L., Chen, D. T. and Wong, A. F. L. (1999). Computer anxiety and its correlates: A meta-analysis. *Computers in Human Behavior*, 15, 609–623.

de Haan, J. (2003). IT and social inequality in the Netherlands. *IT & Society*, 1(4), 27–45.

DiMaggio, P., Hargittai, E., Celeste, C. and Shafer, S. (2004). From unequal access to differentiated use. In K. Neckerman (ed.) *Social Inequality*. New York: Russell Sage Foundation, 355–400.

Dutta-Bergman, M. (2005). Access to the Internet in the context of community participation and community satisfaction. *New Media and Society*, 17, 89–109.

Finn, S. and Korukonda, A. R. (2004). Avoiding computers: Does personality play a role? In E. Bucy and J. Newhagen (eds.), *Media access: Social and psychological dimensions of new technology use*. London: LEA, 73–90.

Hargittai, E. (2002). The second-level digital divide: Differences in people's online skills. *First Monday*, 7(4). Retrieved from http://firstmonday.org/htbin/cgiwrap/bin/ojs/index.php/fm/article/view/942/864

Horrigan, J. and Rainie, L. (2002). Getting serious online: As Americans gain experience, they pursue more serious activities. Washington DC: Pew Internet and American Life Project. Retrieved August 28, 2004, from http//:www.pewinternet.org

Hudiburg, R. A. (1999). Preliminary investigation of computer stress and the big five personality factors. *Psychology Reports*, 85, 473–480.

Katz, J. E. and Rice, R. E. (2002). Social consequences of Internet use, access, involvement, and interaction. Cambridge, MA, US: MIT Press.

Lenhart, A., Horrigan, J., Rainie, L., Allen, K., Boyce, A., Madden, M. and O'Grady, E. (2003). The ever-shifting Internet population: A new look at Internet access and the digital divide. Washington, DC: Pew Internet and American Life Project. Retrieved August 28, 2004, from http//:www. pewinternet.org.

Merritt, K., Smith, D. and Renzo, J. C. D. (2005). An investigation of self-reported computer literacy: Is it reliable? *Issues in Information Systems* 6(1), 289–295.

Norris, P. (2001). Digital divide, civic engagement, information poverty and the Internet worldwide. Cambridge, UK: Cambridge University Press.

NTIA (National Telecommunications and Information Administration). (2000). Falling through the Net II: Toward digital inclusion. Retrieved September 29, 2004, from http://www.ntia.doc.gov/ntiahome/fttn00/contents00.html

NTIA (National Telecommunications and Information Administration). (2002). A nation online: How Americans are expanding their use of the Internet. Retrieved September 29, 2004, from http://www.ntia.doc.gov/ntiahome/dn/index.html.

Park, H. W. (2002). The digital divide in South Korea: Closing and widening divides in the 1990s. *Electronic Journal of Communication/Revue de Communication Electronique*, 12(1 & 2). Retrieved September 28, 2004, from http://www.cios.org/www/ejc

Rockwell, S. and Singleton, L. (2002). The effects of computer anxiety and communication apprehension on the adoption and utilization of the Internet. *Electronic Journal of Communication/Revue de Communication Electronique*, 12(1). Retrieved June 12, 2004, from http://www.cios.org/www/ejc

Rojas, V., Straubhaar, J., Roychowdhury, D. and Okur, O. (2004). Communities, cultural capital and the digital divide. In E. Bucy and J. Newhagen (Eds.), *Media access: Social and psychological dimensions of new technology use*. London: LEA, 107–130.

Stanley, L. (2001). Beyond access. Retrieved March 11, 2004, from www. mediamanage.net/Beyond_Access.pdf

Steyaert, J. (2000). Digitale vaardigheden: Geletterdheid in de informatiesamenleving [Digital skills: Literacy in the information society]. The Hague, Netherlands: Rathenau Instituut.

Steyaert, J. and de Haan, J. (2001). Geleidelijk digital: Een nuchtere kijk op de sociale gevolgen van ICT. Den Haag, Netherlands: Sociaal en Cultureel Planbureau.

Talja, S. (2005). The Social and discursive construction of computing skills. *Journal of the American Society for Information Science and Technology*, 56(1): 13–22.

Tichenor, P. J., Donohue, G.A. and Olien, C.N. (1970). Mass media flow and differential growth in knowledge. *Public Opinion Quarterly*, 34(2): 159–170.

Tilly, C. (1999). *Durable Inequality*. Berkeley, CA, US: University of California Press.

UCLA, University of California, Los Angeles, Center for Communication Policy. (2003). The UCLA Internet report: Surveying the digital future, year three. Los Angeles: UCLA. Retrieved March 2, 2004, from http://www.ccp.ucla.edu/pages/internet-report.asp

United Nations Statistics Division. (2004). Millennium indicators database: Personal Computers and Internet users per 100 population (ITU estimates). Retrieved March 11, 2004, from http://millenniumindicators.un.org/unsd/ mi/mi_indicator_xrxx.asp?ind_code=48

van Deursen, A. (2010). *Internet skills, vital assets in an information society.* Doctoral Thesis: Enschede: University of Twente, Netherlands.

van Deursen, A. and van Dijk, J. (2010). *Trendrapport computer en Internetgebruik 2010, een Nederlands en een Europees perspectief* (Trendrapport Komputer und Internet Benutzung, Ein Niederländisches und Europeïsches Perspectiv). Enschede: Universtity of Twente. Available: www.cfes.nl.

van Deursen, A. and van Dijk, J. (2011). *Trendrapport computer en Internetgebruik 2011, een Nederlands en een Europees perspectief* (Trendrapport Komputer und Internet Benutzung, Ein Niederländisches und Europeïsches Perspectiv). Enschede: Universtity of Twente. Available: www.cfes.nl.

van Deursen, A. and van Dijk, J. (2013). *Digital skills: The key to the information society.* Thousand Oaks, CA, US: Sage.

van Dijk, J. (1999). *The network society: Social aspects of new media,* 1st Edition. London: Sage.

van Dijk, J. (2003). A framework for digital divide research. *Electronic Journal of Communication/Revue de Communication Electronique,* 12(1). Retrieved September 30, 2004, from http://www.cios.org/getfile/vandijk

van Dijk, J. (2005). *The deepening divide: Inequality in the information society.* London: Sage.

van Dijk, J. (2006a). Digital divide research, achievements and shortcomings. *Poetics, 34,* 221–235.

van Dijk, J. (2006b). *The network society: Social aspects of new media,* 2nd Edition. London: Sage.

van Dijk, J. (2012). *The network society: Social aspects of new media,* 3rd Edition. London: Sage.

van Dijk, J., Liset, J., de Haan, J. and Rijken, S., (2000). *Digitalisering van de leefwereld: Een onderzoek naar informatie en communicatietechnologie en sociale ongelijkheid* [Digitization of everyday life: A survey of information and communication technology and social inequality]. The Hague, Netherlands: Sociaal en Cultureel Planbureau.

van Dijk, J. and van Deursen, A. (2012). A social revolution online? The digital divide shifts to gaps of usage. Paper presented at the 62nd Annual Conference of the International Communication Association, May 24–28, 2012, Phoenix, US.

Warschauer, M. (2003). *Technology and social inclusion: Rethinking the digital divide.* Cambridge, MA, US: MIT Press.

Wellman, B. and Berkowitz, S.D. (Eds.). (1988). *Social structures, A network approach.* London: JAI Press.

Zillien, N. and Hargittai, E. (2009). Digital distinction: Status-specific Internet uses. *Social Science Quarterly,* 90(2): 274–291.

Note

1 This is an adapted version of a chapter that appeared as "Digitale Spaltung und digitale Kompetenzen" in the German book "*Informationsgerechtigkeit*" (A. Schüllerr-Zwierlein and N. Zillien (Eds.), 2012). Berlin, Germany: De Gruyter.

Section 2

Highly developed nations and regions

3 The digital divide in Europe

Nicole Zillien
University of Trier

Mirko Marr
Publicitas AG

Social inequality and the Internet

Sociologist Theodor Geiger's work on social inequalities argues that social strata and individual action and perception correlate, outlined as the concept of mentality. Mentality is a psychic predisposition, an immediate imprint on a person by their social world and the experiences made in and radiating from it (Geiger, 1932/1972, p. 77). That is, social position and mentality do not necessarily refer to each other, but there are status-typical mentalities. Accordingly, there is a cover ratio between external structures and individual psyche, which suggests that similar objective characteristics promote the development of similar subjective characteristics. Thus, Geiger thinks in categorical defined inequalities, without leaving aside questions of lifestyle and inner conditions. The French sociologist Pierre Bourdieu (1979/1982) follows a similar principle, when he defines class-specific cultural forms and from this develops his concept of habitus. Using correspondence analysis, Bourdieu verified the existence of class-specific patterns of taste by clustering preferences in music, cooking, art, literature, and so on. As the habitus incorporates both the impact of external conditions and individual practices, the concept represents a link between social structure and individual way of life. Geiger's concept of mentality as well as Bourdieu's concept of habitus can be useful to explain different practices in everyday life. Drawing on these concepts, this chapter suggests that people's incorporation of digital media into their everyday lives does not happen independent of the constraints and advantages of their existing surroundings; rather, the Internet is just one component of people's lives in which numerous social factors interact with each other.

For differences in media use to be considered as a type of social inequality, it has to be the case that the different types of media use entail social advantages or disadvantages. From its beginning in the mid-1990s, the idea that differences in access and usage of the Internet would result in social inequalities accompanied the upcoming spread of the Internet. Those disparities became socio-politically charged by their interpretation against the background of the high priority given to the promotion of digital technologies by European politics in the beginning of the second millennium. This priority was driven by the belief "that the benefits of these technologies and access to the world of information that is contained within them is a benefit that no citizens in the twenty-first century should be without, certainly not at least in the developed world" (Cullen, 2001, p. 311). Reports from the European Union called this vision into question by showing that the diffusion of digital technologies was anything but a sure-fire success: Internet diffusion encountered limitations with just those social groups, that were considered as "information have-nots" in the analog world, whereas already privileged groups made the leap into the digital age with seemingly much less effort. In the long run, the resulting access gaps were interpreted as harbingers of a new two-class society in the dawning age of information. This social-threat scenario had a considerable influence on the debate (Marr, 2005) – the idea of the digital divide caused a change in thinking on the priorities of the promotion of digital technologies, which in the early 1990s were mainly operated under the premise of economic development and IT-oriented policy. The rethinking found its most visible expression in a downright competition for initiatives – in Germany for example under the catchy slogan "Internet für alle" ("Internet for everybody") – and the patronage of major political representatives, targeting the elimination of existing barriers and securing a population-wide network. In the years that followed, these political measures against the digital divide were confronted with three points of criticism (Marr and Zillien, 2010):

1 Necessity: The first point of criticism expounds the problems of the initiated measures under the aspect of necessity. Especially at the end of the 1990s, it was asked if the current disparities in Internet access might only be a snapshot of the diffusion process at a given moment in time. Critics argued that though the Internet diffusion will proceed at different speeds within different social strata, sooner or later it will amount to a near saturation in all segments, so there was no necessity for targeted promotion.
2 Appropriateness: A second point of criticism questions whether Internet access for all is sufficient to prevent digital divides. Critics argue that processes of social disadvantage cannot be eliminated, but rather might be enhanced by reaching the objective. That is because status-specific forms of Internet usage make a significant difference when it comes to the potentials of new technologies.
3 Relevance: Finally, the third criticism is directed at the implicit equation of Internet access and social privileging. Critics suggest that it is not proven that access disparities or usage differences are weighty in terms of the distribution of social resources. It is asked to what extent there is a capital-enhancing effect of the Internet.

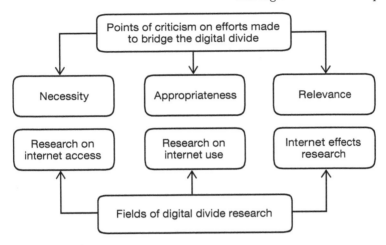

Figure 3.1 Digital divide – points of criticism and research questions

These points of criticism correspond with three fields of digital divide research:

1 Research on Internet access: Digital divide research in the early 1990s drew attention to technology diffusion and focused on the causes, extent and development of social cleavages in terms of access to Internet technology.
2 Research on Internet usage: Later research on the digital divide focused on the different forms of Internet usage regarding technology use, skills and content.
3 Internet effects research: Recent research on the digital divide usually draws on the findings of the access and usage research, without foregrounding technology-related disparities, but rather their influence on the distribution of capital-enhancing resources.

In the following the three sketched lines of research to investigate the digital divide are elaborated and, with regard to the European Union, explained in more detail.

Internet access, usage and effects

Research on Internet access

The main focus of research on Internet access is on the diffusion of the Internet in different social groups. There is no lack of representative longitudinal data concerning the observation of the Internet's spread in Europe, especially in the European Union. Corresponding studies have been and are undertaken in many countries. However, problems are caused by the fact that the central construct of Internet access is operationalized very differently. Following diffusion research (Rogers, 2003), the individual adoption of a technological innovation is considered to be completed only when five different stages of adoption have been successfully passed through: An innovation must not only be known, accepted and tried, but its use has to be habitualized and also integrated into everyday life. If this criterion of diffusion research is transferred to the spread of the Internet, access had to be linked to a regular usage over a long period of time. Research on Internet access is rarely meeting this requirement. Considering this, it can be said that a complete penetration of the population by the Internet is still far away. Even if one applies the rather soft criterion of at least using the Internet at home two or three times a month, at present only 60 percent of the adult population in the European Union can be classified as Internet users (see Table 3.1). Decisive for the question of the digital divide, in terms of access research is the fact that these access rates across different social groups and different countries still vary considerably. An analysis of recent Eurobarometer data shows that four European countries stand out with the highest rates of Internet access at home: the Netherlands (94 percent), Sweden (90 percent), Denmark (88 percent), and Finland (78 percent). Generally, there are higher rates of Internet use in northern and western countries of the European Union. Fewer than half of the population has Internet access at home in Hungary (48 percent), Bulgaria (43 percent), Cyprus (43 percent), Romania (39 percent), Greece (38 percent) and Portugal (35 percent) (Special Eurobarometer 362, 2011, p. 48).

The binary concepts of users and non-users of the Internet, is frequently criticized as being of limited analytical utility. This simple concept assumes that either all users use the Internet in the same way or that usage differences are irrelevant. Selwyn (2004, p. 345) thus came to the conclusion that a binary understanding of the digital divide is "limited and rudimentary." Jung, Qui and Kim (2001, p. 509) accused the concept of technological determinism and Webster (2002, p. 97) noted: "[T]he model lacks sufficient sociological sophistication." Taking this criticism into account, subsequent studies about digital divide tried to cover inequalities of Internet usage in a more differentiated way.

Research on Internet usage

All in all, research on Internet usage analyzes the differences between Internet users in three fields: 1) differences in terms of technology usage, such as the applied Internet equipment, or the frequency of Internet use; 2) differences in skills, for example, the skills to operate a computer or the ability to research specific information through a search engine; 3) differences in terms of used Internet content, such as information or entertainment content.

Differences in terms of technology usage

The Eurobarometer surveys on the information society technologies and services – which started in 1995 and to date have been repeated more than forty times – for example, ask for the places of Internet access (at home, at work, at school, at university, in a friend's house, at a public Internet access point, on the move from a laptop, on the move from a mobile phone, and so on) and for the frequencies of Internet use. Table 3.1 shows that in the European Union 44 percent of the population use the Internet at home (almost) everyday. There are considerable status-related differences: While 57 percent of high-status persons use the Internet (almost) everyday, only one third of low-status persons do so. Besides this there are also remarkable differences in using the Internet daily depending on age and education. Also, the gender gap still exists to date, since 49 percent of men but only 40 percent of women use the Internet on a daily base at home (see Table 3.1).

Table 3.1 Internet use at home in the European Union (as a percentage)

	Everyday/ Almost everyday	Two or three times a week	About once in a week	Two or three times a month	Less often	Never	No Internet access
EU27	44	11	4	1	2	25	13
Sex							
Male	49	11	4	1	2	22	11
Female	40	11	4	1	2	28	14
Age							
15–24	74	10	2	–	1	8	5
25–39	60	13	4	2	2	12	7
40–54	42	15	6	2	3	23	9
55+	21	7	4	1	2	43	22
Education (end of)							
15–	13	6	3	1	1	50	26
16–19	39	14	5	2	3	25	12
20+	65	13	4	1	2	10	5
Still studying	85	6	2	–	1	3	3
Self-positioning on the social staircase							
Low	32	8	3	1	2	27	12
Medium	44	12	5	1	2	25	11
High	57	12	5	1	2	16	7

Source: Special Eurobarometer 359: 79, Europeans aged 15 and over (N= 26,574), November–December 2010

Another differentiated examination of varieties in technology use is, for example, made by Davison and Cotten (2003), who analyze the use of the Internet, depending on the type of Internet connection. They note that users with broadband connections, compared to those who are connected to the Internet through a dial-up connection, display different usage habits. Thus, from the type of Internet connection further layers of the digital divide can be derived. In the European Union 55 percent of all households have broadband access, and persons living in households of three or more and those from large towns are more likely to be broadband users (Special Eurobarometer 359, 2011, p. 58). The current issue of the German *(N)Onliner-Atlas* (TNS Infratest, 2011), an annual publication since 2001, shows that there is also a broadband gender gap: 63.5 percent of men, but only 42 percent of women have a broadband connection; furthermore, the proportion of broadband connections, especially in the East German area, is notably below the national average.

Such work on differences in terms of technology usage is certainly more meaningful than the mere distinction between user and non-user, but the focus is still on the use or non-use of Internet technology. How differently Internet technologies are integrated into everyday life, however, depends essentially on the Internet skills of the user, so the analysis of online skills represents a central area of research on Internet usage.

Differences in skills

Following the Special Eurobarometer 362 (2011, p. 54) 7 percent of those who do not have Internet access at home give as a reason that they do not know exactly what the Internet is. This lack of knowledge is greatest in Spain (20 percent), Belgium (19 percent) and Malta (19 percent), while interviewees from France (3 percent), Germany (3 percent) and the Netherlands (1 percent) almost never mention this rationale for their non-usage. In general, Eurostat data documents that the level of Internet skills across Europe is rising. Here, Internet skills are measured using a self-assessment approach, where respondents were asked whether they 1) use a search engine to find information; 2) send an e-mail with attached files; 3) post messages to chat rooms, newsgroups or any online discussion forum; 4) use the Internet to make telephone calls; 5) use peer-to-peer file sharing for exchanging movies, music and so on; 6) create a web page. Persons who have carried out one or two of these activities are labeled as Internet users with skills on a basic level. Those who have carried out three or four activities relate to the group of Internet users who have skills on a medium level and those who have carried out five or six of the six items are on a high level. In the year 2005, 22 percent of the interviewees were classified as users on a medium or high level, six years later, 43 percent correspond to this group (see Table 3.2).

Table 3.2 Level of Internet skills in the European Union (as a percentage)

	2005	2006	2007	2010	2011
Never used	47	45	40	28	27
Basic level	31	30	29	32	30
Medium level	17	19	23	30	32
High level	5	6	8	10	11

Source: Eurostat data 2012, representative for persons in the EU 27 aged 16 to 74

But it is questionable if self-reports are valid measurements of actual Internet skills. Technically speaking Internet skills can only be validly measured by experimental tests in a controlled environment. Hargittai (2002) emphasized early, that it was important to study differences in Internet-related skills, as these provided the basis for the Second-Level Digital Divide. For empirical analysis of relevant differences, test persons were asked to search the Internet for local cultural events, particular pieces of music or tax forms until they had found the information. The extent of the usage competencies was here operationalized as "the ability to efficiently and effectively find information on the Web" (Hargittai 2002: 2), whereby the search success and the time spent for searching represented the key criteria. In summary, it was found that the age of the respondents was negatively correlated with their capabilities for use, while the Internet experience and formal education had a positive effect. Correspondingly, Alexander van Deursen shows that socio-demographic characteristics are strongly related to Internet skills: "The most important factor – determining all types of Internet skills – is the level of educational attainment. The higher educated the subject, the better they perform on operational, formal, information, and strategic Internet skills" (van Deursen, 2010, p. 195). Another Dutch sociologist, Jan van Dijk, points to the strategic importance of digital skills, which should be defined as "capacities to use computer and network sources as the means for particular goals and for the general goal of improving one's position in society" (van Dijk, 2005, p. 88).

Differences in terms of used Internet content

Research on Internet usage focuses primarily on different types of Internet usage in a descriptive form without testing the individual effects of the particular types of usage as information, communication, transaction and entertainment. Based on Eurostat data Brandtzæg, Heim and Karahasanović (2011) build a typology of Internet users in Europe and identify five distinct user types: Non-Users (42 percent), Sporadic

Users (18 percent), Instrumental Users (18 percent), Entertainment Users (10 percent), and Advanced Users (12 percent). The Advanced Users show a very broad Internet behavior and they are rather oriented towards utility or instrumental activities than towards entertainment-related online activities. Furthermore Zillien and Hargittai (2009) show for Germany that an information related Internet use is positively correlated with the socio-economic status of the users:

> Overall, we find that a user's social status is significantly related to various types of capital-enhancing uses of the Internet, suggesting that those already in more privileged positions are reaping the benefits of their time spent online more than users from lower socioeconomic backgrounds (Zillien and Hargittai, 2009, p. 287).

However, while research on Internet usage only marginally discusses or even statistically tests short- and long-term effects of status-specific Internet use, this is the focus of Internet effects research.

Internet effects research

Internet effects research on digital divide follows the idea that not the differences in access and usage of the Internet itself, but the resulting impacts should be the focus of analysis. DiMaggio and colleagues (2004) addressed the question of whether access to the Internet leads to privileges in the following way: "Are people who have access to the Internet any better off – especially with respect to economic welfare (education, jobs, earnings) or social participation (political participation, community engagement, or receipt of government services and other public goods) – than they would be without the Internet" (DiMaggio *et al.*, 2004, p. 381)? In the opinion of DiMaggio *et al.* the presumption that the Internet facilitates access to education, job opportunities, better health and political participation is a central requirement to determining whether the digital divide should be of concern to scholars of social stratification. That is, if we were to find no relationship between occupying a more privileged position in society and benefitting from Internet usage then "there would be little to debate other than percentage point difference in access and usage over time for various groups" (Mason and Hacker, 2003, p. 41). Selwyn (2004) states, in his theoretical work, that Internet use positively influences productive, political, social, security-related and consumptive participation in society. Corresponding Internet effects were examined for example in terms of labor market integration (Boes and Preißler, 2005), political information (see Marr, 2005, 2007), civic engagement (Mossberger, Tolbert and McNeal, 2007) and income effects (DiMaggio and Bonikowski, 2008). Since these activities are not about optional aspects of life, using the Internet for certain core essential tasks can no longer be seen as simply a luxury good (Hargittai, 2008). Thus, it is mainly in the domain of capital-enhancing user routines that we can speak of digital inequality as a phenomenon of social inequality, and therefore as a relevant object of investigation.

This is especially true for health-related Internet usage, which has the potential to inform and empower patients. A study on European citizens' use of E-health services (Andreassen *et al.*, 2007) states that a total of 44 percent of the joint population of the seven countries used the Internet for health purposes. This means, that 71 percent of the Internet users used the medium for health-related activities, with significant differences between the northern (74 percent), East-European (72 percent) and southern countries (60 percent), despite the high rate in Poland (79 percent). In general, with respect to the health-related use of the online medium, socio-structural differences become apparent: younger, higher educated, high earning, professionals and city residents are more likely to be users of online health information (Murray *et al*,. 2003, Dumitru *et al.*, 2007, Ybarra and Suman 2008). It is noteworthy that almost all such studies show a significantly higher health-related Internet use by women compared to men. At large, socio-structural differences in health-related Internet use, however, are in line with the general patterns of digital inequality. Those groups who use the Internet less, in general and in the specific case of health information – the elderly, low educated, those on low income – are simultaneously exposed to greater health risks, named by a French study as a double divide:

> We found that people who would need the Internet the most as a potential source of health information – to compensate for a lack of information or for remoteness from the health-care system (difficult economic circumstances, social isolation, health problems) – are also those who use it the least (Renahy *et al.*, 2008, p. 9).

Those who could benefit most from a health-related Internet use belong, therefore, to a lesser extent to the users of the respective offerings. In another context Everett M. Rogers (1995) put forward the idea of the "innovativeness-needs paradox." That is, "[t]he individuals or other units in a system who most need the benefits of a new idea (the less educated, less wealthy, and the like) are generally the last to adopt an innovation" (Rogers, 1995, p. 295). Since, there is evidence for positive correlation between the Internet search for health information and the subjective health (Wangberg *et al.*, 2008), it is likely that a self-reinforcing effect occurs: "[I]t seems likely that Internet use may exacerbate existing socioeconomic status differences in health" (Wangberg *et al.*, 2008, p. 70). Accordingly, the Internet effects research shows that availability of the Internet rather leads to positive effects on the part of the already privileged. In other words: "This paradoxical relationship between

64   *Nicole Zillien and Mirko Marr*

innovativeness and the need for benefits of an innovation tends to result in a wider socioeconomic gap between the higher and lower socioeconomic individuals in a social system" (Rogers, 1995, p. 295).

Conclusion

Regarding the development of social inequalities, differences in Internet access and use theoretically either may lead to rising social inequalities, to shrinking social inequalities or all in all there will be no relevant effects of the Internet on social stratification (Hargittai and Hsieh, in press). Even if there is anecdotal evidence for all of these models, digital divide research empirically proves the existence of digital inequalities which result in rising social inequalities. As we have pointed out, for health-related Internet usage in Europe, that those with more resources – whether technical, financial, social, or cultural – end up using the web for more beneficial purposes. This pattern suggests that the adoption and use of the Internet highly depends on the mentality (Geiger, 1932/1972) and respective habitus (Bourdieu, 1979/1982) of the agents. The incorporation of new media into people's everyday lives does not happen independent of the constraints and advantages of existing surroundings. Rather, the adoption and use of the Internet is just one component of people's lives in which numerous social factors interact with each other. The particular uses to which status-high persons put the Internet give them even more resources through which they can improve their positions. At the same time, those in less privileged positions to a lesser extent perform potentially beneficial uses of the Internet. In consequence there will be fewer positive payoffs for people from less privileged backgrounds, which means that the Internet will reinforce or even increase existing social inequalities. That is to say, what knowledge gap research forty years ago generally ascertained is true for the Internet: "[T]he mass media seem to have a function similar to that of other social institutions: that of reinforcing or increasing existing inequities" (Tichenor *et al.*, 1970, p. 170).

References

Andreassen, H. K., Bujnowska-Fedak, M. M., Chronaki, C. E., Dumitru, R. C., Pudule, I., Santana, S., Voss, H. and Wynn, R. (2007). European citizens' use of e-health services: A study of seven countries, *BMC Public Health*, 7, 1–7.
Boes, A. and Preißler, J. (2005). Digitale Spaltung, in SOFI, IAB, ISF and INIFES (ed.), *Berichterstattung zur sozioökonomischen Entwicklung in Deutschland – Arbeit und Lebensweisen. Erster Bericht* (pp. 523–48). Wiesbaden, Germany: VS Verlag für Sozialwissenschaften.
Bourdieu, P. (1979/1982). *Die feinen Unterschiede. Kritik der gesellschaftlichen Urteilskraft.* Frankfurt am Main, Germany: Suhrkamp.

Brandtzæg, P., Heim, J. and Karahasanović, A. (2011). Understanding the new digital divide. A typology of Internet users in Europe. *International Journal of Human-Computer Studies*, 69, 123–138.

Cullen, R. (2001). Addressing the digital divide. *Online Information Review*, 25, 311–320.

Davison, E. and Cotten, S. R. (2003). Connection discrepancies: Unmasking further layers of the digital divide. *First Monday* 8 (3).

DiMaggio, P. and Bonikowski, B. (2008). Make money surfing the Web? The impact of Internet use on the earnings of U.S. workers. *American Sociological Review*, 73, 227–250.

DiMaggio, P., Hargittai, E., Celeste, C. and Shafer, S. (2004). From unequal access to differentiated use. In K. Neckerman (ed.) *Social Inequality* (pp. 355–400). New York: Russell Sage Foundation.

Dumitru, R. C., Bürkle, T., Potapov, S., Lausen, B., Wiese, B. and Prokosch, H. (2007). Use and perception of Internet for health related purposes in Germany: results of a national survey. *International Journal for Public Health*, 52, 275–285.

Geiger, T. (1932/1972). Die soziale Schichtung des deutschen Volkes. Soziographischer Versuch auf statistischer Grundlage. Stuttgart, Germany: Ferdinand Enke.

Hargittai, E. (2002). Second-level digital divide: Differences in people's online skills. *First Monday* 7 (4).

Hargittai, E. (2008). *The digital reproduction of inequality*. In D. Grusky, *Social Stratification*. Boulder, CO, US: Westview Press, 936–44.

Hargittai, E. and Hsieh, Y.P. (in press). Digital inequality. In W. H. Dutton (ed.) *Oxford handbook of Internet studies* (pp.129–150), Oxford, UK: Oxford University Press.

Jung, J., Qui, J. L. and Kim, Y. (2001). Internet connectedness and inequality. Beyond the "divide." *Communication Research*, 28, 507–535.

Marr, M. (2005). *Internetzugang und politische Informiertheit. Zur digitalen Spaltung der Gesellschaft*. Konstanz, Germany: UVK Verlag.

Marr, M. (2007). Das Internet als politisches Informationsmedium. In K. Imhof, R. Blum, O. Jarren and H. Bonfadelli (eds.), *Demokratie in der Mediengesellschaft*. *Mediensymposium Luzern Band 9* (pp. 261–284). Wiesbaden, Germany: Verlag für Sozialwissenschaften.

Marr, M. and Zillien, N. (2010). Digitale Spaltung. In W. Schweiger and K. Beck (eds.): *Handbuch Onlinekommunikation* (pp.257–282). Wiesbaden, Germany: VS Verlag.

Mason, S. M. and Hacker, K. L. (2003). Applying communication theory to digital divide research. *IT and Society*, 1, 40–55.

Mossberger, K., Tolbert, C. J. and McNeal, R. S. (2007). *Digital citizenship: The Internet, society, and participation*. Cambridge, Mass, US: MIT Press.

Murray, E., Lo, B., Pollack, L., Donelan, K., Catania, J., White, M., Zapert, K. and Turner, R. (2003). The impact of health information on the Internet on health care and the physician–patient relationship: Patient perception. *Archives of Internal Medicine*, 163, 1727–1734.

Renahy, E., Parizot, I. and Chauvin, P. (2008). Health information seeking on the Internet: a double divide? Results from a representative survey in the Paris metropolitan area, France, 2005–2006. *BMC Public Health*, 8: 69.

Rogers, E. M. (1995). *Diffusion of innovations*, 4th edition. New York: Free Press.

Rogers, E. M. (2003). *Diffusion of innovations*, 5th edition. New York: Free Press.

Selwyn, N. (2004). Reconsidering political and popular understandings of the digital divide. *New Media and Society*, 6, 341–362.

Special Eurobarometer 359. (2011). "Attitudes on data protection and electronic identity in the European Union." Brussels: European Commission, Directorate-General for Communication.

Special Eurobarometer 362. (2011). "E-communications household survey report." Brussels: European Commission, Directorate-General for Communication.

Tichenor, P. J., Donohue, G. A. and Olien, C. N. (1970). Mass media flow and differential growth in knowledge. *Public Opinion Quarterly*, 34, 159–170.

TNS Infratest. (2011). *(N)Onliner Atlas 2011*. Berlin: Initiative D21.

van Deursen, A.J.A.M. (2010). *Internet skills. Vital assets in an information society*. Enschede, the Netherlands: University of Twente.

van Dijk, J. (2005). *The deepening divide*. London: Sage.

Wangberg, S. C., Andreassen, H. K., Prokosch, H., Santana, S. M., Søren-sen, T. and Chronaki, C. E. (2008). Relations between Internet use, socio-economic status (SES), social support and subjective health. *Health Promotion International*, 23, 70–77.

Webster, F. (2002). *Theories of the information society*, 2nd edition. New York: Taylor and Francis.

Ybarra, M. and Suman, M. (2008). Reasons, assessments and actions taken: sex and age differences in uses of Internet health information. *Health Education Research*, 23, 512–521.

Zillien, N. and Hargittai, E. (2009). Digital distinction. Status-specific types of Internet usage. *Social Science Quarterly*, 90, 274–291.

4 The Internet and social inequalities in the U.S.

James Witte
Marissa Kiss
Randy Lynn
George Mason University

In just over forty years the Internet has evolved from an eclectic network of a handful of users, focused on developing a rudimentary means of communication, to a vast worldwide web for transferring, storing and, above all else, sharing an enormous quantity and variety of information. The Internet and web have not only become a medium for social and asocial use, networking and communication, but also an everyday opportunity for cultural expression through the online activities in which an individual engages.

However, with the development and sophistication of technology and the Internet, opportunities to take advantage of these new technologies are not equally distributed. As the other chapters in this volume detail, there is a global element to Internet inequality. In this chapter, the emphasis is on the U.S., where the digital divide remains a real and persistent phenomenon, despite a relatively long history of Internet use and high degree of Internet penetration.

The initial section of this chapter discusses aspects of the relationship between the Internet and inequality from the perspective of cultural sociology. Beginning with the work of Max Weber, the intent is to consider why the Internet needs to be seen as more than a significant technological development. Through its impact on individuals' lifestyles – not simply in what they own or the activities they participate in, but also in the fundamental orientation as to how they conduct their lives – use of the Internet has emerged as a critical aspect of social stratification in contemporary U.S. life. Next, as a fundamental component of lifestyle, the Internet's link to the creation and maintenance of social capital is discussed as a mechanism, whereby the Internet offers advantage to some, while denying it to others.

The empirical section of this chapter begins with a description of the digital divide in the U.S. through early 2011. The empirical analyses go on to examine differences among the types of communities in which Internet users and non-users live – in terms of the size of the community and duration of residence, but also in the manner by which Internet users and non-users obtain information about their local communities. This is followed by a discussion of the extent to which Internet users and non-users participate in different types of groups as an organizational context for the creation and maintenance of the social ties critical to social capital.

Cultural perspectives on inequality

Cultural perspectives on inequality have their roots in the sociology of Max Weber, who argued that a proper understanding of society required due attention to the independent force of ideas. From this common Weberian root, several distinct approaches to inequality have developed within the cultural perspective. This section briefly describes those common roots and discusses one particularly relevant branch, with an eye to clarifying the relationship between the Internet and inequality from this theoretical perspective.

To begin with, the most obvious difference between Marx and Weber's theories of stratification is found in Weber's recognition of class, status and power as analytically distinct bases of stratification within society. Weber claimed that one can speak of a class when a group of people share a "... specific causal component of their life chances" (Weber, 1946, p. 181). Defined in this way, classes – as groups of similarly situated individuals – are determined in the marketplace. Though Weber identifies "property" and "lack of property" as the basic categories of all class situations, he identifies two further grounds for class distinction: "acquisition classes" and "social classes." While property classes are defined by the type of property owned and its potential to yield a return in the market, acquisition classes may be traced back to the types of skills and services individuals can offer on the market. Social classes, on the other hand, are composed of a range of class statuses sharing a common intra- and intergenerational mobility space (Weber, 1947).

Weber distinguished status stratification from class because the former rests on a subjective sense of community, reflecting stratification according to consumption rather than production. Moreover, the expectation of a certain style of life on the part of group members is often linked, according to Weber, to restrictions on social intercourse that set status group members apart from non-members. Weber points to the potential of status stratification to place restrictions on social intercourse as a primary source of tension between class and status. These combine to yield a rich and complex stratification system, which is associated with differences in life chances and life styles. These, in turn, yield different and exclusionary patterns of social interaction.

The work of Manuel Castells, particularly *The Rise of the Network Society: The Information Age: Economy, Society and Culture, Volume I* (1996, 2000, 2010), represents a variant of contemporary neo-Weberian sociology with particular relevance for the topic at hand. With reference to Weber's *The Protestant Ethic and the Spirit of Capitalism*, Castells describes "the spirit of informationalism," which has altered but not replaced capitalism as the dominant mode of production.

Two aspects of Castells' work warrant emphasis here. The first is the nature of the transformation. Castells argues that business networks, information and communication technologies, and global competition have combined in an historical moment to give rise to the network society. Castells describes a unique culture: "a culture of the ephemeral, a culture of each strategic decision, a patchwork of experiences and interests, rather than a charter or rights and obligations as the ethical foundation of the network society" (Castells, 2010, p. 214). Intertwined with this culture, just as bureaucracy and rational capitalist economic organizations were intertwined with capitalism, is the dominance of a new standard for economic and social organization. Castells argues, for the first time in history, the basic unit of economic and social organization is not an individual or collective subject (e.g., a class, corporation or state), but rather "... the unit is the network, made up of a variety of subjects and organizations, relentlessly modified as networks adapt to supportive environments and market structures" (Castells, 2010, p. 214).

The second particularly relevant aspect of Castells' treatment of the network society is his recognition that not everyone participates equally in the network society: "The new economy affects everywhere and everybody but is inclusive and exclusionary at the same time, the boundaries of inclusion varying for every society, depending on institutions, politics and policies" (Castells, 2010, p. 161). The dynamics of inclusion and exclusion have several implications for power and inequality in several ways. Most obviously – and this is the focus of the empirical section of this chapter – there are real and significant costs to being excluded from networks. Moreover, as the advantages of inclusion are growing, the disadvantages associated with exclusion may be growing at an even faster rate. Furthermore, even among those included within the boundaries of a network, the rules for participation, as well as the tangible and intangible benefits of inclusion may not be of equal import for all members of a network (Witte and Mannon, 2010).

Within the cultural perspective on inequality, an emphasis on differential life chances and patterns of social interaction are common themes that are directly relevant to the relationship between the Internet and inequality. The Internet has become an increasingly important medium of social interaction – both in terms of interaction between individuals *and* interaction with intelligent web-based systems based on social information and relationships.

The Internet and social capital

Current conceptions of social capital largely derive from similar – but not identical – articulations by three influential theorists. First, Bourdieu defines social capital as "the sum of the resources, actual or virtual" resulting from one's location in and maintenance of "a durable network of more or less institutionalized relationships of mutual acquaintance and recognition" (Bourdieu and Wacquant, 1992, p. 14). Second, Coleman conceptualizes social capital as an aggregate "of different entities, with two elements in common: they all consist of some aspect of social structures, and they facilitate certain actions of actors – whether persons or corporate actors – within the structure." "Productive" and "not completely fungible," it is unique among forms of capital in that it "inheres in the structure of social actors and among actors" (Coleman, 1988, p. S98). Third, Putnam (1993, p. 35) initially defines social capital as "features of social organization, such as networks, norms, and trust that facilitate coordination and cooperation for mutual benefit [that enhance] the benefits of investment in physical and human capital." In *Bowling Alone*, Putnam defines social capital as "connecting among individuals... social networks and norms of reciprocity and trustworthiness that arise from them" (2000, p. 19).

Most broadly, then, social capital encompasses relational resources: assets inherent in and arising from our social relationships and networks. Because relational processes enable social capital (Portes, 1998), social relations can be viewed as investments from which social capital is the return (Lin, 1999; Resnick, 2002). Although some theorists – especially Bourdieu – emphasize social capital's prominent role in processes of domination, most interpretations construe social capital as a positive phenomenon, associated with such wide-ranging benefits as increased health (Adler and Kwon, 2002), employment (Lin, 2001), and psychological well-being (Morrow, 1999).

The relationship between Internet use and social capital has been a topic of considerable debate. Studies arguing that Internet use negatively impacts social capital (Kraut *et al.*, 1998; Nie, 2001; Coget, Yamauchi and Suman, 2002) usually rely on some variant of Putnam's time displacement hypothesis, in which increased Internet use is positively correlated with decreases in other modes of communication (Williams, 2006). These studies assert that the Internet is used largely for non-interactive purposes, such as employment-related tasks or interactions with weaker ties, displacing more beneficial face-to-face interactions and ties to organizations or communities.

Displacement arguments are often linked to a broader assertion of a recent historical or ongoing decline of social capital or the size and quality of the social networks in which social capital is embedded (Putnam, 2000; McPherson, Smith-Lovin and Brashears, 2006), although the methods and conclusions of these broader studies have been subject to considerable scrutiny and criticism (Thomson, 2005; Wang and Wellman, 2010; Hampton, Sessions and Her, 2011).

Unlike other media linked to the decline of social capital (e.g., network television), there are ways that the Internet may enable social interactions and the maintenance of social ties. Moreover, Internet technologies may enable the formation of networks and new forms of social capital not possible in offline contexts or from the use of other media (Lin, 1999; Wellman *et al.*, 2001; Resnick, 2002). As a result, researchers have called for a theoretical and methodological understanding of Internet use that is multifaceted and acknowledges varied activities, motives, and gratifications (Shah, Kwak and Holbert, 2001; Bargh and McKenna, 2004; Zhao, 2006).

The extent to which offline interactions that increase social capital are displaced by online activities that do not is mitigated by two complementary aspects of Internet use: on one hand, by the novel or enhanced networking opportunities presented by digital technologies, and on the other hand, by positive displacement effects whereby offline activities that do not increase social capital (e.g., watching television) are displaced by online activities that do (Resnick, 2002; Valenzuela *et al.*, 2009). In this context, online and offline interactions cannot be assumed to represent mutually exclusive categories: online interactions may supplement other modes of communication that maintain social ties and encourage social capital (Wellman *et al.*, 2001; Quan-Haase *et al.*, 2002; Russell *et al.*, 2008; Vergeer and Pelzer, 2009), while ties that are initially formed in online contexts may be continued in offline contexts (Kavanaugh *et al.*, 2005; Best and Krueger, 2006; Goodsell and Williamson, 2008).

Data from the Pew Internet and American Life Project

Data for this chapter comes from the Pew Internet Project, arguably the most complete and comprehensive source of data about Internet use in the U.S. (http://www.pewinternet.org/Static-Pages/About-Us/Project-History. aspx). The Pew Project is made up of an ongoing series of nationally representative telephone surveys of the U.S. population. The Project fielded its first survey about the general role of the Internet and email in people's lives in March 2000. Since that initial survey, the Pew Project has conducted two to three such surveys each year, each drawing on a new sample of respondents. In this chapter we combine data from over 50,000 interviews conducted as part of twenty-five different Pew data collection efforts extending through January 2011.

Trends in Internet use 2000–2011

A primary finding of Witte and Mannon (2010) was that through the first years of the twenty-first century, there still was a significant digital divide in the U.S., particularly with regard to education and income. To set the stage for this chapter, it is important to consider the most recent data available to see if this situation has been mitigated or remains the same.

The digital divide based on education and income

Figure 4.1 uses time series data from the Pew Internet and American Life project to summarize the percentage of U.S. adults who have ever used the Internet according to each respondent's highest level of educational attainment. In March of 2000, 72.4 percent of those with a college degree said they had used the Internet, as compared to 16.5 percent of those with less than a high school degree. By January of 2011 these figures had increased to 94.9 percent and 46.4 percent, respectively. Even using the peak estimate of Internet use among those with a high school degree, 52.1 percent from several months earlier, the difference remains over 40.0 percent. Moreover, as Figure 4.2 shows, when one considers the percentage of respondents who used the Internet in the day previous to their Pew interview it appears that the gap according to educational attainment has grown over time. Seen in this way, the digital divide in the U.S. according to educational attainment grew from 40.1 percent in 2000 to 52.7 percent in 2010.

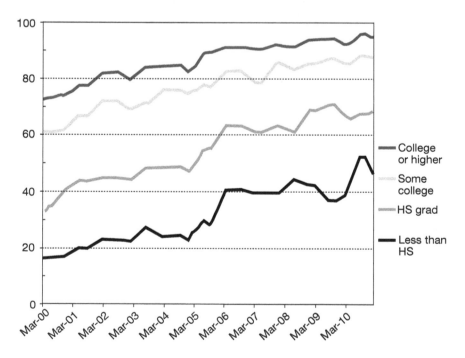

Figure 4.1 U.S. adults who ever used the Internet according to education (2000–2011)

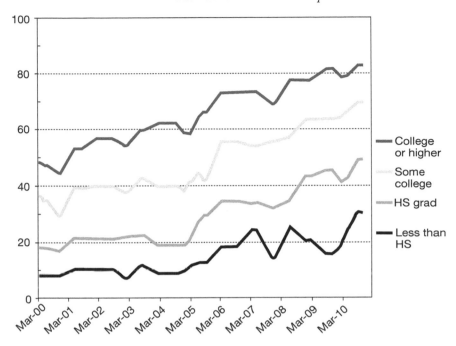

Figure 4.2 U.S. adults who used the Internet yesterday according to education (2000–2010)

A similar pattern is seen in Figures 4.3 and 4.4 that illustrate the digital divide as tied to household income. Beginning in 2000 and continuing through 2010/2011 there has been a significant gap between individuals in households with low and high incomes when it comes to those who report ever having been online (see Figure 4.3) and those who report that they went online the day before their interview (see Figure 4.4). Clearly in this regard, the digital divide has not gone away, though it has narrowed: between 2000 and 2010 the gap in the percentage of individuals in households with incomes less than $20,000 compared to those in households with incomes greater than $75,000 has gone from 53.5 percent to 40.0 percent (see Figure 4.3). However, it is perhaps more important to consider the percentages of individuals who reported going online on the day before they were interviewed, as this may be a better measure of the degree to which the Internet is part of an individual's everyday life. Seen in this way, the gap between individuals in households with the lowest incomes compared to those in households with the highest incomes has actually grown from 42.0 percent to 46.1 percent between 2000 and 2010 (see Figure 4.4).

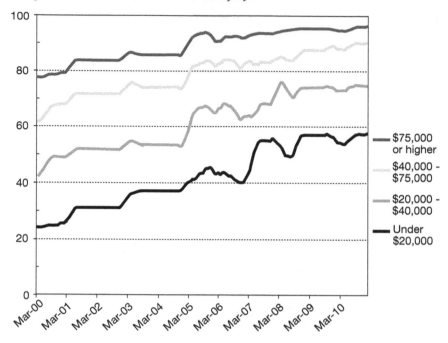

Figure 4.3 U.S. adults who ever used the Internet according to household income (2000–2010)

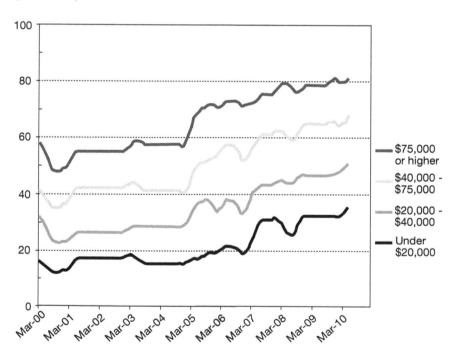

Figure 4.4 U.S. Adults who used the Internet yesterday according to household income (2000–2010)

The digital divide based on education and income controlling for other characteristics

In the previous section we have seen how education and income as significant aspects of the digital divide were not only manifest in the early years of the Internet, but continue to leave their mark on Internet use up through the present. Moreover, as we look at recent data from May 2010, we see that significant differences in Internet use can also be seen according to other salient social categories.

This pattern is summarized in Table 4.1, where Columns [a] and [c] describe, for particular social and demographic characteristics, the percentage of individuals who have ever used the Internet [a] and the percentage who reported using it on the day prior to being interviewed [c]. So, for example, the results show that 79.3 percent of men and 78.7 percent of women have ever used the Internet; however, this small difference is not statistically significant. Looking at other demographic characteristics, on the other hand, there are significant differences in percentages according to age, race and ethnicity.

But these percentages only look at a single demographic characteristic at a time and may be misleading since the various demographic characteristics are also related to one another. In an effort to sort this out, logistic regression results are reported in Columns [b] and [d] of Table 4.1, which provide the exponentiated log of the odds obtained when ever having used the Internet and having used it yesterday are regressed on these social and demographic characteristics. These results indicate that in a multivariate framework, the significant effects of race and ethnicity fall away, while gender is significant for having ever used the Internet, but not for having used it yesterday. Age, education and income, by contrast, are highly significant both for ever having used the Internet and having used it yesterday. Having established that differences in Internet use persist in the U.S., it is important to take a closer look at the consequences of those differences.

Internet use, community type and sources of local information

One aspect of lifestyle that clearly distinguishes non-Internet users from Internet users is their residential pattern and the type of communities in which they tend to live. Table 4.2 indicates that non-Internet users are more likely to have lived in their neighborhoods for a longer time, while a relatively large proportion of Internet users tend to be relative newcomers to the neighborhoods they live in. In addition, nearly half of all non-Internet users (44.2 percent) have lived in their neighborhoods for twenty years or more as compared to under a third of Internet users (30.0 percent). Table 4.2 also shows that non-Internet users tend to live in small cities, towns and rural areas (72.4 percent), while Internet users live disproportionately in large cities and suburbs (47.0 percent).

Table 4.1 Social and demographic patterns of Internet use

	Ever used the Internet		Used the Internet yesterday	
	[a] percentage	[b] exponentiated log of odds	[c] percentage	[d] exponentiated log of odds
Gender				
Male	79.3	—	62.2	—
Female	78.7	1.611**	60.5	1.23
Age				
18–24	95.5**	—	77.1**	—
25–34	93.3	0.457*	75.2	0.646*
35–44	87.6	0.178**	74.1	0.529**
45–54	81.3	0.107**	60.3	0.231**
55–64	75.6	0.085**	54.7	0.157**
65 and older	42.4	0.018**	29.0	0.074**
Race				
White	79.6**	—	61.9**	—
Black	72.4	0.696	55.1	0.863
Asian	91.1	1.097	83.9	1.711
Other/mixed race	79.4	0.992	54.5	0.871
Ethnicity				
Hispanic	81.4**	1.035	60.5	0.744
Non-Hispanic	78.8	—	61.5	—
Education				
Less than HS	51.9**	0.072**	29.8**	0.168**
HS graduate	67.7	0.099**	48.7	0.262**
Some college	88.0	0.298**	69.2	0.546**
College or higher	95.9	—	82.6	—
Income				
Less than $10,000	47.7**	—	30.2**	—
$10,000–$20,000	63.3	—	42.9	—
$20,000–$30,000	73.0	—	52.2	—
$30,000–$40,000	77.6	1.475**	53.1	1.33**
$40,000–$50,000	90.2	—	68.9	—
$50,000–$75,000	88.8	—	72.1	—
$75,000–$100,000	94.3	—	83.6	—
$100,000 and above	95.7	—	82.7	—

* $p < 0.05$, ** $p < 0.01$. May 2010 Pew Internet and American Life Survey. – indicates reference category.
1) Constant = 36.586 Nagelkerke Pseudo R2 = 0.487
2) Constant = 3.293 Nagelkerke Pseudo R2 = 0.368

Table 4.2 Neighborhood and community characteristics according to Internet use

	Never used the Internet (%)	Ever used the Internet (%)
*How long living in the neighborhood******		
Less than one year	5.5	10.4
One to five years	22.6	26.8
Six to ten years	11.6	17.6
Eleven to twenty years	16.1	20.1
Twenty years or more	44.2	30.0
*Type of community******		
A large city	18.7	23.0
A suburb near a large city	8.8	24.0
A small city or town	45.5	35.0
A rural area	26.9	18.0

* p < 0.05, ** p < 0.01. January 2011 Pew Internet and American Life Survey

It is no surprise that, when compared to Internet users, those who do not use the Internet are more likely to be long-time residents of small cities and towns or to live in rural areas, but there are surprising aspects of how they inhabit their environments. In January 2011, the Pew Project asked a series of questions about where respondents received information about their local community. Comparing the upper and lower panels of Table 4.3, there are significant differences between those who have or have never used the Internet across all three sources of information. Non-Internet users are more likely to read a print version of a local newspaper every day (26.2 percent) and to watch a local television news broadcast every day (64.2 percent) than Internet users, 20.7 percent of whom read a local newspaper and 45.4 percent of whom watch the local television news every day. Non-Internet users are also more likely to never read a local newspaper; thus, local television is their primary source of news. Interestingly, non-Internet users are significantly *less likely* to rely on word of mouth as a source of local information: they are less likely to receive such information everyday (22.1 percent) than Internet users (25.2 percent), but they are also more likely to never receive local word of mouth information (16.1 percent) than Internet users (6.7 percent). Thus, it appears that non-Internet users are already at a disadvantage when it comes to multiple sources of local information, not just those that are Internet based.

Table 4.3 Sources of local information according to Internet use

How often do you get local information from...	Source of information (%)			
	Print version of a local newspaper**	A local television news broadcast**	A local radio broadcast**	Word of mouth from friends, family, co-workers and neighbors**
Never used the Internet				
Every day	26.2	64.2	28.9	22.1
Several times a week	17.8	17.8	13.2	26.3
Several times a month	10.7	3.8	6.2	15.8
Less often	12.6	5.7	11.3	19.7
Never	32.7	8.6	40.4	16.1
Total	100.0	100.0	100.0	100.0
Ever used the Internet				
Every day	20.7	45.4	34.7	25.2
Several times a week	18.4	23.1	17.5	32.1
Several times a month	17.5	9.5	8.7	22.7
Less often	18.0	10.9	13.3	13.2
Never	25.4	11.2	25.8	6.7
Total	100.0	100.0	100.0	100.0

* p < 0.05, ** p < 0.01. January 2011 Pew Internet and American Life Survey

Moreover, as Table 4.4 suggests, Internet users already have a variety of online resources that they use to obtain particular types of local information. Column [a] of Table 4.4 indicates that local weather is the most commonly sought type of local information, as 88.7 percent of all respondents reported seeking information of this type. Of all those who sought information on the local weather, Column [b] shows that 43.2 percent used the Internet and/or a mobile device to get this information, while among those who sought this information and were Internet users Column [d] reports that 53.9 percent used the Internet and/or a mobile device to get information on the local weather. Table 4.4 also reveals interesting variation in the degree to which the Internet and mobile devices are used for local information according to the type of information. So, for example, local breaking news is the second most commonly sought type of local information (Column [a]); however, only

Table 4.4 Obtaining local information

Individuals who seek information of the following type:	Use the Internet or mobile phone to get information		
	[a] (%)	% of all individuals [b]	% of Internet users only [c]
Local weather	88.7	43.2	53.9
Local breaking news	80.0	21.3	26.6
Local politics, campaigns and elections	67.0	26.7	33.9
Local arts and cultural events, such as concerts, plays, and museum exhibits	60.0	28.4	34.7
Other local government activity, such as council meetings, hearings or local trials	41.8	15.3	19.2
Local job openings	38.8	44.8	55.7
Local social services that provide assistance with things like housing, food, health care, and child care	35.4	19.5	26.7
Local zoning, building and development	30.5	12.8	16.1

January 2011 Pew Internet and American Life Survey. Based on Form B respondents [N=1,164]

26.6 percent of all Internet users said they used the Internet and/or mobile devices to get this type of information. By contrast, relatively few respondents reported looking for information on local job openings 38.8 percent (Column [a]); but, 55.7 percent of Internet users stated that they used the Internet or mobile devices to get this type of information.

Taken together, the materials found in Tables 4.3 and 4.4 indicate that as information and communication technology has developed, matured and become increasingly social and mobile, access to online and offline local information resources is another way in which lifestyle differences characterize the digital divide.

Internet use and social ties

As noted above, there has been an ongoing debate about the extent to which Internet use is likely to increase or decrease the types of social ties that are associated with social capital. December 2010 data from the Pew Survey Project speaks directly to this point. All respondents were asked about their active participation in fourteen different types of groups.

Results from this question are summarized by the radar graph found in Figure 4.5, in which the filled-in area shows the percentages of Internet and non-Internet users who are active in each type of group. For twelve of the fourteen types of groups, a greater percentage of Internet users than non-users were active members. Veterans groups or organizations, such as the American Legion or the Veterans of Foreign Wars, and farm groups were the only two types of groups in which non-users were more likely to be active than Internet users. These were also the two types of groups that attracted the smallest percentages of participants. Overall, the average Internet user belonged to 2.6 types of groups, while the average non-user belonged to only 1.3 types of groups.

As is the case with Internet use (see Table 4.1), a variety of social and demographic factors are associated with participation in different types of groups and not just whether or not one is an Internet user. Column [a] in Table 4.5 presents results from Ordinary Least Squares (OLS) regression of the number of types of local groups, in which an individual is active, on the same set of demographic and social characteristics that were used as predictors of the probability of Internet use in Table 4.1. Column [a] of Table 4.5 shows that women, older individuals, non-Whites (with the exception of Asians), and those in households with higher incomes belong to significantly more types of groups. Meanwhile those with less than a college degree belong to significantly fewer types of groups. In Column [b] of Table 4.5, the model is expanded to include whether or not an

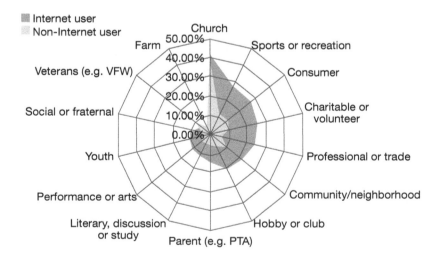

Figure 4.5 Participation in social groups: adult Internet users and non-Internet users in the United States. Source: Pew Internet & American Life Survey, December 2010.

Table 4.5 Active participation in types of groups regressed on demographic characteristics

	Unstandardized regression coefficients		
	[a] *base model active group participation*	[b] *expanded model active group participation*	[c] *expanded model all group participation*
Gender			
Male	—	—	—
Female	0.271**	0.251*	0.139
Age			
18–24	—	—	—
25–34	0.003	0.053	0.036
35–44	0.623**	0.709**	0.683*
45–54	0.494**	0.603**	0.807**
55–64	0.618**	0.740**	1.190**
65 and older	0.605**	0.860**	1.555**
Race			
White	—	—	—
Black	0.622**	0.638**	0.940**
Asian	−0.200	−0.180	0.037
Other/mixed race	0.839**	0.838**	1.217**
Ethnicity			
Hispanic	−0.222	−0.198	−0.079
Non-Hispanic	—	—	—
Education			
Less than HS	−1.830**	−1.646**	−2.371**
HS grad	−1.419**	−1.333**	−2.127**
Some college	−0.984**	−0.971**	−1.539**
College or higher	—	—	—
Income			
	0.229**	0.205**	0.254**
Internet use			
Internet user	—	0.560**	1.168**
Non-user	—	—	—
Constant	1.568**	1.083**	1.921**
Adjusted R2	0.195	0.200	0.191

* $p < 0.05$, ** $p < 0.01$. May 2010 Pew Internet and American Life Survey. – indicates reference category.

individual is an Internet user. Adding this variable does little to change the relationships established in Column [a], while establishing, all other things being equal, that *there is a positive and significant relationship between Internet use and the number of community oriented groups to which an individual belongs.*

In addition, Pew respondents were asked to consider their active participation in any other groups, not just those with an obvious community orientation. When both sets of groups are combined, the average Internet user participated in a total of 3.9 types of groups as compared to an average of 2.0 for non-users. Further, as Column [c] of Table 4.5 indicates this significant difference remains even after controlling for other individual characteristics, while the effects of these other characteristics are essentially the same as with the smaller subset of community groups.

Conclusion

In sum, the theoretical perspectives and empirical analyses presented in this chapter suggest that despite tremendous changes in the content available online and the ways that users access content, there has actually been little change in the fundamental relationship between the Internet and inequality in the U.S. in recent years. Particularly with regard to educational attainment and income, there has been no closing of the digital divide. Further, as the informational resources available through the Internet have become more valuable, especially with the increase in fine-grained content that is highly relevant and valuable to specialized groups, including geographically defined community groups, then the relative costs and consequences of exclusion increase as well.

References

Adler, P.S. and Kwon, S-K. (2002). Social capital: prospects for a new concept. *Academy of Management Review* 27(1), 17–40.
Bargh, J.A. and McKenna, K.Y.A. (2004). The Internet and social life. *Annual Review of Psychology, 55*, 573–590.
Best, S.J. and Krueger, B.S. (2006). Online interactions and social capital: Distinguishing between new and existing ties. *Social Science Computer Review, 24*(4), 395–410.
Bourdieu, P. and Wacquant, L.J.D. (1992). *An Invitation to reflexive sociology.* Chicago, U.S. and London: University of Chicago Press.
Castells, M. (1996, 2000, 2010). *The rise of the network society: The information age.* Oxford, U.K.: Blackwell.
Coget, J.F., Yamauchi, Y. and Suman, M. (2002). The Internet, social networks and loneliness. *IT & Society, 1*(1), 180–201.
Coleman, J.S. (1988). Social capital in the creation of human capital. *American Journal of Sociology, 94*(Supplement), S95–S120.

Goodsell, T.L. and Williamson, O. (2008). The case of the brick huggers: The practice of an online community. *City & Community, 7*(3), 251–271.

Hampton, K.N., Sessions, L.F. and Her, E.J. (2011). Core networks, social isolation, and new media." *Information, Communication & Society, 14*(1), 130–155.

Kavanaugh, A., Carroll, J.M., Rosson, M.B., Zin, T.T., and Reese, D.D. (2005). Community Networks: Where Offline Communities Meet Online. *Journal of Computer-Mediated Communication, 10*: 00. doi: 10.1111/j.1083-6101.2005.tb00266.x

Kraut, R., Patterson, M., Lundmark, V., Kiesler, S., Mukopadhyay, T. and Scherlis, W. (1998). Internet paradox: A social technology that reduces social involvement and psychological well-being? *The American Psychologist, 53*(9), 1017–1031.

Lin, N. (1999). Building a network theory of social capital. *Connections, 22*(1), 28–51.

Lin, N. (2001). *Social capital: A theory of social structure and action.* New York, NY: Cambridge University Press.

McPherson, M., Smith-Lovin, L. and Brashears, M.E. (2006). Social isolation in America: Changes in core discussion networks over two decades. *American Sociological Review, 71*(3), 353–375.

Morrow, V. (1999). Conceptualising social capital in relation to the well-being of children and young people: a critical review. *Sociological Review* 47 (4), 744–765.

Nie, N.H. (2001). Sociability, interpersonal relations, and the Internet: Reconciling conflicting findings. *American Behavioral Scientist, 45*(3), 420–435.

Portes, A. (1998). Social capital: Its origins and applications in modern sociology. *Annual Review of Sociology, 24*(1), 1–24.

Putnam, R.D. (1993). The prosperous community: Social capital and public life. *American Prospect, 13*, 35–42.

Putnam, R.D. (2000). *Bowling alone: The collapse and revival of American community.* New York: Simon & Schuster.

Quan-Haase, A., Wellman, B., Witte, J.C. and Hampton, K.N. (2002). Capitalizing on the Net: Social contract, civic engagement, and sense of community. In B. Wellman and C. Haythornwaite (Eds.), *The Internet in everyday life.* London, U.K.: Blackwell, 291–324.

Resnick, P. (2002). Beyond bowling together: SocioTechnical capital. In J. Carroll (ed.), *HCI in the new millennium.* New York: Addison-Wesley, 247–272.

Russell, C., Campbell, A. and Hughes, I. (2008). Ageing, social capital and the Internet: Findings from an exploratory study of Australian "silver surfers." *Australasian Journal on Ageing, 27*(2), 78–82.

Shah, D.V., Kwak, N. and Holbert, R.L. (2001). "Connecting" and "disconnecting" with civic life: Patterns of Internet use and the production of social capital. *Political Communication, 18*(2), 141–162.

Thomson, I.T. (2005). The theory that won't die: From mass society to the decline of social capital. *Sociological Forum, 20*(3), 421–448.

Valenzuela, S., Park, N. and Kee, K.F. (2009). Is there social capital in a social network site?: Facebook use and college students' life satisfaction, trust, and participation. *Journal of Computer-Mediated Communication, 14*(4), 875–901.

Vergeer, M. and Pelzer, B. (2009). Consequences of media and Internet use for offline and online network capital and well-being: A causal model approach. *Journal of Computer-Mediated Communication, 15*(1), 189–210.

Wang, H. and Wellman, B. (2010). Social connectivity in America: Changes in adult friendship network size from 2002 to 2007. *American Behavioral Scientist, 53*(8), 1148–1169.

Weber, M. (1947). *The theory of social and economic organizations.* Edited by T. Parsons. New York: The Free Press.

Weber, M. (1946). *From Max Weber.* Translated by H.H. Girth and C.W. Mills. New York: Oxford University Press.

Wellman, B., Quan-Haase, A., Witte, J. and Hampton, K. (2001). Does the Internet increase, decrease, or supplement social capital?: Social networks, participation, and community commitment. *American Behavioral Scientist, 45*(3), 436–455.

Williams, D. (2006). On and off the Net: Scales for social capital in an online era. *Journal of Computer-Mediated Communication, 11*(2), 593–628. doi:10.1111/j.1083-6101.2006.00029.x

Witte, J. and Mannon, S. (2010) *The Internet and social inequalities,* London: Routledge.

Zhao, S. (2006). Do Internet users have more social ties? A call for differentiated analyses of Internet use. *Journal of Computer-Mediated Communication, 11*(3), 844–862.

5 Missing in the midst of abundance

The case of broadband adoption in Japan[1]

Mito Akiyoshi
Senshu University

Motohiro Tsuchiya
Keio University

Takako Sano
Ministry of Internal Affairs and Communications

Broadband technology and social and economic outcomes

The advent of broadband technology provides societies with new communicative opportunities and challenges. The deployment of broadband is expected to spur economic growth (ITU/UNESCO, 2011). It is not clear whether or how broadband technology achieves positive economic and social outcomes, however. In fact, the literature on media history, the social shaping of science and technology, social constructivism theories, and Actor Network Theory attest to the complex relationship between technology and society (Grint and Woolgar, 1997). The growing field of research on the distribution of access to and use of information technology is most commonly known under the rubric of digital divide.

Researchers working on the issue of the digital divide rediscover the coevolution of technology and society, a phenomenon underscored in research of a constructivist persuasion. Contrary to the initial anticipation that the Internet would serve as a great social equalizer by democratizing the production, dissemination, and use of information, it has become clear that individuals bring different levels of skills and different needs to the Internet. Instead of democratizing communications, the Internet may perpetuate or even exacerbate inequality as economic and social returns to using the Internet differ across the population (van Dijk, 2006; Witte and Mannon 2010). While the concept of digital divide primarily focuses on differences between individuals with Internet access and without, it becomes increasingly evident that social inequality is manifest at the level of different uses among those who have access. The term digital inequality is often used to turn our attention away from the simplistic dichotomy of having or not having Internet access to the unequal distribution of various resources deployed for appropriation of information communication technology. Digital inequality is becoming a serious issue for research on social stratification because inequality in digital technology use translates into inequality in other domains of life. For example, web use is positively associated with earnings growth by enhancing human capital, by providing superior access to job information, and by signaling socially valued aspects of the user's identity (DiMaggio and Bonikowski, 2008).

The present chapter examines how the propagation of broadband technology is facilitated or curtailed by the differential distribution of economic and social opportunities in Japan in order to understand the dynamics of social stratification processes mediated by the appropriation of technology. The chapter is organized in six sections. The second section introduces and motivates the research problem. The third section provides an overview of key concepts with a special focus on broadband use and social inequality. The fourth section details the data and methods. The fifth section presents our findings. By way of conclusion, the sixth section deals with the relationship between access, skills, and broadband adoption barriers.

Broadband in Japan

Broadband policy development

This section provides an overview of Internet and broadband access in Japan in order to contextualize and historicize our research problem. The broadband penetration rate to households in Japan increased around 2001 (see Figure 5.1). In November 2000, the government unveiled its "IT Basic Strategy" with a goal of making high-speed Internet access (30 to 100 Mbps) available to its citizens by 2005. To implement the strategy, "IT Basic Law" was enacted in January 2001.

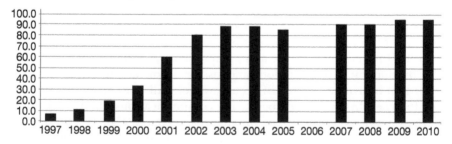

Figure 5.1 Household Internet penetration rates

Note: As the data format for the year 2006 is different from the one for other years, the data for 2006 was dropped.

Source: The Ministry of Internal Affairs and Communications of Japan

Services providers were faced with the choice of DSL (Digital Subscriber Line) or optic fibers. Yahoo! BB, a major Internet service provider aggressively promoted DSL. NTT (Nippon Telegraph and Telephone), the privatized former state monopoly, was reluctant to accept DSL requests from Yahoo! BB and other DSL operators, because it thought that the use of old coppers for DSL would hinder the deployment of new optic fibers. Ambivalent, NTT started offering DSL services while accelerating the deployment of optic fibers (Bleha, 2009; Tsuchiya and Thierer, 2002).[2] The competition between DSL and fiber optics presented a good bargain for potential customers. By 2009 optic fiber subscriptions surpassed those of DSL subscriptions (see Figure 5.2). By 2007, Japan boasted "the cheapest and fastest" broadband services (Orbicom, 2007). Japan's price for broadband per megabit per second is the lowest among OECD member countries (OECD, 2011a) as of September 2011 (see Figure 5.3). In 2010 a 1Mbps connection cost 0.08 dollars in Japan; it cost 0.19 dollars in Korea; and 1.10 dollars in the United States.

The growth of broadband technology applications in Japan

Three issues are of great interest as to the growth of Internet and broadband technology applications in Japan. First, Japan started out as an "underperformer" on Internet connectivity rates during the 1990s and later it transformed itself into a leader of broadband technology after 2000. Second, much of Japan's Internet traffic is mediated by the web-enabled mobile phone. Third, unlike other industrialized societies, where gender gaps in computer-based Internet access were present in the 1990s but disappeared around 2000, the gender gap in computer-based Internet access persisted in Japan.

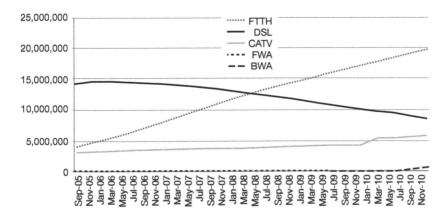

Figure 5.2 Type of broadband subscription in Japan

Source: The Ministry of Internal Affairs and Communications of Japan

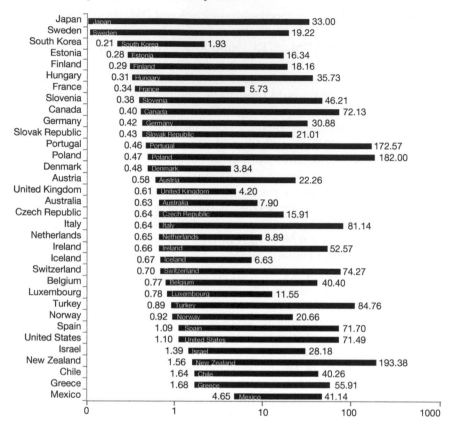

Figure 5.3 Broadband prices per megabits per second of advertised speed, Sept. 2011 – USD PPP

Source: OECD (2011a) The OECD broadband portal http://www.oecd.org/dataoecd/22/42/39574970.xls

From underperformer to leader of broadband adoption

It has been stated that a nation's Internet connectivity rate or the proportion of Internet users in the population is mainly explained by its GDP, the percentage of population with higher education, and quality of existing telecommunication infrastructure (Norris, 2001). According to these indices, Japan was an underperformer during the first decade of Internet diffusion. That is, the actual percentage of Internet users was below what was predicted by models. In 2000, 34 percent of Japanese households had access to the Internet while 48 percent of Swedish households and 42 percent of US households were online (OECD, 2011b). The slow diffusion of the Internet in Japan is attributed to several factors such as limited English proficiency among the population, the introduction of computer and QWERTY keyboards without a natural transition from the typewriter, and exorbitant telephone charges in the days of dial-up.

The IT Basic Strategy was a response to the lagged expansion of Internet connectivity. It prioritized the provisioning of affordable broadband access. The expansion of broadband capacity is a chicken-and-egg problem. There must be strong demand for broadband services to justify investment, but without services already in operation, it is difficult to create sufficient demand. The strong commitment combined with coordinated efforts on the part of the government to update network infrastructure meant that the initial dilemma was eased by policy measures.

In Japan, fiber optic cable is the leading platform. Fiber-To-The-Home (FTTH) connections are available among 86.5 percent of households (see Figure 5.4). Availability of broadband technology does not necessarily entail actual use, however. The OECD average of broadband subscriptions per 100 inhabitants was 5.1 in 2011. Japan is ranked sixteenth with 27.0 subscriptions per 100 inhabitants (see Figure 5.5). The striking contrast between abundant technological capabilities and limited actual use constitutes the puzzle the present chapter addresses.

Mobile Internet access

Web-enabled mobile phones are widely used in Japan. Akiyoshi and Ono (2008) observe that mobile phones serve as a viable alternative to computers for those who have limited resources. The wide acceptance of web-enabled mobile phones may suppress broadband Internet access from the computer. There is evidence that there exist mobile phone users who exclusively use mobile phones to access the Internet (Akiyoshi and Ono, 2008).

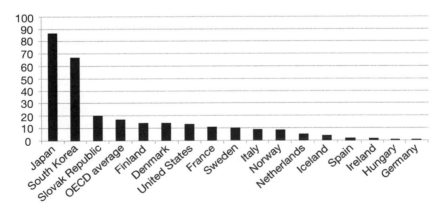

Figure 5.4 FTTH/B household availability

Source: OECD (2011a) The OECD broadband portal http://www.oecd.org/dataoecd/47/3/44435611.xls

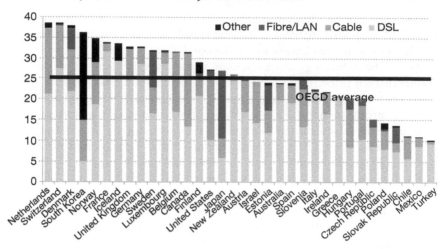

Figure 5.5 OECD fixed (wired) broadband subscriptions per 100 inhabitants, by technology, June 2011

Source: OECD (2011a) The OECD broadband portal http://www.oecd.org/dataoecd/21/35/39574709.xls

Digital divide in Japan

As is the case with other industrialized societies, Internet access and use are unevenly distributed across the population in Japan (Akiyoshi and Ono, 2008). The significance of gender is peculiar to Japan: in other industrialized societies, the early Internet users tended to be men. By 2000, women caught up with men in terms of Internet use in most industrialized societies. Figures from as late as the late 2000s show that gender remains a significant variable in Japan.

Lost in technological bliss? The puzzle

Why does broadband adoption remain suppressed in Japan even as the essential infrastructure is available in most parts of the country? With its high-quality broadband infrastructure already in place, the case of Japan's broadband adoption or the lack thereof represents the quintessential challenges faced by industrial societies as they seek to make the most of new technological opportunities to address a variety of issues including economic development, education, environmental conservation, social and health services, and community-building. To anticipate the conclusion, we found that differences in cultural capital can be carried over to the digital realm. Those endowed with high levels of cultural capital are the ones who are willing and able to unlock the potential of broadband technology. They employ broadband Internet access to do things they have been doing and to try new types of activities. On the other hand, those with limited cultural capital are less informed about new broadband applications. Even when they do use broadband, they tend to be "univore" users.

Omnivorous use of broadband

Definitions of broadband

In order to identify key determinants that are associated with broadband adoption, a clear definition of the concept of broadband is required. The Broadband Commission for Digital Development of ITU/UNESCO proposes three types of definition: a definition based on quantitative indicators, a definition based on qualitative indicators, and a definition that combines quantitative and qualitative indicators (ITU/UNESCO, 2011). The present chapter adopts the third approach and defines broadband as connections that have download speeds equal to or faster than 1Mbps delivered by DSL, cable modem, FTTH/FTTB, satellite, fixed wireless, and power line communication. As for qualitative indicators, we restrict the definition of broadband to computer-based connections because computer-based Internet access and mobile phone access differ in affordances.

Becoming a broadband user

Digital technology access is a cumulative and recursive process. The full process of technology appropriation is achieved when successive kinds of access are achieved. Van Dijk suggests that in addition to material access, motivational access and skills access are integral to the process of technology appropriation (van Dijk, 2006).

Motivational access can be conceptualized as a multistage concept. It does not always assume a linear order. Sometimes it begins with knowledge about a particular service followed by interests and intent. Alternatively, serendipity might have its way and a potential user might stumble on a product or service that in retrospect, she or he regards essential to achieving their goals. Social network may matter as well. "Becoming a broadband user" is an achievement comprised of multiple steps.

Acknowledging the presence of multiple paths that lead to sustained use and applications, we attempt to examine the distribution of knowledge about services and applications delivered by broadband. Knowledge may not initiate the process of technology appropriation but it shapes the structure of opportunities available to the potential adopter. Knowledge gaps were identified in European societies in Internet use gaps (Bonfadelli, 2002; van Deursen and van Dijk, 2010). We expect that there exist substantial knowledge gaps in Japan as well.

Usage applications and users

Our inquiry begins with an observation that Japan's strong broadband infrastructure in and of itself does not bring about actual use on the part of its citizens. One of the fruitful approaches to examine a set of variables that influence the success or failure of a technology is to look into users. Different types of social groups have different levels of skills and different preferences for applications (Witte and Mannon, 2010). The present chapter shows that the classical debates among perspectives on causes and consequences of inequality are relevant to an understanding of stratification process in an era in which access to or mastery of new technologies influences access to jobs, government services, and opportunities for social and political participation (DiMaggio and Bonikowski, 2008). Those classical perspectives on social inequality include the conflict perspective, the cultural perspective, and the functionalist perspective (Witte and Mannon, 2010).

The conflict perspective explains the existence of social inequality as a function of class relations. The cultural perspective seeks the origin of social inequality not only in economic factors, but also in non-economic ones such as lifestyle, social status, and political power. The functionalist perspective suggests that observed inequality is a result of a division of labor, a sine qua non for the functioning of society. A focus on usage applications and users reveals that sources of digital inequality are multiple and cannot be reduced to variation in economic resources. As such, it supports the cultural perspective. As Max Weber analyzed, distinctive worldviews and lifestyles produce complex systems of stratification (Weber, 1991; Witte and Mannon, 2010). Specifically, education and the consumption of "old" media such as TV and books predict knowledge and use of various broadband applications. Therefore, the seeming mystery of lack of avid use of broadband technology is explained by the significance of non-economic resources in technology use. Availability of affordable broadband technology does not mean the narrowing of digital inequality or productive use of technology because technology adoption is a function of cultural resources.

Types of activities supported by broadband technology

A literature review reveals that the Internet has become indispensable to users in their everyday lives. It is used to help people cope with illness, pursue training, make financial decisions, look for a new place to live, and switch jobs. Productive or work-related uses are generally distinguished from activities associated with entertainment or consumption (DiMaggio and Bonikowski, 2008). It has been suggested that usage of narrowband versus broadband connections affect usage time and the type and range of applications (van Dijk, 2006). Types of application enhanced by broadband connections include online learning, live streaming, video-on-demand, and downloading/uploading digital media content.

Omnivorous use

Different levels of skills and different motivations that individuals bring to the Internet can be conceptualized in terms of cultural capital. It is a useful notion to deal with subdued use of broadband in a society where material access is achieved in principle because it calls our attention to lifestyle differences that are not fully explained by the absence of material means. Cultural capital refers to cognitive resources, knowledge, tastes, and dispositions involved in the production and reproduction of class distinctions. It is supposed to affect labor market outcomes along with human capital and social capital (Bourdieu, 1984, 1986).

Two issues need to be elaborated on to apply the concept of cultural capital to analyze differences in adoption and usage of broadband technology. First of all, it has become increasingly clear that a higher level of cultural capital is associated with being "omnivorous," or being able to consume and enjoy a wide variety of cultural expressions. Bourdieu suggests a one-to-one correspondence between the level of cultural capital and the preferred genre of cultural products. He believed that, for example, the upper class prefers opera and the working class likes popular music. Nevertheless, empirical studies on cultural consumption repeatedly found that cultural capital "haves" are more capable of appreciating multiple genres than cultural capital "have-nots" (Erickson, 1996; Peterson, 1992; Chan and Goldthorpe, 2007). Those endowed with higher levels of cultural capital like Stravinsky *and* Sting while those with limited cultural capital assets like only Sting. The distinction lies not between opera lovers and rap fans but between omnivores and univores.

Second, the universe of consumption fields encompasses not only art, but multiple realms of pursuits such as hobbies, socializing, food, interior décor, fashion, and media use (Holt, 1998). The roll-out of broadband implies the emergence of yet another domain where differences in cultural capital are reflected in differences in interests and activities. Media use is a domain of cultural practice where *habitus*, or a collection of patterns of thought, behavior, and taste is manifested and enacted. Just as those with a high level of cultural capital enjoy multiple genres of art, they are omnivorous in media use. In fact, recent studies on Internet use saw the rise of a "broadband elite" that uses the connection for ten or more online activities on a typical day (Horrigan and Rainie, 2006).

The slow take-up of broadband technology presents a difficult conundrum for researchers. The concepts of cultural capital and habitus can be fruitfully applied to answer why the Japanese do not use broadband technology when affordable, high-quality access is widely available. The theoretical answer drawn from the theory of cultural capital is that it is because only those with the right kind of cultural capital and habitus know enough to use broadband technology for a wide range of online activities. It is crucial to investigate the link between usage applications and characteristics of users in terms of the distribution of cultural capital to examine whether empirical data lends support to the theoretical claim.

Hypotheses

To recap the key concepts and propositions in the previous sections, the present chapter responds to a call for an approach which would expand the scope of inquiry beyond material access and would incorporate more multifaceted aspects of digital inequality. We do so by examining characteristics of users and actual behaviors rather than speculating about intrinsic properties of broadband technology. We draw on the theory of cultural capital to relate different modes of access and uses to different levels of skill, different motivations and different interests.

We hypothesize that the stagnant adoption rate of broadband connection in Japan is attributed to the uneven distribution of cultural capital. Those with limited cultural capital are likely to be unaware of the availability of new applications even when high-quality broadband technology is within their reach. When they do know of new applications, they tend to be univore users. Formally, our hypotheses are as follows:

Hypothesis 1: Those endowed with limited cultural capital resources are less likely to be aware of new applications delivered by broadband technology than those with higher levels of cultural capital.

Hypothesis 2: The omnivore/univore distinction is observed in terms of the number of applications. Those with higher levels of cultural capital use more applications and services than those with limited cultural capital assets.

The next section discusses data and methods to test these hypotheses.

Data and methods

Data analysis is made possible by the Broadband Adoption and Usage Survey (BAUS). The BAUS was designed to address a range of questions about the socioeconomic characteristics of broadband users and their online behaviors. The data was collected by an online survey in March 2011. The population of BAUS is individuals with computer-based Internet access aged between 16 and 65 living in a household in 44 prefectures in Japan.[3] 99,684 were randomly chosen from the roster of possible respondents maintained by a polling organization and invited to take part in the survey. 3,571 valid observations were obtained. The characteristics of the respondents were compared with comparable survey data to ensure that respondents were not significantly different from non-respondents.

Dependent variables

In order to test our hypotheses, we looked at 12 types of broadband applications (see Table 5.1). Figure 5.6 cross-tabulates types of Internet and broadband applications with user responses (see Figure 5.6). The original variables about knowledge of broadband applications have three categories. We asked the respondent whether she or he (1) knew that a particular type of application was available and she or he had used it, (2) knew that the service was available but she or he had never used it, or (3) did not know that the service was available. Binary variables to indicate whether the respondent knew about applications were created from these variables. Those who did not know about availability of a particular application were coded as one in the new "don't know" variable.

Independent variables

Key variables that are known to affect usage patterns are included in the models. Female is a binary variable. Age is a continuous variable. Indicator variables were used to code the level of education, hours spent watching TV on a typical day, the number of books the respondents read per month, marital status, employment status and living with a child. Education, the number of hours spent watching TV, and the number of books read were treated as proxies of cultural capital.

Table 5.1 Types of broadband application

Types of application	Observed variables
Education	Online learning
Transaction	Transactions with government agencies
Video streaming	Diet and local assembly sessions Press conferences Stock-holder meetings
Medical services	Making a medical appointment Seeking health advice online
Consumption	Grocery shopping Auctioning
Entertainment	Downloading music Downloading novels Video on demand

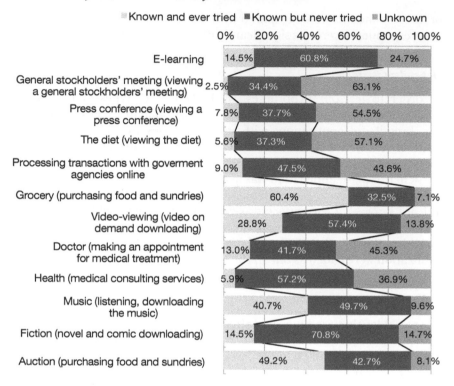

Figure 5.6 Internet and broadband applications

Source: BAUS

Findings

A series of indicator variables to distinguish those who did not know about services were created to test Hypothesis 1. By regressing "don't know" variables on independent variables, their influence and statistical significance were estimated. The results of logistic regression are summarized in Table 5.2. The dependent variable was coded as one if the respondent did not know about an application. A negative sign suggests that the pertinent independent variable suppresses the log odds of being ignorant of an application. For example, the positive and significant effect of being female in Model 2 (0.471) indicates that women are 1.6 (=$e^{0.471}$) times as likely as men to state that they don't know that they can use the computer to complete transactions with government agencies.

In addition to proxies of cultural capital, other "usual suspects" variables show interesting patterns. Gender turned out to be significant in 6 applications out of 12. Those include transactions with government agencies, viewing information about diet and local assembly sessions,

Table 5.2 Logistic regression models predicting don't know responses

		(1) learning	(2) transaction	(3) diet	(4) press conference	(5) stock-holder meeting	(6) appointment	(7) advice	(8) grocery	(9) auction	(10) music	(11) novel	(12) video on demand
Female		0.150 (0.1007)	0.471*** (0.0000)	0.701*** (0.0000)	0.613*** (0.0000)	0.580*** (0.0000)	0.0266 (0.7323)	-0.0737 (0.3589)	-0.169 (0.2581)	0.0482 (0.7330)	0.152 (0.2560)	0.368*** (0.0010)	0.321** (0.0051)
Education	Junior college	-0.207* (0.0380)	-0.200* (0.0292)	-0.251** (0.0077)	-0.159 (0.0863)	-0.291** (0.0029)	-0.198* (0.0286)	-0.126 (0.1746)	-0.186 (0.2920)	0.00889 (0.9562)	-0.0876 (0.5583)	-0.0733 (0.5505)	-0.0502 (0.6927)
	University	-0.616*** (0.0000)	-0.394*** (0.0000)	-0.336*** (0.0001)	-0.355*** (0.0000)	-0.408*** (0.0000)	-0.344*** (0.0000)	-0.184* (0.0355)	-0.177 (0.2752)	0.0438 (0.7749)	-0.0416 (0.7705)	-0.100 (0.4036)	-0.0712 (0.5639)
TV	< one hour	0.0398 (0.8672)	-0.0398 (0.8443)	-0.305 (0.1319)	0.135 (0.4982)	-0.120 (0.5661)	-0.195 (0.3240)	-0.288 (0.1493)	-0.305 (0.3006)	-0.437 (0.1330)	-0.473 (0.0947)	-0.318 (0.2138)	-0.00994 (0.9702)
	< two hours	0.0182 (0.9362)	0.106 (0.5836)	-0.212 (0.2757)	0.218 (0.2519)	-0.0704 (0.7254)	-0.204 (0.2824)	-0.153 (0.4214)	-0.617** (0.0304)	-0.563* (0.0409)	-0.505 (0.0575)	-0.503* (0.0390)	-0.184 (0.4722)
	< three hours	0.0136 (0.9529)	-0.127 (0.5188)	-0.173 (0.3820)	0.272 (0.1622)	-0.0768 (0.7067)	-0.290 (0.1336)	-0.374 (0.0550)	-0.776** (0.0099)	-0.852** (0.0032)	-0.796** (0.0041)	-0.637** (0.0107)	-0.451 (0.0886)
	three or more hours	0.0618 (0.7868)	0.0785 (0.6886)	-0.0796 (0.6869)	0.322 (0.0956)	-0.0136 (0.9467)	-0.265 (0.1670)	-0.371 (0.0547)	-0.788** (0.0076)	-0.867** (0.0022)	-0.866** (0.0015)	-0.530* (0.0303)	-0.372 (0.1514)

Table 5.2 continued

		(1) learning	(2) transaction	(3) diet	(4) press conference	(5) stock-holder meeting	(6) appointment	(7) advice	(8) grocery	(9) auction	(10) music	(11) novel	(12) video on demand
Books	< three books	-0.520*** (0.0000)	-0.485*** (0.0000)	-0.481*** (0.0000)	-0.424*** (0.0000)	-0.436*** (0.0000)	-0.406*** (0.0000)	-0.529*** (0.0000)	-0.587*** (0.0001)	-0.692*** (0.0000)	-0.548*** (0.0000)	-0.646*** (0.0000)	-0.682*** (0.0000)
	< five books	-0.736*** (0.0000)	-0.697*** (0.0000)	-0.623*** (0.0000)	-0.573*** (0.0000)	-0.589*** (0.0000)	-0.632*** (0.0000)	-0.699*** (0.0000)	-0.344 (0.1926)	-0.651* (0.0139)	-0.543* (0.0276)	-0.834*** (0.0001)	-0.757*** (0.0005)
	five or more books	-0.716*** (0.0001)	-0.952*** (0.0000)	-0.591*** (0.0000)	-0.584*** (0.0000)	-0.725*** (0.0000)	-0.418*** (0.0027)	-0.693*** (0.0000)	-0.991** (0.0029)	-0.403 (0.1029)	-0.426 (0.0757)	-0.631** (0.0022)	-0.528* (0.0109)
Household income		-0.234*** (0.0000)	-0.184*** (0.0000)	-0.194*** (0.0000)	-0.199*** (0.0000)	-0.218*** (0.0000)	-0.175*** (0.0000)	-0.176*** (0.0000)	-0.235*** (0.0009)	-0.180** (0.0069)	-0.139* (0.0284)	-0.158* (0.0030)	-0.215*** (0.0001)
N		3571	3571	3571	3571	3571	3571	3571	3571	3571	3571	3571	3571

P-values in parentheses.
* $p < 0.05$ ** $p < 0.01$ *** $p < 0.001$
Notes: Employment status, age, network size, mobile phone ownership, marital status and living with a child are controlled. Coefficients for the controls are now shown. The reference category for education is high school or less, the reference category for TV is zero, and the reference category for the number of books is zero.

viewing press conferences, viewing stockholder meetings, downloading novels and comics, and video viewing including on-demand services. On the other hand, there are no gender differences in knowledge about online learning, grocery shopping, making an appointment for medical treatment, medical consulting, downloading music, and auctioning. Rather than having uniform effects, the effect of gender varies across types of application. It is beyond the scope of the present chapter to determine what produces observed differential effects, but it seems that the effect of gender is insignificant in activities traditionally popular among women (e.g. learning and grocery shopping). Further research is needed to examine the effect of gender in terms of the relevance of an application.

Household income has negative effects on the log odds in all models. Negative signs suggest that those who are in affluent households are likely to know about a wide variety of applications. Even though shopping and auctioning are common applications used by the majority of the respondents (see Figure 5.6), the sizable effects of household income on these two dependent variables suggest that there exist households that are deficient not only in disposable income but also in knowledge of online shopping. Unlike gender, household income is significant in all the models. The unequal access to and use of information and communication technology may not be a distinct or new type of inequality. Rather, the results suggest that it is closely related to traditional inequality issues such as unequal distribution of household incomes.

At the same time, variables associated with the level of cultural capital have remarkable effects. The adoption of broadband technology cannot be reduced to economic difference. As for institutionalized forms of cultural capital, the indicator for junior college or for vocational school is significant in five models. The indicator for university or for four-year college is significant in seven models. Interestingly, the two education indicators are not significant in models regarding consumption and entertainment. It implies that education makes differences in more consequential areas of activity. In particular, the effect of university-level education on online learning is remarkable. Those with university degrees are the first to know about online learning opportunities.

In summary, our first hypothesis is supported by data. Those endowed with limited cultural resources are less likely to be aware of new applications delivered by broadband technology than those with higher levels of cultural capital. Differential use practices are produced by different levels of cultural capital as well as by socioeconomic status and demographic attributes.

To test Hypothesis 2, a zero-inflated Poisson (ZIP) model is constructed. The dependent variable is the number of applications known and tried by the respondents. It is constructed by adding up the values of indicators for knowing and having used applications. Because there are 12 applications, the maximum possible value is 12 and the minimum is 0. All the independent variables used in logistic regression analysis are included in the model.

Contrary to logistic regression models regarding the lack of knowledge, a positive coefficient in the current ZIP model indicates that it is positively associated with the number of applications (see Table 5.3). The first set of coefficients refers to the Poisson model for those who have used at least one application. The second set of coefficients refers to the binary model to classify the individual into either the "always zero" group or the "not always zero" group.

Table 5.3 Zero-inflated Poisson regression predicting the number of applications ever used

(a) Count Equation			(b) Binary Equation		
Female		−0.0500 (0.0564)	Female		−0.328* (0.0407)
Education	Junior college	0.0804** (0.0098)	Education	Junior college	−0.171 (0.3900)
	University	0.107*** (0.0002)		University	−0.0646 (0.6964)
TV	< one hour	−0.00165 (0.9789)	TV	< one hour	0.262 (0.4099)
	< two hours	−0.0783 (0.1939)		< two hours	−0.0296 (0.9249)
	< three hours	−0.0313 (0.6107)		< three hours	−0.0229 (0.9441)
	three or more hours	−0.0800 (0.1967)		three or more hours	−0.426 (0.2233)
Books	< three books	0.169*** (0.0000)	Books	< three books	−0.336* (0.0319)
	< five books	0.216*** (0.0000)		< five books	−0.300 (0.2680)
	five or more books	0.221*** (0.0000)		five or more books	−0.232 (0.4012)
Household income		0.0689*** (0.0000)	Household income		−0.174* (0.0211)
			N		3571

P-values in parentheses.
* p < 0.05   ** p < 0.01   *** p < 0.001
Notes: Employment status, age, network size, mobile phone ownership, marital status, and living with a child are controlled. Coefficients for the controls are now shown. The reference category for education is high school of less, the reference category for TV is zero, and the reference category for the number of books is zero.

The result is consistent with our hypothesis that the omnivore/univore distinction is observed in terms of the number of applications. Education and the number of books read are positively associated with the number of applications ever used. The highly educated and the well-read are likely to try different applications. Household income has a positive influence on the number of applications as well. On the other hand, cultural capital proxies are not significant in the bottom half of the output. Cultural capital proxies do not change the odds of being in the always zero group compared with the not always zero group.

To summarize, data analysis confirmed that our hypotheses are supported. They together suggest that usage applications are systematically related to cultural capital assets. Holding socioeconomic conditions and demographic attributes constant, those endowed with higher levels of cultural capital are likely to know about available broadband applications and are likely to try some of them. Our analysis also supports the omnivore/univore distinction. These findings are interesting for two reasons: (1) they show that patterns of broadband applications are successfully analyzed in terms of the production of distinction (in Bourdieu's sense); and (2) they reveal that there are strong connections among seemingly unrelated individual traits and activities (reading books and auctioning online, for example).

Conclusion

The present chapter has raised a number of intriguing questions about what explains the sub-optimal use of broadband capability in Japan. It employs the cultural perspective to uncover the roots of inequality in Internet use. As it turned out, successful usage presupposes not only material access, but motivational access and knowledge. Basic digital and informational skills such as touch typing and using a search engine are relevant. Yet the challenge of effective broadband adoption and usage cannot be trivialized to the issue of technology per se. Our analysis shows that traditional inequality issues are of much importance. Drawing on the concept of omnivore derived from the critique of Bourdieu's theory, we demonstrated that individuals rich in cultural capital use a wide variety of broadband applications. Some individuals are excluded from newly emerging communicative possibilities by choice or by circumstance not because they do not have access to a computer, but rather because they do not have the right cultural tools. Socioeconomic factors and demographic characteristics remain influential as well.

The first and foremost contribution of the present chapter is to address the serious omission of current research on broadband adoption and application, namely, the lack of conceptual elaboration, definition, and theory. It began with simple yet central questions such as what exactly having access to broadband Internet is and who are likely to be unaware of available broadband applications. Drawing on the classical sociological traditions of cultural perspectives (Weberian theory) in general and cultural capital in particular, it identifies multiple paths through which differences in cultural capital translate into differences in use and application. Second, the chapter empirically examines socioeconomic and behavioral variables and mechanisms involved in broadband adoption in under-studied communities of broadband users. Japan is among the leaders of broadband deployment in the world. Detailed analyses of broadband adoption patterns have been much needed but yet they have been hard to come by thus far partly because of the lack of data. The present chapter is a first step to fill in the lacuna in our knowledge with newly available data.

References

Akiyoshi, M. and Ono, H. (2008). The diffusion of mobile Internet in Japan. *The Information Society*, 24(5), 292–303.

Bleha, T. (2009). *Overtaken on the Information Superhighway: How the U.S. lost Internet leadership and what to do about it*. Charleston, SC, US: Booksurge.

Bonfadelli, H. (2002). The Internet and knowledge gaps. *European Journal of Communication*, 17(1), 65–84.

Bourdieu, P. (1984). *Distinction : A social critique of the judgment of taste*. Cambridge, MA, US: Harvard University Press.

Bourdieu, P. (1986). The forms of capital, (R. Nice, trans.). In J. G. Richardson (ed.) *Handbook of theory and research for the sociology of education* (241–258). New York: Greenwood Press.

Chan, T.K. and Goldthorpe, J.H. (2007). Social Status and Newspaper Readership. *American Journal of Sociology*, 112(4), 1095–1134.

DiMaggio, P. and Bonikowski, B. (2008). Make money surfing the web? The impact of Internet use on the earnings of US workers. *American Sociological Review*, 73(2), 227–250.

Erickson, B. (1996). Culture, class, and connections. *American Journal of Sociology*, 102(1), 217–251.

Grint, K. and Woolgar, S. (1997). *The machine at work: Technology, work and organization*. Cambridge, UK: Polity.

Holt, D. B. (1998). Does cultural capital structure American consumption? *Journal of Consumer Research*, 25(1), 1–25.

Horrigan, J. B. and Rainie, L. (2006). The Internet's growing role in life's major moments. Pew Internet and American Life Project, Washington, DC. Retrieved August 5, 2011. http://www.pewinternet.org/Reports/2006/The-Internets-Growing-Role-in-Lifes-Major-Moments.aspx

ITU/UNESCO. (2011). Broadband: A platform for progress. Retrieved October 23, 2012 from http://www.unesco.org/new/fileadmin/MULTIMEDIA/HQ/CI/CI/pdf/broadband_commission_report_overview.pdf

Norris, P. (2001). *Digital divide: Civic engagement, information poverty, and the Internet worldwide*. Cambridge, UK: Cambridge University Press.

OECD. (2011a). Broadband Portal. Retrieved August 5, 2011 from http://www. oecd.org/document/54/0,3746,en_2649_34225_38690102_1_1_1_1,00.html

OECD. (2011b). OECD Telecommunications and Internet Statistics, (database). Retrieved August 5, 2011 from http://www.oecd-ilibrary.org/science-and-technology/data/oecd-telecommunications-and-internet-statistics_data-00170-en

Orbicom. (2007). *Digital Review of Asia Pacific 2007/2008*. Ottawa, Canada: IDRC.

Peterson, R. A. (1992). Understanding audience segmentation: From elite and mass to omnivore and univore. *Poetics*, 21(4), 243–258.

Tsuchiya, M. and A. Thierer. (2002). Is America exporting misguided telecommunications policy? The U.S.-Japan Telecom Trade Negotiations and beyond. *CATO Institute Briefing Papers*, 79.

van Deursen, A. J. A. and van Dijk, J. A. G. (2010). Internet skills and the digital divide. *New Media & Society*, 13(6), 893–911.

van Dijk, J. A. G. M. (2006). Digital divide research, achievements and shortcomings. *Poetics*, 34(4–5), 221–235.

Weber, M. (1991). *From Max Weber: Essays in sociology*, London: Routledge.

Witte, J. C. and Mannon, S. E. (2010). *The Internet and social inequalities*. New York: Routledge.

Notes

1 An earlier version of this chapter appeared as a presentation at TPRC 2011 (Arlington, VA, US on September 24, 2011). The first two authors are grateful to the Institute for Information and Communication Policy for financial support. We also received helpful advice from Massimo Ragnedda and Glenn Muschert, the editors of this volume.

2 NTT was also reluctant to open up optic fiber facilities, because the fiber networks were, NTT claimed, established after its privatization in 1985 and thus it had proprietary rights over them. NTT's bifacial approach (responding to DSL requests and deploying optic fibers) enabled a swift transition to broadband technology.

3 Originally, BAUS was designed to include a nationally representative sample. One day prior to the scheduled survey start date, the Great Eastern Earthquake struck Japan. The survey was suspended and was eventually conducted a few weeks later dropping four hardest-hit prefectures, namely, Ibaraki, Iwate, Miyagi, and Fukushima.

Section 3

Rapidly developing large nations – the BRIC nations

6 The digital divide in Brazil
Conceptual, research and policy challenges

Bernardo Sorj
Edelstein Center for Social Research

Introduction

The digital divide refers to the social consequences of the unequal distribution of access and users' capabilities of information and communication technologies among countries and within societies. In this article we discuss some theoretical, research and policy challenges posed by the digital divide within national societies, that is, how the different levels of access to products, services, and benefits of new information and communication technologies affects different segments of the population. The Brazilian case will be used to exemplify the general argument.

Communication and information technologies (C&IT) include an array of products (radio, TV, cable TV, fixed and mobile phones, computers, the Internet) and, although they are converging technologies, each one of them creates its own digital divide. In this study we will focus mainly on the digital divide related to the unequal access to computers with Internet connection (telematics).

From a sociological perspective, the main theoretical question posed by the digital divide is how it is related to and affects existing forms of social stratification. To answer this question social scientists need to clearly conceptualize the issues involved and to produce or have access to data that can inform theoretical efforts. From a policy perspective the challenge is to ensure that telematics diminish rather than increase social inequality.

Social stratification and the Internet

Classical sociological theories on stratification are a necessary, but limited, starting point to understand how the Internet is disseminated and used. Marxist theories can be extremely useful to understand the capital accumulation dynamics and the formation of dominant groups in the communications sector, but are rather unhelpful for the understanding of how they disseminate and impact society, other than the general statement, which is not rigorously Marxist, that the richer have more and better access (at home, work and school) than the poorer.

Weberian theory of social status is relevant to the extent that there is a strong correlation between level of education and the capacity to transform Internet information into knowledge. However, Weber's concept of status, while it includes education, is much broader. Finally, the Durkheimian concept of division of labor could be developed to explain changes in the labor market structure (job creation and destruction, job qualifications) produced by telematics, but is less insightful regarding the ways by which new technologies disseminate among different social strata.

In the preceding decades conceptual debates in sociology shifted their focus. The most important change was toward the analysis of global forms of stratification instead of national forms. While national studies are more sensitive to the symbolic and political dimensions of social classes, globalization theories tend to have a narrower economic perspective. This is a natural result of the level of abstraction needed to generalize about global trends. The paradoxical effect is that sociological research, even when intended to be critical of dominant trends, tends to converge with the dominance of economic thinking on social stratification. This not only applies to the digital divide but in general studies on social stratification become strongly influenced by economics and policy making, which is translated in focusing mainly on the issues of social inequality and poverty.

In fact a great number of academic studies and, even more, reports on the digital divide made by international bodies which command enormous resources and research capabilities are mostly made by economists or strongly influenced by the economic perspective. For sociologists the best source for data on social trends in telematics would be that of research firms serving major telecom communication, but their data is not publicly available.

Understanding the impact of the Internet in social stratification is therefore a complex and still unresolved question. The problem obviously surpasses the specificities of the impact of the Internet on society, which we will describe, and is related to general changes in late capitalism. Classical theories of stratification were developed in Europe, before the welfare state, economies of mass consumption, and service-based economies. From Marx to Bourdieu, theories of social stratification were conceived in European societies in which social classes were relatively self-contained subcultures, from taste to politics. This is no longer the case, even in Europe, and was always less so in the USA and many other nations like, for instance, Brazil. Given the strong influence of the economic perspective on the debates on the digital divide, sociologists can at least contribute by qualifying the issues, by analyzing the social dimensions of telematics impact on different social groups, while working on reshaping the problems and concepts posed by classical theories of social stratification.

What are the specific characteristics of the Internet's impact on social stratification? Social stratification refers to individuals' relative position in society within a continuum distributed according to criteria of higher or lower access to economic, political or symbolic resources. The digital divide, in principle, is not a continuum but a binary distribution of the population between those who have (access) and those who have not,[1] although this opposition masks the enormous variation among those that have access – in particular quality and time of access and the capacity to make the best use of the possibilities of the media, mainly dependent on the educational qualifications of the users (see Witte and Mannon, 2010).

Telematics also represents a tool that enhances previous social networks and social capital. The more diversified the number and quality of professional contacts the higher the potential of the Internet as a medium to enhance professional and work opportunities. Therefore its potential as a communication instrument is greater among high income users since most probably all the members of their network have access to the Internet, while this is not the case for the low-income users. This is even truer in the case of international contacts, because low-income sectors are very unlikely to have an international social network (with the relevant exception of poor families with members working abroad, often illegally, for whom the Internet offers cheap communication and contact with their native land and families).

One of the characteristics that make the relationship between the digital divide and other forms of stratification particularly elusive is the poly-functional character of the Internet. Access doesn't indicate the type of uses. It can be used for leisure and amusement, as a communication tool, a source of information, an instrument for access to knowledge or part of a job definition. Therefore having Internet access and knowing the basics of computing does not necessarily mean that it enhances people's life chances. It is the *uses* of information technology that are the most important criterion for evaluating its impact on social structures. These uses depend on the capabilities and creative appropriation of the new technology by the different social actors.

While there are correlations between having access and level of income, literacy is a *sine qua non* precondition for using the Internet. The "old" communication technologies (phone, radio, TV) are part of the family of "illiterate friendly" products – that is, products that can be used by individuals who have little or no literacy – while computers and the Internet not only demand basic educational skills but their relevance and potential increase in direct proportion to previous intellectual skills.[2] Differently from other forms of stratification, telematics has decisive generational determinants: the older the person the higher the chances of having difficulties to adapt to the use and possibilities of the new technologies.[3]

As the Internet is spreading very rapidly, the digital divide should be analyzed in a diachronic and dynamic perspective, as a case of the social *product cycle,* in which initially a product is introduced in small quantities with a high price and later it is mass-produced permitting access by a large part of the population. A new product initially reaches only those at the highest income levels and later, with mass production and price reduction, is disseminated throughout all sectors of the population. Thus, the dynamics of technological innovation always reinforce social inequality in the initial stages, when the product reaches only the highest income sectors of the population. At a later stage of mass production, the product is disseminated through the lower social classes in a process that can be more strongly affected by public policy.

Since richer sectors of society are the first to have access to new products, they have the benefit of initial competitive advantage in using and mastering them. At the same time, those who are excluded face new disadvantages. Therefore new ICT products increase, in principle, the social gap and social exclusion. Therefore, as we will see below, the main aim of digital inclusion policies is to diminish the negative impact of new ICTs on wealth distribution and life chances.

The digital divide in Brazil

Existing data on Brazil's digital divide is quite sophisticated. Still, it hardly allows for a more detailed sociological analysis.[4] Nonetheless, what do the existing data show (the latest being from 2010)?

1) Access is distributed unequally among regions. The poorer the region the lower the percentage of people with Internet access at home. The North and the Northeast regions, the poorest of the country, have, respectively, 17 percent and 15 percent of homes with Internet access, while the Southeast has 39 percent and the South 32 percent.

2) Access is related not only to income, but geographical location. While the urban areas' national average is 31 percent, the rural areas' average is 6 percent, with a slower rate of growth. Although the rural population is poorer than the urban, the enormous difference between them is due to the fact that a large number of rural areas have no access to Internet servers. Therefore regional differences are also related to the fact that the poorest regions also have the highest percentage of the rural population. For private telecom enterprises serving sparse populations is not profitable and universalization of infrastructure access depends on public policies that subsidize or make mandatory connecting all parts of the territory. In spite of the Brazilian government's plans to make service universal, the goal is still far from being achieved.

3) The growth of households with Internet access did increase exponentially in recent years. It went from a national average of 13 percent in 2005 to 31 percent in 2010. Price reduction for computers, with government tax exemptions for the cheapest models, undoubtedly played an important role, but for the poorer groups the major bottleneck is the high monthly cost of subscribing to Internet services or phone bills.

4) A division of the population in five classes of strata[5] (A, B, C, D, E) shows 90 percent of the highest strata had Internet access in 2010, compared to 65 percent of group B, 24 percent of group C, and 3 percent of groups D and E. While the growth in the number of persons with access from group A remained stagnant in recent years, having arrived at the near saturation point, the most important growth happened in group C.

5) Access to broadband Internet is also distributed unequally between social classes and regions, although it tends to increase in all of them.

6) If we include other forms of access (work, LAN-houses, houses of other people, and school) the number of persons with Internet access in total went from 30 percent in 2005 to 49 percent in 2009. The percentage of the population using LAN-houses for Internet access increased from 18 percent in 2005 to 34 percent in 2010, indicating that for the poorest strata LAN-houses are a main source of access and are responsible for an important part of the growth of Internet access for this group.[6] Twenty-seven percent cited the houses of others as their main source of access, which confirms our own research that, among the poor, houses of friends or family are a central source of access (see Sorj and Guedes, 2005). Work was also indicated by 22 percent as the main site of access, which probably follows the same pattern of being an alternative for those that do not have access at home. School was indicated by 14 percent as being the main source of access, a number that should grow with the expected increase of technology labs in public schools, still poorly served (see Sorj and Lissovsky, 2010). Finally, free public access in LAN-houses represented 4 percent.

7) Communication is the most important Internet activity (94 percent), followed by searches for information (87 percent) and education (66 percent), with only 17 percent using it for financial services. Participation in blogs, discussion lists and Twitter is higher among the richer, the most educated, the younger, and in the wealthier regions.

8) The use of the Internet through mobile phone is only relatively widespread among class A (21 percent), decreasing to 10 percent in class B, 5 percent in class C and 1 percent in classes D/E.

The findings presented above mainly confirm general trends observed in developing countries. Still they have limited relevance for understanding the relative importance of the Internet in life quality and life chances for different social groups: how e-literacy (or the lack of it) affects the labor market, job opportunities, social mobility, job searches, income, consumption, access to relevant information, social participation and news of the world. In this sense more sociological research is needed, in particular comparative case studies that focus on particular social groups and environments (work, school, job qualifications/salary, school, etc.). This is not a task easy to quantify. For instance, quantifying the impact of telematics on children's school performance among different social backgrounds is far from obvious if we consider that there is no clear consensus on the impact of telematics on education in general.[7]

Statistical studies – in particular those on developing countries – have a central parameter: the division between those who have and those who do not have access to computers and to the Internet. Although central, this measurement is insufficient to understand the different processes of social *appropriation by the actor*: the capacity for making sense, interpreting and using the information available on the Internet, both by individuals and communities. Case studies are extremely useful but mostly they refer to exceptions rather than rules.[8] More qualitative and quantitative study is needed on the relationship between content production and content appropriation among the different sectors of society.

It is important to differentiate between the social impact of new technologies as presented in statistical data and the concrete way that those technologies are experienced by the users. Personal affect does not figure in aggregate data or theoretical concepts, but is based on comparing their current with their previous situation. In the case of the digital divide, the experience in Brazil and other developed countries is that the widespread dissemination of mobile phones made it possible for a large proportion of the population to have access, for the first time, to a phone line, in spite of use limitations from difficulty to pay mobile fees. In addition, many case studies indicate that the use of telematics improves the quality of life of poor communities. This may be the case, but it does not mean that social inequality is decreasing, considering the appropriation of the new technologies by the dominant groups of society who generally have more access and superior skills to use digital technologies, compared with less affluent groups.

Digital divide policies

Social stratification, and in particular social inequality, cannot be dissociated in contemporary capitalism from the role of the state. Either through legislative and regulatory measures, or by distributive public policies, state intervention affects income and access to public goods; influencing social inequality and the life conditions of the poorest sectors of the population. Both in academic research and policy reports, the relationship between the Internet and social stratification has as its main focus its impact on social inequality and poverty. However poverty is not an objective category. It is defined by common sense and/or political fiat, and it changes according to the level of cultural/economic/technological/ political development of each society. The introduction of a new category of products for consumption that become a condition of "civilized" life (be it a telephone, electricity, a refrigerator, radio or TV) raises the minimum standard of living which defines poverty.

Although many authors and policy think tanks present the new communication technologies as a panacea, the introduction of new "essential" products tend to increase inequality and feelings of social deprivation (see Sorj, 2005). Policies related to reducing the digital divide as a tool in the fight against poverty, do not necessarily diminish social inequality or change existing forms of social stratification. Furthermore, under conditions of economic growth it is possible to reduce poverty indicators (the size of the population below a set poverty line), while simultaneously increasing social inequality. Thus the fights against inequality and poverty have some convergences but are not synonymous.

Internet access is now considered a public social good in most countries and public policies include, *inter alia*, assuring that access is available to the more isolated regions, distributing laptops to students, tax exemptions to diminish the cost of computers, creating computer labs at public schools and opening free access LAN-houses.

The search for miraculous solutions to solve social problems is a constant in developing countries. The Internet is too important to be brought into the cycle of miracle cures that later are abandoned for not meeting unrealistic expectations. Policies aimed at reducing the digital divide are a necessary component of social policy but they are an insufficient answer to social and economic problems. The same is true in relation to e-education and to the problems of school performance.

Social policies related to the digital divide cannot be dissociated from education policies. The ability to use the information available on the Internet as a source of knowledge, and intellectual and professional development depends on the users' prior skills. This qualification assumes basic literacy and abilities acquired within the school system. Thus social inequality as expressed in educational inequity is reproduced and increases with use of the Internet. As long as much of the population of the developing world continues to struggle with illiteracy and semi-literacy, universal access to the Internet will be an illusory goal.

Training in the use of the computer and the Internet (called digital literacy or e-literacy) can be offered through formal courses in school or at work, private courses, or courses promoted by non-governmental organizations, or in contexts (schools, work or home) where the Internet is used and people nearby are able to offer assistance when needed. Children, in particular, tend to learn to use computers and the Internet through play almost without direct orientation. However the probability of having the type of access that allows this kind of learning by osmosis, either at home or work, is lower in low-income sectors where the chances of owning a home computer or having access to a computer in the work place are extremely low.

The increasing complexity associated with the fight against social inequality creates new challenges for strategic planning of governmental actions and for the development of social policies in which sociological sensibility can be extremely useful. The urgency to resolve the problem of the digital divide cannot justify hasty pharaonic investments in areas that demand experimental pilot programs, adequate local conditions, user training, systems of evaluation and technical support. This is particularly true of the installation of Internet access in schools, which should be distinct from viewing the school as place in which deprived children can have access to the Internet as an educational tool. ICTs should not be transformed overnight into a privileged instrument for the educational system. The adaptation of professors to this new instrument is a long process that cannot be disassociated with the general improvement of professional development. Developing adequate software, adapting pedagogical systems, and developing critical teaching techniques on the use of ICTs will be a necessarily long term learning process in the majority of developing countries. Until that time, the role of ICT labs in schools should be to introduce students to these instruments and their uses and provide them training on basic programs, in order to motivate them and to facilitate future integration in the job market.

Finally, the fight against the digital divide depends, above all, on the capacity of state action to use market impulses and the experiences of civil society, non-governmental organizations and private initiatives to assure that poor sectors of the population are integrated into and participate in the construction of the global society. For instance, the experience in several Latin American countries indicates that NGOs or state free public tele-centers in poor neighborhoods have a pioneer role in opening a niche which is generally rapidly overtaken by the private initiative of locals that offer good services with very low tariffs.

Conclusions

The consequences of the Internet on social stratification are a disputed terrain in the sociological literature. While there are reasonable arguments for considering the Internet as a tool to diminish social distance, democratizing knowledge, and social participation, it can be equally argued that it increases centers of power, state and corporate social control (e.g., among the "optimist" scholars, see Castells, 2009; Benkler, 2006; or for critical stances, see Grewal, 2008; Zittrain, 2008; Carr, 2010). Both sides reflect different aspects of social reality and the main criticism that both perspectives deserve is that the Internet is but one dimension of social dynamics. Thus, the final impact of the Internet will depend in large measure on a dynamic that is outside of the technological realm; or more properly, on unintended consequences and the economic, social and political factors that are shaped also, but not only, by the Internet.

In developing countries, where Internet access is not available to large portions of the population its initial social impact is to increase social inequality because it reaches first the wealthiest sectors of the population. Thus, the fight against the digital divide is not so much a fight to diminish social inequality in itself as it is an effort to prevent inequality from increasing because of the advantages that those groups of the population with more economic resources and education enjoy as a result of exclusive or better access to telematics. Sociological analysis can be particularly helpful in understanding the different impact of the Internet on different social strata and age-groups, the ways it impacts on users and the different forms of appropriation of the technology.

From a policy perspective the struggle for digital inclusion is a struggle against time. New information technologies increase existing social inequalities; therefore policies for digital inclusion are nothing more than a struggle to re-align the possibilities for access to the job market and life chances of the poorer groups. But promoting access is only a step. The true value of information depends on the user's ability to interpret it. To be useful, information must be meaningful, must be transformed into knowledge through a process of socialization and practices that build analytical capacities. Therefore confronting the digital divide cannot be separated from confronting the educational divide.

E-social development does not substitute for other kinds of social development, nor does the fight against the digital divide supplant the set of measures necessary for facing poverty, social inequality, and one of their most terrible consequences, urban violence. Policies to universalize access to the Internet in developing countries will not be successful if they are not associated with other social policies, in particular those relating to education. Obviously, this does not mean that we must wait until we are able to eradicate illiteracy in order to develop digital inclusion policies. The demands of the economy and the labor market require interrelated policies that work with different social sectors and different rhythms in order to universalize the Internet as a public service.

References

Benkler, Y. (2006). *The wealth of networks*. New Haven, CT, US: Yale University Press.
Brazilian Steering Committee. (2011). Survey on the use of information and communication technologies in Brazil: ICT Households and ICT Enterprises – 2010. Retrieved July 17, 2012 from http://op.ceptro.br/cgi-bin/indicadores-cgibr-2010?pais=brasil&estado=rj&academia=academia&age=mais-de-60-anos&education=pos-doutorado&purpose=pesquisa-academica.

Carr, N. (2010). *The shallows: What the Internet is doing to our brains.* New York: W.W. Norton.

Castells, M. (2009). *Communication power.* Oxford, UK: Oxford University Press.

Christensen, C., Johnson, C.W. and Horn, M.B. (2008). *Disrupting class: How disruptive innovation will change the way the world learns.* New York: McGraw-Hill.

Grewal, S. (2008). *Network power.* New Haven, CT, US: Yale University Press.

Schacter, J. (1999). *The impact of education technology on student achievement: What the most current research has to say.* Retrieved July 21, 2012 from http://www.eric. ed.gov/PDFS/ED430537.pdf

Sorj, B. (2005). *Information societies and digital divides: An introduction.* Milan, Italy: Polimetrica.

Sorj, B. and Guedes, L.E. (2005). *Internet y pobreza.* Montevideo, Uruguay: Editora UNESCO, Ediciones Trilce.

Sorj, B. and Lissovsky, M. (2010). Internet in Brazilian public schools: Policies beyond politics, *IRIE – International Review of Informatics Ethics,* 14, 41–63.

Witte, J.C. and Mannon, S.E. (2010). *The Internet and social inequalities.* New York: Routledge.

Zittrain, J. (2008). *The future of the Internet and how to stop it.* New Haven, US: Yale University Press.

Notes

1 It can be argued that Marxist classical class theory was also dualistic, opposing the owners of the means of production to workers. However, Marx himself and the Marxist tradition recognize the existence of other social classes (lumpenproletariat, petit bourgeoisie, peasantry, etc.).

2 In the future the convergence of technologies will increase the need to process written information, even to manipulate a cell phone, creating an internal digital divide among users according to their literacy.

3 For instance, in a study we have done on the use of telematics by Brazilian public schools teachers we concluded that the older the teacher the more difficulties they have in adapting to the use of telematics as a teaching tool.

4 The Brazilian national institute for statistics (IBGE) is responsible for collecting data on the digital divide which is periodically elaborated in detail by the Brazilian Steering Committee. (See Brazilian Steering Committee, 2011).

5 This division is based on using as the main criteria household facilities, appliances, and level of education. For statistical reasons groups D and E were fused.

6 Seventy-five percent of users of LAN-houses declared that they had no Internet access at home.

7 See, for instance, the studies online provided by Learning Point Associates: http://www2.learningpt.org/catalog/. For a good summary of evaluations carried out through 2005 see *Critical issue: Using technology to improve student achievement.* http://www.ncrel.org/sdrs/areas/issues/methods/technlgy/te800. htm (retrieved March 6, 2011). The major studies carried out in the 1990s were summarized by John Schacter (1999). *The impact of education technology on student achievement: What the most current research has to say.* http://www.eric.ed.gov/ PDFS/ED430537.pdf (retrieved March 6, 2011). The argument that new technologies require a radical change in teaching methods in order to be effective is proposed by C. Christensen, C.W Johnson. and M.B. Horn (2008).

Disrupting class: How disruptive innovation will change the way the world learns. New York: McGraw-Hill.

8 Years ago we analyzed a publication by the World Bank of successful stories of tele-centers in developing countries. None of the experiences survived the end of support given by foreign donors to the "benchmark".

7 Digitizing Russia

The uneven pace of progress toward ICT equality

Inna F. Deviatko
National Research University
Higher School of Economics

This chapter addresses major dimensions of Internet-related inequalities in contemporary Russia including relevant regional, urban/rural, income, gender, occupation and age-related predictive variables commonly used in order to operationalize differences in socioeconomic positions of individuals and families and, correspondingly, in their access to the Internet. The analysis is based on multiple data sources – from 2007–2010 Russian Federal State Statistics Service Household Budget Survey data[1] to the Public Opinion Research Foundation (FOM) Internet Use Survey (2002–2011) and other opinion and market research agencies' data on Internet coverage among different population groups. In addition to examining causes of a gap in access to the Internet using computers and mobile phones, current policies aimed at closing the digital divide as well as prospects and possibilities of convergence between different groups of population in patterns of information technologies usage will be briefly analyzed.[2]

Talking about the various dimensions of digital divide in Russia, I will demonstrate the explanatory relevance and great theoretical promise of a neo-functionalist approach to future research of stratification in the digital sphere. As the question "Are there any social classes at all?" arises all the more insistently in the field of stratification research (Weeden and Grusky, 2005), an alternative account based on what is sometimes called "a retooled Durkheimian approach to class analysis" (Grusky and Galescu, 2005, p. 53) originating mostly from *The Division of Labor in Society* (Durkheim, 1984 [1893]) and based on tracing the differences between *gemeinschaftlich* occupational groupings looks more viable at least when it goes about explaining micro-level variability in individual attitudes, lifestyles and behaviors (Grusky and Galescu, 2005) not excluding Internet-based activities and preferences.

Inequality of possibilities and/or inequality in outcomes: A preliminary overview

By Internet access equality, we mean the idea of equal opportunities for people to use Internet-based services and information sources in their work, educational activities and during their leisure time. One has to note immediately that the researcher is generally not expecting to discover identical patterns of Internet usage including such individual-level indicators as usage time and location of a principal Internet access device, Internet navigation skills, exact amount of perused content in native and foreign languages and so on. Variables describing varying patterns of Internet use, at least analytically, pertain rather to inequalities in outcomes than to unequal possibilities and a lot of research should be done before one is able to single out "pure" effects of the initial inequality of possibilities on outcomes related to Internet use from relevant effects of varying individual preferences, abilities, occupation-determined needs and efforts, life styles and so on. Moreover, the idea of Internet equality implicitly touches upon the question of whether people have *rights* to equal opportunity of Internet access, the positive answer to which could be reasonably disputed (Cerf, 2012). In order to avoid the outlined conceptual and analytical difficulties I will discuss differences in Internet access available to subpopulations and major socio-demographic groups in Russia mostly in a descriptive way focusing primary attention on the equality of opportunities and avoiding overtly axiological judgments.

In comparative perspective, Russia currently ranks thirty-sixth on the Household Download Index from Speedtest.Net[3] which is "comparing and ranking consumer download speeds around the globe. The value is the rolling mean throughout in Mbps over the past 30 days where the mean distance between the client and the server is less than 300 miles" (Net index by Ookla, 2012).

Other possible comparative estimates include the BCG e-Intensity Index which comprises different measures of Internet activity across nations. It is computed as a weighted sum of three sub-indices: 1) *enablement* (quality of infrastructure in terms of broadband penetration and availability of access – 50 percent), 2) *expenditure* (money spent on online retail and online advertising – 25 percent), and 3) *engagement* (extent of Internet use by businesses, governments and consumers – 25 percent). The index is calculated by The Boston Consulting Group which recently published a report on Internet influence upon the Russian economy which gives a BCG e-Intensity Index value of 52 for Russia which could be compared to 53 for Brazil, 41 for China and 140 for Denmark, currently heading the BCG rating (The Boston Consulting Group, 2011, pp. 13–17).

For the third quarter of 2011, the monthly Internet audience in Russia (the number of people over 18 years old, living in Russia and going online at least once a month during the analyzed period) reached 44.98 percent – an estimate based mainly on data from the Public Opinion Research Foundation (FOM) Internet Use Survey (as cited by Russian Internet statistics service Russian Domains at: http://statdom.ru/internet#29: level=2). Internet penetration for Moscow and Saint Petersburg during the same period supposedly exceeded 69 percent. In June 2011 iKS-Consulting claimed that the penetration of broadband access to Internet in Russia for households reached 36 percent with 19 million private consumers (iKS-Consulting Agency, 2011). The household-level data on growth in possession of personal computers and PDAs from 2001 to 2009, shown in Figure 7.1, clearly demonstrate the dramatic increase in technical opportunities of getting access to the Internet, corroborating the general conclusion of the recent expansion of the Internet audience in Russia.

The picture of augmentation in Internet use in the last decade can be supplemented by data on the purposes of Internet use (Table 7.1). Predictably, purposes of "personal communication and information exchange in social networks, e-mailing relatives and friends" and "downloading movies, music, games; playing online games" are gaining a lead but "reading the news, getting information from electronic libraries, encyclopedias" is third in popularity among respondents of the Russian Federation Federal State Statistics Service household budgets survey. The evident differences in patterns of Internet use between urban and rural households emphasize the importance of the geographic dimension of digital inequality and related differences in infrastructural possibilities and living standards.

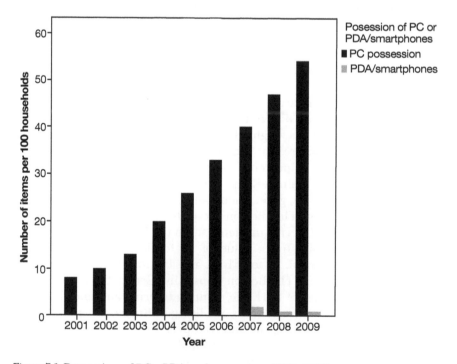

Figure 7.1 Possession of PCs, PDA and computers, 2001–2009

(Based on data from: Russian Federation Federal State Statistics Service. Central Statistical Data Base. http://www.gks.ru/dbscripts/Cbsd/DBInet.cgi)

Table 7.1 Patterns of Internet use: Percentage of urban and rural households using the Internet for different purposes in 2010

Purpose of Internet use (for all households having Internet access in a group):	*All households using the Internet* (100.0)	*Urban households* (100.0)	*Rural households* (100.0)
Finding a new job or performing paid work, mailing information	9.4	10.5	3.9
Finding information, drawing up documents, performing paperwork on and the websites of government institutions and state agencies	18.8	20.4	10.2
Searching for information on products and services, buying/ordering goods, booking services, putting up personal advertisements on sale of personal belongings or real estate	37.7	41.1	19.6
Banking online (making payments, money transfers, etc.)	12.2	13.9	3.3
Distance learning (compulsory or optional educational programs)	12.3	12.5	11.0
Reading the news, getting information from electronic libraries, encyclopedias, etc.	72.6	74.9	60.7
Personal communication and information exchange in social networks, e-mailing relatives and friends	83.5	84.3	79.4
Discussion of social and political issues, participation in Internet-based campaigns and public opinion polls, etc.	10.3	11.6	3.5
Downloading movies, music, games; playing online games, etc.	78.2	79.1	73.5
Other purposes	9.4	8.4	14.7

(*Source*: Household incomes, expenses and consumption in 2010, based on the household budgets survey of the Russian Federation Federal State Statistics Service.)

Geography matters? Regional and urban/rural differences in ICT access

Being the largest country in the world (with a total area reaching 17,098,242 sq. km) and comprising immense, sparsely populated territories with uncongenial climates (the average population density being about 8.3 people per km² as can be seen from the 2011 Federal State Statistics Service of Russian Federation data). Russia has always been a kind of challenge for major infrastructural projects. Providing equal possibilities of access to digital communications to a population dispersed over the vast territories has proved to be a difficult task (see Figure 7.2).

As data on urban and rural households having access to Internet (Tables 7.1 and 7.4) show, the differences between the general levels of Internet usage and specific activities remain strongly pronounced due to

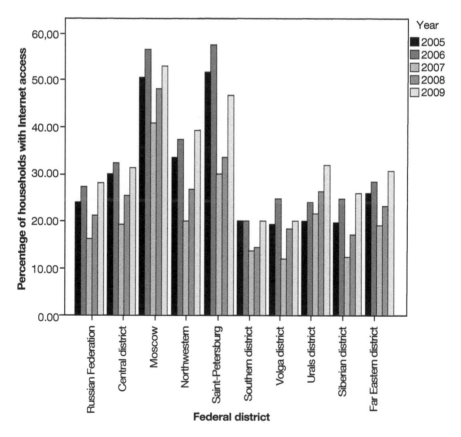

Figure 7.2 Percentage of households having Internet access by federal districts, 2005–2009

(Based on data from: Russian Federation Federal State Statistics Service, Central Data Base, household budgets survey indicators, http://www.gks.ru/dbscripts/Cbsd/D)

the higher costs of providing fixed access for rural households. However, some recent data from the FOM Internet in Russia: Penetration Dynamics. Summer 2011 survey (FOM (Public Opinion Foundation), 2011) hint at the possibility of mobile broadband access superseding the fixed access for the rural population.[4]

Table 7.2 demonstrates interregional differences in Internet coverage roughly reflecting the general population settlement patterns: the Central Federal District ranking first among major administrative regions (i.e. federal districts) in population density (57 people per km²) and third in percentage of households having Internet access; the Southern Federal District (including the North Caucasian District in 2009) being at the bottom of the list with rural population predominant in some of the North Caucasus upland regions (Dagestan, Chechnya, Ingushetia, and Karachay-Cherkessia).

Yet the influence of income on Internet access cannot be fully isolated from "purely" geographical factors like population distribution and spatial allocation of big cities and large industrial areas. Predictably, a perfect correlation is observed between average per capita monthly incomes and Internet-access levels for federal districts.[5] In a following section the influence of per capita income on Internet access is examined more thoroughly.

Table 7.2 Percentage of households having Internet access by federal districts, 2008–2009

	2008	*2009*
Central Federal District[i]	25.3	31.4
Moscow	48.2	53.0
Northwestern Federal District[ii]	26.6	39.4
Saint Petersburg	33.2	46.8
Southern Federal District (until 2009)	14.1	19.9
Volga Federal District	18.2	24.6
Urals Federal District	26.2	31.8
Siberian Federal District	17.0	25.9
Far Eastern Federal District	23.1	30.6

i Including Moscow.
ii Including Saint Petersburg.
iii HBS question: "Do your household members have access to the Internet at home?" (Yes, no).

(*Source*: Based on data from the Russian Federation Federal State Statistics Service, Central Data Base, household budgets survey indicators, http://www.gks.ru/dbscripts/Cbsd/DBInet.cgi)[iii]

Income inequalities and inequalities in Internet access: A progressive convergence?

As the Russian Federation Federal State Statistics Service data show, income remains a major influence upon the possibility of using the Internet (see Table 7.3), but a comparison between rates of households having Internet access in income deciles for years 2008 and 2010 shows some tendency for the initial gap to be bridged. Diminishing costs of getting Internet access have led to a reduction of the difference between the first and the tenth deciles from 33.1 to 24.5 percentage points. The 2010 data also shed some light on differences in purposes for using the Internet among income groups. Here we cite only *minimal* and *maximal* percentage values for using the Internet in educational and work-related purposes:

- finding a new job or performing paid work – 4.4 percent in the lowest decile and 15.9 percent in the fourth decile;
- finding information, drawing up documents, performing paperwork on the websites of government institutions and state agencies – 6.9 percent in the lowest decile and 29.8 percent in the ninth decile;
- searching for information on products and services, buying/ordering goods, booking services, putting up personal advertisements for sale of personal belongings or real estate – 25.5 percent in the sixth decile and 49.4 percent in the ninth decile;
- distance learning – 7.2 percent in the highest decile and 21.2 percent in the fourth decile.

These data defy a possibility of a straightforward Marxist interpretation of income inequality as derivative of inequality in possession of the means of production: Internet use for purposes related to production does not neatly follow the dividing lines between income groups and vice versa. Particularly, data on using the Internet for distance learning in low-income deciles as compared to the highest decile do not give direct support to the idea of alienation of lower-income groups from their work and educational prospects. Lower-income groups demonstrate the tendency to control at least some aspects of their lives and freely develop their individuality through Internet-based access to educational facilities without having to wait until the revolution "puts the conditions of free development and movement of individuals under their control" (Marx and Engels, 1970, p. 85). However, currently available data do not allow us to check a more complicated model differentiating between occupation, income, class and ways of using the Internet for production purposes (including knowledge production and human capital accrual).

Recent governmental efforts directed at promotion of wider Internet use for educational and production related purposes (through direct

Table 7.3 Internet access by income decile in 2008 and 2010 compared

Group	The lowest decile	2nd	3rd	4th	5th	6th	7th	8th	9th	The highest decile
Percentage of households having Internet access (of all households in a decile) in 2008/2010	11.3/31.0	18.2/38.9	22.1/40.6	25.6/41.7	30.1/44.6	33.5/45.5	44.7/54.1	49.3/60.8	44.6/59.1	44.4/55.5
Including:										
• from a home PC	6.0/25.5	11.0/32.2	14.6/33.8	16.7/35.8	20.3/37.2	24.6/38.8	34.7/47.2	38.8/53.3	34.1/50.9	29.8/47.2
• from an office computer	3.9/7.7	5.9/9.4	7.4/8.9	8.9/9.5	10.2/14.1	13.5/16.0	17.5/20.0	21.2/23.5	23.0/25.0	23.9/25.4
• from a place of study (school, etc.)	2.6/3.9	3.1/3.7	3.5/3.4	3.4/3.8	4.1/3.5	4.2/3.1	4.4/3.7	2.7/3.0	2.0/1.7	3.3/1.6
• from an Internet-cafe	0.6/0.2	1.2/0.7	0.7/0.7	0.9/3.1	1.1/0.4	0.9/0.3	1.0/0.4	0.7/0.2	1.0/0.2	1.3/0.0
• other	0.3/1.0	0.7/1.2	0.6/1.2	0.8/0.7	1.0/0.6	1.3/0.7	1.0/1.0	1.1/1.2	0.8/0.8	1.5/0.9

(*Source:* Based on data from the Russian Federation Federal State Statistics Service, the sample survey on households' budgets (http://www.gks.ru/free_doc/new_site/population/urov/urov_635.htm and http://www.gks.ru/bgd/regl/b10_102/IssWWW.exe/Stg/god/03-06.htm)

communication infrastructure investments and money transfers to corresponding state and municipal agencies) are epitomized in two major programs: the Digital Russia Program (2002–2010) and the Digital Government Program (from 2008 on), which succeeded it. The Russian Ministry of Information and Communications reported recently (ITAR-TASS News Agency, 2011) that the United State and Municipal Services Portal (http://www.gosuslugi.ru/ru/), launched in 2008 under the aegis of the Digital Government Program, now serves 1.3 million individual users with an average monthly increase of 100,000 newly registered clients. Besides this, the federal budget now funds the publicly available Internet connection program for primary and secondary schools which currently covers about 90 percent of Russian regions (RIA Novosti News Agency, 2010).

Gender, occupation and age-related differences in Internet access

Recent data from a TNS Web Index Report (TNS Russia, 2011) shows that a gender balance in Internet use – 51 percent males and 49 percent females – is now approaching the general proportion of females and males among Russian adults, following a period of moderate male predominance among Internet users (the later fact could be at least partly attributed to moderate male predominance among younger age groups which are better represented among Internet users).[6] Though, it should be kept in mind that the Web Index data are gathered and combined from two sources: a regular offline survey based on telephone interviews with urban dwellers aged over 12 (from cities with populations over 100,000) and an online Internet-access panel survey. The nature of the data currently defies the possibility to evaluate the statistical validity of this and other conclusions in any direct way (however TNS Russia recently advertised the creation of a supplementary "user-centric" panel which should make the task easier).

The other source of our data is the Russia Longitudinal Monitoring Survey (RLMS) which provides, in particular, high-quality individual data on Internet use. The only serious restriction on comparability of the RLMS data[7] on Internet use stems from the exact wording of questions on Internet usage, technical devices used for getting access to Internet, locations and purposes of use: relevant questions define the period of interest as "the past 12 months" (e.g., *Have you used the Internet in the past 12 months?*). Nevertheless we can use RLMS data for some comparisons with regards to the socio-demographic features of Russian Internet users. Most recent data (RLMS 19th Round, 2011, available at: http://www.hse.ru/rlms/spss) on gender composition of Internet users give a slightly different picture: among those 80 percent of adult individuals who have used the Internet in the previous 12 months, there were 45.5 percent males and 54.5 percent females. Even being mindful of the intricacies of comparing heterogeneous data, the existing empirical evidence allows us to detect the rapid closing (or even possible disappearance) of the gender digital gap in Russia, which can be compared with similar trends among American adults (Witte and Mannon, 2010, p. 27). Data on the purposes of Internet use by gender obtained from the same data source demonstrate few statistically significant differences at the 0.05 level, in particular, for using the Internet for entertainment (83.4 percent of males and 74.1 percent of females who used the Internet answered positively) and work (41 percent of males and 47 percent of females) – a fact which purportedly reflects some remaining gender role-specific differences in occupational structure and leisure time.

The TNS Web Index Report (TNS Russia, 2011) gives some clue as to the occupational structure of the Internet audience in Russia: approximately 13 percent were managers, 28 percent were professionals (including specialists and white-collar workers), 20 percent were students, 17 percent were workers, 8 percent were housewives and 14 percent were under the unspecified label "others" among Russian Internet users in November, 2011. RLMS data for 2011 provide a more detailed, though somewhat discrepant, picture of shares of major occupational groups

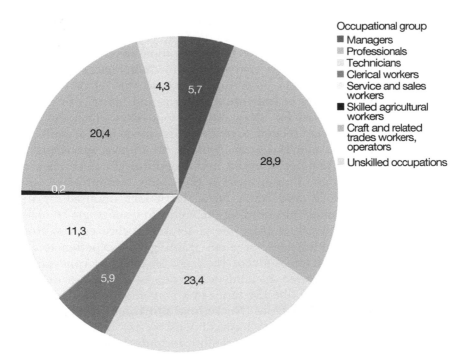

Figure 7.3 Major occupational groups in yearly Internet audience (% of all respondents who used Internet during the past 12 months) (Based on: RLMS, 2011)

among the general yearly Internet audience in Russia, as shown in Figure 7.3. Professionals and technicians account for 28.9 percent and 23.4 percent respectively among Internet users[8] which harmonizes well with a functionalist vision of Internet use intensity in professions based on expert knowledge but skilled industrial, construction and technical workers and machine operators now also form a considerable share of the Internet audience.[9]

Different age groups are represented unequally among Russian Internet users. Younger groups (especially those between 16 and 35) are much more active in using the Internet and, generally, people of productive age are more active than the elderly (Tables 7.4 and 7.5). This gap is narrowing rather slowly following a path similar to the one observed among American adults (Witte and Mannon, 2010, pp. 28–29) though recent data from FOM Internet penetration research reveals a 10 percent share of Internet users for Russian adults aged over 55 (FOM (Public Opinion Foundation), 2011) which doubles the 2009 estimates (Table 7.4).

General discussion and some conclusions

It is now slightly more than a decade since P. DiMaggio and E. Hargittai called for "an expanded paradigm" to describe new digital inequalities typical for the epoch of rising Internet penetration level (DiMaggio and Hargittai, 2001, p. 4). But perplexing methodological problems immediately arise when one is trying to expand the list of variables predicting the subtleties of individual patterns and benefits of use by simply adding indicators for inequalities of outcomes which describe individual-level Internet-related activities (like inequality of skills or purposes (DiMaggio and Hargittai, 2001, p. 8)) without specifying *ab origin* major dimensions of unequal initial opportunities like class or occupational structure. This strategy is potentially overburdened with explanatory circularity and often faces restrictions imposed by the nature of data available, thus limiting the ability to disentangle complex effects of "true" inequalities (like intergenerational class effects) from effects caused by preferences, previous training and experience, etc. Unfortunately, the current state of the basic sociological concepts of class and status (when even an analytical review of recent research on inequality prefers to describe the latter in a non-antagonistic language of observed economic disparities (Neckerman and Torche, 2007)) makes the task of revealing the most basic dimensions of "true" inequality rather formidable.[10] It becomes even more formidable in the effort of interpreting consequences for stratification systems and attendant new inequalities (or even equalities) in education, work and leisure of those rapid and massive social and economic transformations which have been taking place in post-Soviet societies since the late 1980s.

Table 7.4 Age-related differences in regular Internet access for rural and urban households (percentage of the total number of household members in a relevant age group, for age groups under 74)

| | All Households | | Households: | | | |
| | | | Urban | | Rural | |
	2008	2009	2008	2009	2008	2009
Regular users ratio for household members under 74	16.0	22.6	19.9	27.5	5.1	9.6
Regular users ratio for household members by age groups:						
Under 16	10.2	16.0	12.7	18.7	4.4	9.4
16 – 35	28.7	38.2	35.2	45.5	8.8	16.8
36 – 55	13.2	20.5	16.6	25.6	4.3	7.5
56 – 74	2.4	4.2	3.0	5.5	0.7	0.5

(*Source*: Households incomes, expenses and consumption in 2009, based on the household budgets sample survey of the Russian Federation Federal State Statistics Service.)

Table 7.5 Age-related differences in occasional Internet access for rural and urban households (percentage of the total number of household members in a relevant age group, for age groups under 74)

| | All Households | | Households: | | | |
| | | | Urban | | Rural | |
	2008	2009	2008	2009	2008	2009
Occasional users ratio for household members under 74	5.6	6.2	6.6	7.2	2.9	3.5
Occasional users ratio for household members by age groups:						
Under 16	2.9	3.2	3.3	3.8	1.9	1.6
16 – 35	6.8	6.1	7.3	6.5	5.1	4.9
36 – 55	7.5	9.4	9.3	11.3	2.7	4.3
56 – 74	1.9	2.7	2.4	3.3	0.5	1.0

(*Source*: Households incomes, expenses and consumption in 2009, based on the household budgets sample survey of the Russian Federation Federal State Statistics Service)

The validity of generalizations one may find in authoritative sources on digital inequalities – e.g., "In today's information-based economy, Internet access and use can be understood as an asset used to maintain class privilege and power" (Witte and Mannon, 2010, p. 81) – is to a considerable degree threatened by social scientists' inability to define "big classes" otherwise than through differences in income, wealth and, to a degree, education, all of which could be treated as effect-indicators of class affiliation in any cogent interpretation of a Marxist imagination of class, defining classes strictly in terms of their relationship to the means of economic production (not just wealth or "assets" treated too loosely by some New Left theorists who forget that what can count as an asset depends on what kind of person is granted this asset).

Available data on gender, occupation and income related differences in Internet use among Russian adults do not provide decisive evidential support to theoretical visions of Internet inequalities inspired either by Marx or by Weber. The basic conclusion of a prevailing importance of household income in predicting inequalities in rates of access to the Internet is compatible with both accounts, although it was demonstrated that data on using the Internet for purposes related to production does not follow neatly the division lines between income groups – a fact which could be considered as undermining the possibility of the straight-line Marxist interpretation. However, whatever the deepest reasons for income disparities are, the data obtained show some tendency for convergence in rates of access for different income groups which could be attributed both to recent trends in diminishing income inequalities among Russian households and to diminishing costs for Internet access due to the concerted yet unintentional action of recent technological changes and market forces. The geographic dimension of inequality turned out to be equally important with the effects of technological constraints, economic underdevelopment, population distribution and regional average incomes resisting disentanglement in the survey data currently available.

The revealed influence of occupational structure on Internet inequality gives some distinct (but not yet definitive and consistent) evidence supporting the leading positions of professionals and white-collar workers among Russian adult Internet users. This conclusion may give a second breath to the least articulated and underestimated version of stratification theorizing in sociology dating back to Durkheim and promoted in Parsons' writing on modern professions and occupational groupings (Parsons, 1940; 1971). As already noted at the beginning of this chapter a kind of neo-Durkheimian approach to analysis of *gemeinschaftlich* "micro-classes" (Grusky and Galescu, 2005) could be helpful for explaining sources of observed differences in the occupational structure of the Internet audience in Russia. Our data on differences in Internet use intensity between professionals, technicians and the rest can be accounted for by work-based distinctions stemming, in the final analysis, from the technical division of labor and coming into being at the disaggregate level through the processes of occupational self-selection, repeated social interactions among co-workers, explicit professional training and socialization, etc. (Grusky and Galescu, 2005).

It goes without saying that more substantive evidence in support of all these preliminary conclusions depends on both elucidation of our theoretical formulations of deeper causes of inequality and methodological progress in empirical research on qualitative and quantitative disparities in Internet access in Russia.

References

Cerf, V. (2012, January 4). Internet access is not a human right. *The New York Times*, p. A25.

DiMaggio, P. and Hargittai, E. (2001, Summer). From the 'digital divide' to 'digital inequality'. *Princeton University Center for Arts and Cultural Policy Studies Working Paper Series* (#15).

Durkheim, E. (1984 [1893]). *The division of labor in society.* New York: The Free Press.

Federal State Statistics Service of Russian Federation. (2011). *The modern demographic situation in Russia: An analytical report.* Retrieved from http://www.gks.ru/wps/wcm/connect/rosstat/rosstatsite/main/population/demography/.

FOM (Public Opinion Foundation). (2011). *Internet in Russia: Peneration dynamics.* Moscow. Retrieved from http://corp.fom.ru/projects/23.html#1.

Grusky, D. and Galescu, G. (2005). Foundations of a neo-Durkheimian class analysis. In E.O. Wright (Ed.), *Approaches to class analysis* (pp. 51–81). Cambridge, UK: Cambridge University Press.

iKS-Consulting Agency. (2011, July 6). The Big Four consolidate the market (in Russian: «Большая четверка» консолидирует рынок). Retrieved from http://www.iks-consulting.ru/topics/thematic/wideband_access/3844317.html.

ITAR-TASS News Agency. (2011, December 20). *News of Ministry of Information and Communications.*

Marx, K. and Engels, F. (1970). *The German ideology.* C. Arthur, (Ed.) New York: International Publishers, Co.

Neckerman, K. M. and Torche, F. (2007). Inequality: Causes and consequences. *Annu. Rev. Sociol., 33*, 335–57.

Net index by Ookla, 2012. Retrieved 8 january, 2012 from http://www.netindex.com/download

Nisbet, R. A. (1967). *The sociological tradition.* London: Heinemann.

Parsons, T. (1940, May). An analytical approach to the theory of social stratifications. *The American Journal of Sociology, XLV*(6), 841–862.

Parsons, T. (1971). *The system of modern societies.* Englewood Cliffs, New Jersey, US: Prentice-Hall.

RIA Novosti News Agency. (2010, May 31). President Medvedev demands Internet access for 100% of Russian schools. *RIA Novosti.*

Rosstat (Russian Federal State Statistics Service). (2010). *The Demographic Yearbook of Russia.* Moscow: Rosstat.

The Boston Consulting Group. (2011). *Russia online: How Internet is transforming the Russian economy.* Moscow: The Boston Consulting Group, Inc.

TNS Russia. (2011). *TNS Web Index Report*. Moscow. Retrieved from http://www.tns-global.ru/rus/data/ratings/index/.

Weeden, K. A. and Grusky, D. (2005). Are there any big classes at all? In D. Bills (ed.), *The shape of social inequality: Stratification and ethnicity in comparative perspective* (Vol. 22. Research in Social Stratification and Mibility, pp. 3–56). Amsterdam: Elsevier.

Witte, J. C. and Mannon, S. E. (2010). *The Internet and social inequalities*. New York and London: Routledge.

Notes

1 The sample survey on households' budgets has been conducted in all regions of the Russian Federation since 1997 and covers 47.8 thousand households. The returns of the survey are compiled quarterly and for a year as a whole.

2 It should be stated in advance that different Internet-related data sources used in this chapter are sometimes not in complete agreement with each other and in some cases look inconsistent even within themselves (for example, even a cursory glance at data on households' access to the Internet by federal districts in Figure 7.2 based on our most reliable statistical source – Russian Federation State Statistics Service databases – discovers enigmatic yet order-preserving slumps in 2007 and 2008 access rates which can be attributed both to possible methodological changes in exact question wordings and changing definitions of Internet-access regularity). The reasons for these and other discrepancies vary widely and cannot always be easily pinpointed to a specific source like a lack of commonly used methodological conventions in the field of conceptualization and measurement of variables related to digital communications and public and private usage of information technologies. Although detailed discussion of existing threats to reliability and validity of ICT-equality related data lies beyond the scope of this chapter, special attention to any variations and differences in data collection techniques and available estimates will be paid whenever multiple data sources are used.

3 The current value of the Household Download Index for Russia (11.61 Mbps) is calculated for data obtained between December 8, 2011 and January 6, 2012 http(http://www.netindex.com/download/, access date – January 8, 2012).

4 Numerical estimates based on this FOM survey should be treated with caution and compared to other data sources. Consider, for example, the following overblown estimate that 31 percent of the rural population aged over 18 has mobile access (e.g., http://raec.ru/upload/files/pages-from-in-numbers8_1.pdf).

5 Pearson's r=0,995 for 2008 year data, $p < 0.01$ (and r=0.812 for 2009 year data is also significant at the 0.01 level).

6 *The Demographic Yearbook of Russia, 2010* (Rosstat (Russian Federal State Statistics Service), 2010) gives 45.3 percent (53928245) for males and 54.7 percent (65131870) for females aged over 16 in the general population (as could be calculated from Table 1.10 data) with female predominance *only* for age groups over 55 and male predominance in younger age groups.

7 Source: Russia Longitudinal Monitoring Survey, RLMS-HSE, conducted by the National Research University Higher School of Economics and ZAO "Demoscope" together with Carolina Population Center, University of North Carolina at Chapel Hill, and the Institute of Sociology RAS.

8 $p < 0.01$.

9 Among those RLMS 19th Round respondents who were currently employed (N=7792), 4.4 percent were managers, 19.2 percent were professionals, 17.9

percent were technicians, 5.4 percent were clerks, 13.1 percent were service and sales workers, 0.4 percent were skilled agricultural and fishery workers, 28 percent were craft and related trades workers and machine operators, and 11.7 percent were unskilled workers.

10 The shrewd comment formulated by R. Nisbet in the late 1960s remains relevant for the significant part of sociological research in the field of stratification and inequality: "Only after the historic and essential bases of social class in European society had become tenuous and uncertain, had become threatened by forces such as political centralization, citizenship and mass education – forces which would, in the long run, make class the weakest of all traditional social unities under the modern regime – did the study of social stratification burst forth in full brilliance" (Nisbet, 1967, p. 174).

8 The digital divide in India

Inferences from the information and communication technology workforce

P. Vigneswara Ilavarasan
Indian Institute of Technology Delhi

The present chapter examines the digital divide in India using the case of the workforce in the information and communication technology (ICT) industry. It studies the digital divide in access and use of the Internet using a social inequality lens. Social inequality can be explained in multiple ways. The conflict perspective, which originated from Karl Marx, argues that the society is in a continuous friction between two groups over resources. The dominant group in terms of ownership of resources will tend to suppress the other group in order to maintain the status quo over the resources through all possible ways. The institutions in the society will be manipulated to maintain the dominance in a perpetual manner thus resulting in overall social inequality. The other suppressed group explores breaking this dominance with consequent reactions resulting in conflicts. The conflict will be constant, but the nature and form of resources will change. The resources rooted in economic capital can also morph into other forms of capital, like cultural or social (Bourdieu, 1986).

According to the conflict perspective, the ownership of and access to the Internet will also be part of the resources. The dominant class or group will have better ownership of and access to the Internet than the others. The paths to acquire the resources, computer ownership, expertise to use the Internet and the forms of content of the Internet, for example English language, will be controlled by the dominant class to block the entry of the other classes.

The cultural perspective has its origins in the works of Max Weber and deviates from the conflict perspective by bringing forth the importance of "status" in explaining social inequality. The status denotes a distinct set of lifestyles and world views. The individuals come together through a collective understanding of and adherence to lifestyles to form status groups or define status positions. The family background and occupational group are two important factors in deciding ones' status position (Witte and Mannon, 2010). Though there is a possibility of better economic positions conferring higher statuses, not all trajectories are linear. In other words, not all high paying jobs result in higher prestige.

The cultural perspective approaches the Internet as a part of the lifestyle or distinct culture of a restricted group used to differentiate it from others.

Unlike in the US, data on access and use of the Internet across various social groups are unavailable in India for social science research. The extant data on Internet use from the private agencies offers little insights on how various social groups are faring in the digital space. Given these limitations, an occupational group, the workforce in the ICT industry, is examined to understand the digital divide in India. This examination is carried out within the frameworks of two sociological perspectives: cultural and conflict.

This chapter is in five sections. The first section discusses the available statistics on ICTs in India. The second section links the idea of the digital divide and the ICT workforce in the light of sociological discourse. The third section discusses the presence of the digital divide in the ICT workforce. The fourth section seeks to explain the exclusion process that resulted in the digital divide. The fifth section concludes the chapter.

India and ICTs

India is comprised of 28 states and 7 territories and is the largest democracy in the world with 1.2 billion people. It is one of the fastest growing economies in the world and has been adopting liberalization policies since the early 1990s. Despite the fact that the Indian ICT industry is one of the favored destinations for software and business process outsourcing in the world, the ICT infrastructure in India is relatively unimpressive. In a measurement of electronic government by the United Nations (UN, 2010) using an index of three components (online service, telecom infrastructure, and human capital), India was ranked 119 out of 183 countries in the world, inferring weak ICT infrastructure in the country. Out of a wide range of ICTs, mobile phones are predominantly used, but high value functions like mobile Internet penetration or 3G services are still in nascent stages.

In 2011, there were around 771 million wireless phone subscribers. Mobile tele-density is 65 percent for the country with relatively poor tele-density in rural locations (31 percent) when compared to urban locations (143 percent). Internet penetration is low with only 11.21 million broadband subscribers as of 31 Jan 2011 (GoI, 2011). A private research study estimated that mobile Internet usage was 2 million in 2009 (IAMAI, 2009). Rough estimates (IAMAI, 2011) show that the number of cybercafés in India exceeds 10, 000, with these most likely to be located in urban locations. Twenty-four percent of the households use the Internet. These details suggest the urban bias in ICT access in the country.

The extant large scale data on ICTs in India does not permit disaggregated analysis with respect to any social groups and the Internet. The Indian government recognizes the lacuna in the statistical framework and is making efforts to include ICT indicators (OECD, 2007). Given the low penetration of the Internet, there is a possibility that access to the Internet is present only among the privileged groups. Maplecroft (2011) warns that the digital divide in India is severe when compared to other BRIC countries and "most [people] cannot afford ICTs (only 3 percent of households own PCs), lack the education required to use it effectively (India has secondary school enrolment rates of 55 percent and adult literacy rates of just under 63 percent) and are located in geographical areas that have little or no connectivity to ICT services" (Maplecroft.com, 2011, para. 6).

State-level data (GoI, 2012) show that out of 19.7 million Internet subscribers as of December 2011, 19.6 percent are located in Maharashtra, 11 percent are in Tamil Nadu, 9.8 percent are in Delhi, and 8.6 percent are in Karnataka clearly indicating the dominance of developed states in accessing the Internet.

The Indian government is making significant efforts to enhance the overall ICT infrastructure through the National E-governance Plan (for details see DIT, 2011). As a part of this plan, Common Service Centers (CSCs), a variant of the tele-center model, are being established across the country (for details see, http://www.csc-india.org). One CSC in each eight villages will connect all citizens to all public and private services, including the Internet. If this is successful, all citizens will have access to the Internet through the more than 100,000 planned CSCs, thus bridging the digital divide. Currently, there are no studies that directly examine the usage of CSCs by disadvantaged groups. However, studies on tele-centers in the pre-CSC period show that social inequalities are reflected in these initiatives.

The digital divide in India

The social stratification in India is predominantly caste based. The constitution of India classifies the citizens into four categories: scheduled castes (SCs), scheduled tribes (STs), other backward classes (OBCs) and the open category (OC). SCs are depressed classes, and were untouchables in the traditional India. STs are the indigenous people. OBCs are people who have lower social, economic and educational statuses, but better statuses than those of the SCs and STs. The OC includes the rest of the people. This categorization implies that the OC members are from an upper caste/upper class, and have relatively better educational positions in society. Similarly, persons belong to SC/ST categories come from a lower caste/lower class, typically have poor educational backgrounds, and are considered as the disadvantaged groups in India.

The classification of people forms the basis for most of the policy measures in the country. As per the 2001 Census, the literacy rate of SCs and STs was 54.7 percent and 47 percent, respectively, compared to the national level of 64.8 percent. In the public employment and education systems 15 percent, 7.5 percent and 27 percent are reserved for SCs, STs and OBCs, respectively. Despite the reservations, SC/STs and OBCs are underrepresented in the areas of education and employment, with SCs and STs lagging notably behind OBCs (for details see Deshpande, 2006; Mohanty, 2006). This chapter will make an attempt to capture the presence of SC/STs in the digital space in India.

In a study of 132 tele-centers in South India (Kumar and Best, 2006), it was found that usage by SC/STs is relatively lower and locating tele-centers in SC/STs neighborhoods appears to be an important factor in increasing the usage. Their study also pointed out that Internet usage is significantly related to higher literacy, economic status, and youth. Another study on use (Thomas, 2006) found similar trends and reinforced the point that "people's capabilities to use ICTs are associated with the existing level of socio-economic development" (p.130). These findings suggested that policy initiatives might result only in "theoretical access" and not in the "effective access" by which the individual feels able to access (Selwyn, 2004).

The poor or limited access or use of ICTs by SC/STs can be explained through two theoretical perspectives: conflict and cultural. Similar approaches were used by Witte and Mannon (2010) to explain the inequalities in access and use of the Internet in the US Through a review of conflict theories, the authors argue that unequal access to ICTs, especially the Internet, by disadvantaged groups is the result of lower class background conferred by lower parental education, employment status, and family income. This uneven access and use between the ruling (and elite) classes and the ruled (or working) strata will reproduce the class positions of the respective parties, thus maintaining the ongoing social inequality. The ruling capitalists sustain their dominance by keeping the class assets as an advantage in the production process. The class assets include skills to access and use ICTs.

A cultural perspective adds cultural factors to the economic status to explain the inequalities. The elite reinforces its dominant status and the inequalities by its lifestyle and consumption patterns which include things like "membership of the right club, living in the right neighborhood, and being invited to the right parties" (Witte and Mannon, 2010, p.86). The nature of occupations and families are important in determining the nature of access and use of ICTs which in turn determine or maintain the prestige status of the dominant class. The dominant class will be homogeneously situated in positions that access the resources including ICTs. Witte and Mannon (2010) showed that people with better educational and occupational prestige, typically in managerial/professional occupations, perform high-skilled Internet activities, product searching, or online banking and are most likely to use the Internet at work, as compared to low-skilled Internet activities such as emailing or reading blogs, typical of the lower educational and occupational categories.

Given this, in simple words, SC/STs are less likely use CSCs, as they did not have access to ICTs earlier and their children study in schools where there is limited or no access to ICTs. Also, as most of the SC/STs are either landless laborers or hold low level public office positions (Mohanty, 2006), even when they use CSCs, the nature of their activities are most likely to be low-skilled like seeking entitlements such as caste certificates or certifications of poverty status, rather than other high value added services.

This chapter examines the digital divide in India by studying one aspect, SC/STs in the ICT workforce. This is a slight deviation from the existing literature on the digital divide that tends to focus predominantly on access and use of ICTs by the individuals or groups. Earlier, DiMaggio *et al.* (2001) indicated that "few sociologists have examined the Internet's institutional structure, industrial organization, or political economy" (p.329). A study of representations of disadvantaged or minority groups in ICT occupations makes an appropriate site for understanding the digital divide for four reasons. First, on the theoretical level, occupational groups are status groups where use of ICTs is part of lifestyle and might be erecting barriers to the entry of minority groups to maintain the class privileges. An understanding of the composition of the occupational group provides insights into the manifestation of the digital divide. Also, Sassen (2002) argues that digital technologies cannot be studied in isolation and the "digital space is embedded in the larger societal, cultural, subjective, economic, imaginary structurations of lived experience and the systems within which we exist and operate" (pp. 368–369). Second, there is a paucity of large scale data on access and use of ICTs by citizens (OECD, 2007), thus preventing any disaggregated analysis with respect to SC/STs. For instance, IAMAI (2011) has collected data from 19,000 households, 68,000 individuals, 1000 Small and Medium Enterprises, and 500 cybercafés, but does not provide any data on the social categories. Third, ICT occupations directly use, and sometimes produce, the Internet at work thus making them the frontrunners in cyberspace. The attempts to measure "ICT for development" by the international agencies use the size of the ICT workforce as one of the core ICT indicators (see for instance, ITU, 2010). The non-representation of SC/STs will support the case for the digital divide. Fourth, the ICT industry in India is treated "as the most consistent growth driver for the economy" (MIT, 2011) and public policy initiatives aggressively support the industry. It is also important to understand whether this sector is digitally inclusive.

The Indian ICT industry is one of the growing parts of the Indian economy, having grown from US$ 21.6 billion in 2004 to US$ 73.1 billion in 2010 (NASSCOM, 2011). It contributes 6.1 percent to the GDP and was estimated to be employing 2.3 million people directly and 8.2 million indirectly in 2010. The industry is predominantly an exporter of IT and business process services, which together account for 69 percent of the total revenue in the industry. A trade press report aptly summarized the status of ICT workers in India:

> [the ICT sector] started emerging as a role model for the country. IT professionals in India were one of the highest paid, on average, IT was the most sought after area at campus recruitments...IT had the highest number of people to be nominated for civilian honors by the nation. IT leaders and news hogged the limelight in the media for the right and sometimes wrong reasons. IT was the biggest employment generator in the country. It was IT professionals who were travelling the most into and out of the country. IT captains were bagging global awards in business excellence. And as a marriage bureau said, "IT grooms and brides command the highest premium today, after doctors and IAS [Indian Administrative Services] officers" (Dataquest, 2006, p. 16).

The digital divide and the ICT workforce

Researchers of the Indian ICT industry, especially on labor or workforce issues, face serious hurdles as disaggregated data on the composition of the ICT workforce are not available (Ilavarasan, 2008). The industry itself is not open for independent researchers as the ICT companies are bound by the non-disclosure agreements signed with their respective clients. Given this limitation, this chapter is dependent on the author's prior studies and other published studies/secondary data.

Existing small scale survey based studies repeatedly report that participation of SC/STs is either low or absent. In Ilavarasan's (2007) study of 114 ICT workers, there were no SC/STs. This sample corresponded with the industry average on education, gender, years of experience and average age of the workforce. Oommen and Sundararajan (2005) also did not find a single SC/ST worker in their sample of 100, and out of 132 people surveyed there was only one SC/ST in Upadhya and Vasavi's study (2006). Though all these studies had modest samples, the findings are similar. The next social category, OBCs are entering the ICT sector, but in much lower numbers than their representation in the population as a whole would suggest, ranging from ten percent (Ilavarasan, 2007) to 20 percent (Oommen and Sundararajan, 2005).

In addition to non-participation of SC/STs, there are other similar characteristics emerging from the review of existing studies. Regarding parental educational levels, Upadhya and Vasavi (2006) reported that "80 percent of respondents' fathers were graduates or above, and only three respondents had fathers with less than SSLC [Grade ten] level education" (p.37).

In Oommen and Sundararajan's (2005) survey there was only one father without a school diploma, while Krishna and Brihmadesam's (2006) study had 82 percent of the fathers having a bachelor's degree or more, but none had education levels below high school. Accordingly, the occupational status of fathers followed a similar pattern: most of them were either in middle or higher public services, professionals, or businessmen. None of the studies reported a father being a landless laborer or in an occupation from a lower socio-economic category.

All the studies uniformly found that there was a predominance of urban backgrounds among the ICT workers. In Ilavarasan's (2007) study, only 18 percent said that they were from rural places. Similarly, only 12 percent of respondents came from rural locations in Oommen and Sundararajan's (2005) study and slightly more in Krishna and Brihmadesam's (2006) study. It was reported as only 5 percent in an ethnographic study (Upadhya and Vasavi, 2006).

The studies also showed that Hinduism was the dominant religion among the ICT workers in India. Hindus formed 88 percent in Upadhya and Vasavi's (2006) sample. It was 95 percent in Ilavarasan's (2007) study and 74 percent in Oommen and Sundararajan's (2005) survey. Earlier research showed that Muslims, who form 13.4 percent of the population, can be compared on a par with the SC/ST in terms of participation in education and employment (Basant, 2007). Thus, the nature of the ICT workforce can be summarized as follows: a "typical software worker in India ...hails from an urban and a semi-urban locality; follows Hinduism, and belongs to upper socio-economic strata of the Indian society" (Ilavarasan, 2007, p. 818).

Though the existing studies did not have a detailed presentation of the caste breakdown of the samples, they indicated the dominance of Brahmins, a caste of priests and teachers that traditionally occupies the higher order of social stratification in India. Fuller and Narasimhan (2008) reasoned that Brahmins would be dominant in the Chennai ICT cluster as they were among those who were the first to receive Western education before migrating to urban locations. Earlier, Saxenian (2002) cited return migration of Indians to start new IT ventures in India as one of the reasons for the birth and growth of the Indian ICT industry. Taeube (2004) analyzed the names of the interviewees of all major studies and argued that "the majority of the key people in the Indian software industry are located in South India, are Brahmins, and come from a South Indian background in terms of ethnicity or family affiliation" (p. 219).

The process of exclusion

This section will explain the process by which SC/STs are thwarted from entering the ICT workforce. The first part of this exclusion process is the need for an undergraduate degree in engineering or a master's degree in sciences. The abundant availability of engineers during the nascent stages of the sector, the introduction of programs like master's degrees in computer application and efforts to meet the American visa requirements for onsite work have resulted in this pattern (Sharma, 2009). There is direct linkage between the basic training imparted via a college education and the skill sets required for ICT jobs. In India, the majority of the ICT workers have engineering degrees in all possible disciplines, which include textiles, mining and civil, but not necessarily in computer science, software engineering, or ICT. Unlike their Western counterparts, college dropouts would not be able to find a job in the ICT industry in India due to specific hiring practices. The samples of the existing studies clearly support this observation. For instance, Oommen and Sundararajan (2005) and Ilavarasan (2007) do not show a single worker with only high school qualifications or bachelor's degrees in arts and humanities disciplines.

The supply of SC/STs graduate engineers seems to be lagging when compared to the other groups. For instance, the urban SC/STs, who are more likely to be educated than their rural counterparts, have a lower number of engineering graduates (3.4 percent), when compared to their share in the total population, (14.5 percent in 1999–2000). These figures are strikingly lower than the urban Hindu upper castes that comprise 36.9 percent of the population but form 66.8 percent of the engineers (Deshpande, 2006). High school completion, a necessary condition to enter colleges, is low among SC/STs. Hasan and Mehta (2006) reinforced the point that SC/STs are underrepresented in college education. They showed that among urban males aged 17 to 30, only 7.89 percent of SCs and 2.69 percent of STs completed a high school education. As the high school graduation rate is low for these groups, the presence of SC/STs in engineering colleges is limited. The enrollment of SC/STs in disciplines that are directly related to the ICT sector and in the national elite institutions of science and technology are "at best negligible" (Rao, 2006, p.220). A study (Varma and Kapur, 2010) of undergraduate engineering students at Indian Institutes of Technology (IITs), one of the top global schools for engineering education, showed that the "IITs have been catering to predominantly Hindu students from upper and middle castes and classes" (p.715). The aspiring students of IITs take private coaching or tutoring classes to clear the entrance examination which are not affordable to poor students. The cost of tutoring is around INR 100000 (US$ 2000) per annum which is high for a country where more than half the population is living on below US$2 per day.

A second filter in the exclusion process is the entrance exam conducted by ICT firms. The firms hire people directly either at college premises or at private venues. A fresh entrant needs to have a minimum of 70 percent grades in high school, higher secondary, and bachelor's degree education to appear for an entrance exam (Ilavarasan, 2007; Upadhya and Vasavi, 2006). This criterion is strictly enforced for the entry-level positions to reduce the number of people to be called for the next round of recruitment process. The sample of Oommen and Sundararajan (2005) showed only one worker with 60 to 70 percent marks. An SC/ST student who has secured admission to the engineering college due to reservation policies, but who performs below 70 percent during schooling will be unable to compete in the open recruitment process.

Third, the personal interviews conducted as part of the recruitment process serve as a major barrier (Upadhya, 2007). Though some top firms give one-year jobs directly to the successful candidates based on the written tests, conducting two rounds of face-to-face interviews, technical and human resources, is common. Even after assuming that a SC/ST candidate has scored the required 70 percent in school and college, he or she is likely to fail in the interviews. As the Indian ICT sector is catering to the export market, spoken English and good communication skills are expected. During the interview process, candidates are tested on the traits of social skills which favor those from more affluent socio-economic backgrounds who had access to good educational systems (Upadhya and Vasavi, 2006). An analysis of online advertisements for entry-level ICT workers showed that social skill traits like personality, teamwork, and communication skills are identified for possible hiring criteria (Malish and Ilavarasan, 2011). A recent study shows that SC engineering students do recognize this shortcoming and start to explore the public jobs where there is relaxation of marks and no personal interviews (Malish, 2011). Any attempt to introduce reservation policies in the private sector or the ICT sector is met with stiff resistance from the industry (see for instance, Rediff, 2003).

Employee referral programs in ICT firms work as the fourth barrier. It involves an existing worker referring an external candidate for the vacancy and getting an incentive on the successful placement of the candidate (Ghosh and Geetika, 2007). A trade publication reports that the percentage of people hired through this process ranges from 48 to 60 percent (HR World, 2008; Singh, 2004). This process will also typically exclude the SC/STs from ICT employment. Given the dominance of non-SC/STs in this sector, the social networks of the current workforce will prioritize the non-SC/STs. As the workers tend to maximize their opportunities to earn incentives, the chances of SC/STs entering ICT employment via referral would be minimal.

Conclusion

The existing discourses on the digital divide focus on the ownership and consumption of the Internet (Witte and Mannon, 2010). This chapter analyzed the level of participation of disadvantaged groups, specifically SC/STs, in the ICT workforce in India, and concludes that the digital divide prevails.

The exclusion process observed in the ICT industry is a manifestation of social inequalities and the continuation of class privileges. The strategies used by the elite class to maintain the status quo in this emerging sector is a combination of forms of cultural capital – educational qualifications, personality traits, and social networks. These strategies are not completely driven by the market as the industry is moving from *onsite*, where subcontracted work is performed on clients' sites, to *offshore*, where subcontracted work happens in India. Such a recruitment process applies often to non-engineering graduates as well. Currently, the top ICT firms are hiring basic science graduates and training them for the international global production of software (for instance, Chandran, 2011). There is a possibility of disadvantaged groups entering this sector, but they need to negotiate the cultural capital barriers.

The ICT sector enjoys a considerable amount of government support in terms of provision of high-skilled manpower, fiscal incentives, and infrastructure (Balakrishnan, 2006). Recent government initiatives to increase the ready-made talent pool available for the ICT sector through the establishment of 20 more Indian Institutes of Information Technology (IIITs) with private industry support (Livemint, 2011) or through permitting private universities to offer programs in ICT-related areas will increase the existing gap as the cost of education is high when compared to the public institutes.

The findings from the Indian ICT industry are not different from other countries. For instance, in the US women and minorities are underrepresented in computing education and the industry (Simrad, 2009; Varma, 2009). As the production of ICTs are dominated by the dominant class, the resultant outcomes including the Internet will lack the creativity brought by diversity and will eventually perpetuate the digital divide present in the consumption of ICTs. It appears that significant shifts in thinking are required from both government and industry before inroads can be made toward bridging the digital divide in the production space of ICTs.

References

Balakrishnan, P. (2006). Benign neglect or strategic intent? Contested lineage of Indian software industry. *Economic and Political Weekly*, 41(36), 3865–3873.
Basant, R. (2007). Social, economic and educational conditions of Indian Muslims. *Economic and Political Weekly*, 42(10), 828–832.
Bourdieu, P. (1986). The forms of capital. In J. Richardson (ed.) *Handbook of theory and research for the sociology of education*. New York: Greenwood, 241–258.
Chandran, P. (2011). IT firms hire non-engineering graduates to cut cost. *Business Standard*, 4 March. Retrieved from http://business-standard.com/india/news/it-firms-hire-non-engineering-graduates-to-cut-cost/427271/ on 10 June 2011.
Dataquest. (2006). Raising the bar. *Dataquest*, 24(13).
Deshpande, S. (2006). Exclusive inequalities: Merit, caste and discrimination in Indian higher education today. *Economic and Political Weekly*, 41(24), 2438–2444.

DiMaggio, P.J., Hargittai, E., Neuman, W.R. and Robinson, J. (2001). Social implications of the Internet. *Annual Review of Sociology.* 27, 307–336.

DIT. (2011). *India: Journey from knowledge economy to inclusive information society.* New Delhi: Department of Information Technology, Government of India.

Fuller, C.J. and Narasimhan, H. (2008). From landlords to software engineers: Migration and urbanization among Tamil Brahmans. *Comparative Studies in Society and History,* 50(1), 170–196.

Ghosh, P. and Geetika. (2007). Recruitment strategies: Exploring the dimensions in the Indian software industry. *Asian Journal of Management Cases,* 4(1), 5–25.

GoI. (2011). *Draft consultation paper on mobile governance policy framework.* New Delhi: Department of Information Technology, Government of India.

GoI. (2012). State-wise number of broadband and Internet subscribers in India. Lok Sabha unstarred question No 425, dated 14 March 2012.

Hasan, R. and Mehta, A. (2006). Under-representation of disadvantaged classes in colleges: What do the data tell us? *Economic and Political Weekly,* 41(35), 3791–3796.

HR World. (2008). Employee referral bonus jackpots: 15 companies with awesome new-hire incentives. www.hrworld.com. Retrieved from http://www.hrworld.com/features/referral-bonus-jackpot-031108/ on 10 September 2011.

IAMAI. (2009). *Mobile Internet in India. Internet and Mobile Association of India.* Mumbai: Internet and Mobile Association of India.

IAMAI. (2011). *I-Cube 2009–2010 – Internet in India.* Mumbai: Internet and Mobile Association of India.

Ilavarasan, P.V. (2007). Is Indian software workforce a case of uneven and combined development? *Equal Opportunities International,* 26(8), 802–822.

Ilavarasan, P.V. (2008). Occupational classification of the software workforce: Case of India. *Indian Journal of Labour Economics,* 51(1), 105–114.

Livemint. (2011). *Govt. plans 20 new IIITs on PPP basis.* Livemint, 5 August. Retrieved from http://www.livemint.com/2011/08/05194116/Govt-plans-20-new-IIITs-on-PPP.html on 7 June 2011.

ITU. (2010). *Core ICT Indicators, 2010.* Geneva: International Telecommunication Union.

Krishna, A. and Brihmadesam, V. (2006). What does it take to become a software professional? *Economic and Political Weekly,* 41 (30), 3307–3314.

Kumar, R. and Best, M.L. (2006). Social impact and diffusion of telecenter use: A study from the Sustainable Access in Rural India (SARI) Project. *Community Informatics,* 2(2), 116–136.

Malish, C.M. and Ilavarasan, P.V. (2011). Social exclusion in information capitalism: A study of online recruitment advertisements in the Indian software industry. In K. Nicolopoulou, M. Karatas-Ozkan, A. Tatli and J. Taylor, *Global knowledge work: Diversity and relational perspectives.* Cheltenham, UK: Edward Elgar Publishing Limited, 114–139.

Malish, C.M (2011). *Negotiating cultural capital in the knowledge economy of India: An empirical study of scheduled caste engineering students in Kerala.* PhD thesis under progress at Indian Institute of Technology Delhi, India.

Maplecroft.com (2011). Maplecroft ranking highlighting the 'digital divide' reveals India lagging behind Brazil, Russia and China. www.maplecroft.com Retrieved from http://maplecroft.com/about/news/digital_inclusion_index.html on 6 June 2011.

MIT. (2011). *IT software, services and BPO*. New Delhi: Ministry of Communications and Information Technology, Department of Information Technology, Government of India. Retrieved from http://www.mit.gov.in/content/it-software-services-and-bpo on 6 June 2011.

Mohanty, M. (2006). Social inequality, labour market dynamics and reservation. *Economic and Political Weekly*, 41(35), 3777–3789.

NASSCOM. (2011). Executive summary, *IT-BPO sector in India: Strategic review 2010*. New Delhi: NASSCOM. Retrieved from http://www.nasscom.in/Nasscom/templates/NormalPage.aspx?id=58654 on 10 March 2011.

OECD. (2007). *Documenting capabilities for measuring ICT in India: A position paper*. Directorate for Science, Working Party on Indicators for the Information Society. Technology and Industry Committee for Information, Computer and Communications Policy. Organisation for Economic Co-operation and Development.

Oommen, U. and Sundararajan, A. (2005). Social structuring of human capital of the new global workforce. Paper presented to the International Conference on New Global Workforces and Virtual Workplaces: Connections, Culture, and Control, National Institute of Advanced Studies, Bangalore, India, 12–13 August 2005.

Rao, S.S. (2006). Engineering and technology education in India: Uneven spread, quality and social coverage. *Journal of Educational Planning and Administration*, 20(2), 205–225.

Rediff. (2003). Infosys mentor against caste-based reservations. www.rediff.com. Retrieved from http://www.rediff.com/news/2003/apr/15murthy.htm on 7 June 2011.

Sassen, S. (2002). Towards a sociology of information technology. *Current Sociology*, 50(3): 365–388.

Saxenian, A. (2002). The Silicon Valley connection: Transnational networks and regional development in Taiwan, China and India. *Science, Technology and Society*, 7(1), 117–149.

Selwyn, N. (2004). Reconsidering political and popular understandings of the digital divide. *New Media & Society*, 6(3), 341–362.

Sharma D.S. (2009). *The Long revolution: The birth and growth of India's IT Industry*. Noida, London: Harper Collins.

Simrad, C. (2009). *Obstacles and solutions for underrepresented minorities in technology*. Palo Alto, CA, US: Anita Borg Institute for Women and Technology.

Singh, A. (2004). Why HR managers vouch for the referral system. www.itpeopleindia.com. Retrieved from http://www.itpeopleindia.com/20040802/cover.shtml on 11 September 2011.

Taeube, F. (2004). Culture, innovation, and economic development: The case of the south Indian ICT clusters. In S. Mani and H. Romijn, (eds.), *Innovation, learning, and technological dynamism of developing countries* (202–228). New Delhi: Bookwell.

Thomas, J.J. (2006). Informational development in rural areas: Some evidence from Andra Pradesh and Kerala. In G. Parayil (ed.) *Political economy and information capitalism in India*, (109–132). Hampshire, UK: Palgrave Macmillan.

UN (2010). *United Nations e-government survey 2010*. Geneva: Economic & Social Affairs, United Nations.

Upadhya, C. and Vasavi, A.R. (2006). *Work, culture and sociality in the Indian IT industry: A sociological study* (Final Report submitted to IDPAD). Bangalore, India: National Institute of Advanced Studies.

Upadhya, C. (2007). Employment, exclusion, and "merit" in the Indian IT industry. *Economic and Political Weekly*, 42(20), 1863–1868.

Varma, R. (2009). Bridging the digital divide: Computing in tribal colleges and universities. *Journal of Women and Minorities in Science and Engineering*, 15(1), 39–52

Varma, R. and Kapur, D. (2010). Access, satisfaction, and future: undergraduate education at the Indian Institutes of Technology, *Higher Education*, 59(6), 703–717.

Witte, J.C. and Mannon, S.E. (2010). *The Internet and social inequalities*. New York: Routledge.

9 The digital divide in China, Hong Kong and Taiwan

The barriers of first order and second order digital divide

Shu-Fen Tseng
Yuan Ze University

Yu-Ching You
National Taiwan University

Introduction

The International Telecommunication Union (2010) stated that the global number of Internet users had surpassed 2 billion in 2010, of which 1.2 billion users were in developing countries. The rate of Internet access has steadily increased from 394 million to over 2 billion in just over a decade. Despite the significant increase of worldwide Internet users, global distribution of Internet access has been extremely unequal. While an estimated 71 percent of the population in developed countries had access to the Internet at the end of 2010, there was only 21 percent of the population with access in developing countries. Globally, the Internet user divide is significantly influenced by gender, age, education, and income, and there are major differences between urban and rural areas (ITU, 2011).

This chapter follows Marx's central theories regarding the economic relations between capitalists and laborers. Capitalists were defined by their ownership of the means of production that helped capture surplus value in the production and consumption processes. Capital was created through the process of commodities production and exchange. Marx saw capital as part of the surplus value that creates further profit (Lin, 2001). In this scheme of the capitalist society, controlling and possessing the capital, such as tools, technology, and facilities that are associated with production implies ownership of the resources.

Coming with the diffusion of computers, telecommunications, and Internet in the 1970s, the information technology revolution fundamentally restructured capitalism. There has been a shift from material production to information-processing activities in advanced capitalist countries. Through infusion and application of information and communication technologies in the production and consumption, advanced economies increased their productivity and economy growth. The new techno-economic system can be adequately characterized as *informationalism* (Castells, 2000). The diffusion of information technology was highly selective. The process and benefits associated with *informationalism* were uneven throughout the world. In the information era, individuals, firms, institutions, regions, and societies are divided into two groups, those with the material and cultural resources to operate in the digital world, and those unable to adapt to the speed of change (Castells, 2001).

Witte and Mannon (2010) provided a useful overview of theories relevant to understanding inequality in access to and use of the new information technology. They described how the Internet is a major source of creating social inequality and social exclusion. Theoretically rooted in Marx's point of view, one of their aspects suggested that ownership of valuable resources, including skill assets, puts certain social classes at a distinct advantage. Inequality in a capitalist society rests on the ability of a dominant class to use its assets to maintain an advantage in the productive process. Individuals with significant Internet competencies and literacy might enjoy a privileged position in the information society (Witte and Mannon, 2010).

Since the late 1990s, the unequal distribution of Internet access between population segments within a society and across nations has gained recognition among concerned parties, such as scholars, policy makers, and advocate groups. The development of the Internet has been suggested as an enabling technology for transforming society, eliminating power differentials, realizing a free and democratic society, and other benefits. Lack of access to the Internet or information communication technology (ICT) jeopardizes one's opportunity of social participation and thwarts one's life chances. Wider uses of ICTs offer considerable opportunities for those able to take advantage of them, and increased exclusion for those who cannot. At the national level, poor nations without high technological investment suffer a competitive disadvantage compared to their wired rivals in the global economy (Norris, 2001).

Study of the digital divide has focused on the gaps between the population groups in computer and Internet access and unequal distribution of Internet services across regional and geographic areas. Concerning how the national context and political institutions affect individuals' technological access and online engagement, Norris (2001) outlined two contradictory predictions about technological diffusion and its consequence within a society: normalization and stratification models. In a normalization model, the differences between groups only increase in the early stages of adoption. The leading group starts the curve earlier, along with the resources, skills, and knowledge to take advantage of digital technologies. In the long run, differences between groups disappear, as the leading group enters the phase of saturation and the following groups reveal higher expansion rates, the penetration becomes saturated in these societies. The optimistic normalization model assumes that Internet penetration will saturate all groups in society as the Internet becomes user friendly, less expensive, and its benefits become more widely recognized. On the other hand, in the stratification model, the higher and lower social strata start with different resources, while the higher social strata will reach capacity and start saturation earlier in the curve of adoption. The pessimistic stratification model assumes that socially disadvantaged groups will encounter high cost and other obstacles that halt Internet penetration before they reach the perfect saturation. Norris argued that the stratification model provides a more realistic scenario where groups who are already well networked via traditional forms of ICT will maintain their advantage in the diffusion of new technology. A similar argument can be found in van Dijk's (2005) illustration of the "Matthew effect" in new media access, which indicated that those who already have a head start in possessing particular resources benefit more from a new resource than those who are behind and already have some disadvantages.

Much of the research on the digital divide focuses on the first order effects regarding those who have access to ICTs versus those who do not. As Internet access gradually increased worldwide during the past decade, foci on digital inequality studies shifted to the second order digital divide. While the first order effects focus on the inequality in access to ICT, the second order addresses the effects of inequality resulting from the different ways people use ICT technology. Hargittai (2002) argued that as more people start using the Internet, it becomes less useful to merely look at the binary classification of whether one is online or not. Instead, she suggested a need to start looking at the differences in people's online skill and stated that how those who are online use the medium is more important when discussing issues of digital divide.

The second order digital divide stresses a gradual shift of inequality in the information society from ICT access to ICT usage. The shift to ICT usage is important because of its implication for social inclusion in that ICT plays a critical role in all aspects of the new economy and information society (Warschauer, 2003). Recently, research has shown that the different usage of ICT can be related to variability in the risk of marginalization, because differential ICT use can have close interrelations with inclusion or exclusion in the professional sphere, not to mention access to public services, consumption patterns, and personal development (Brotcorne *et al.*, 2010). Scholars argued that unequal attainment of digital skills and the usage of ICT for particular purposes of information, communication, transaction, or entertainment is one of the main reasons for the deepening divide in the information society (van Dijk, 2005). The digital inclusion study of the UK confirmed that there was a strong association between the social disadvantages an individual faces and their ability to access and use digital services. By including users' online activities in the measurement of digital exclusion, the UK study discovered individuals with specific disadvantages appear to be excluded from the applications of technology that could help them most (Helsper, 2008).

By recognizing the capability of ICT to build various types of capital through access to relevant Internet resources, we adopt the Marxist perspective of capital in this chapter. Once individuals have access to ICTs, and have the capacity to use Internet resources effectively in transforming them into economic, political and social capitals, they have more freedom to participate in society in the way they wish to. Those who enjoy the high levels of economic and social superiority also use their dominant positions to acquire ICT resources and maintain existing advantages. Individuals suffering social disadvantages such as low income, less education, and poorer skills, are more likely to be excluded from the information society. In this chapter, earlier Internet adopting economies in Asia, such as Hong Kong and Taiwan, and a fast-growing nation, specifically China, are compared to test the normalization and stratification hypotheses of Internet penetration. Secondary and longitudinal data of national ICT access from the Individual/Household Digital Divide Survey[1] in Taiwan and the Statistical Report on Internet Development in China[2] are collected to examine barriers of the first order digital divides in China, Hong Kong and Taiwan. A longitudinal comparison across different socio-economic groups in each of these regions yields results showing whether the normalization or stratification model better describes Internet penetration over the past decade. Secondly, activities that people do on the Internet, such as searching for information, communication, entertainment, and online consumption, are compared to explore the divides of digital engagement in these regions. The comparative digital divides and the social implications of digital inequality in these regions are discussed in the final section.

The first order divide: Digital access

Early research on the digital divide has focused on inequality in Internet access. It has generally suggested that Internet access penetrates at varying rates between different segments of the population (NTIA, 1995). The gaps generally followed the social inequality lines of gender, age, race, ethnicity, education and geographic location disparities. Digital connectivity is essential as lack of Internet access for individuals implies unequal opportunities for economic mobility and social participation in the information society. As Internet penetration continues to rise worldwide, the important question is: does the gap between groups shrink in the long run as the normalization hypothesis suggested or is the gap is widening as outlined by the stratification model? The answer to this question would lead to an optimistic or pessimistic prediction of Internet diffusion in a society. In this section, trends of the first order divide in Taiwan, Hong Kong and China are presented (see the figures in Appendix 9.1), followed by a cross-regional comparison of digital access in these regions.

Trends of digital access

Internet growth has been significant in Taiwan. The annual national Individual/Household Digital Divide Survey in 2010 illustrated that the individual Internet penetration rate has exceeded 70 percent in Taiwan. The household Internet penetration rate also reached 80 percent in 2010. More than half of the Internet users used wireless and mobile technologies to access the Internet in 2010. The long-term trends showed that the gap of Internet access between men and women disappearing in Taiwan. Almost every young adult below the age of 20 used the Internet in 2010. Internet access in the elder groups was increasing, yet at a slower rate than that of their younger counterparts, thus resulting in huge gaps when compared to the younger groups. Those highly educated (college degree or above) were more likely to access the Internet, and this group showed a saturated Internet connectivity rate. In comparison, less than 20 percent of people with an elementary school education or less were connected to the Internet, thus huge educational gaps persisted. Rural areas generally experienced lower levels of connectivity when compared to metropolitan areas, although these gaps appeared to be shrinking. Well-off households have saturated Internet access and the poor households have gradually increased their Internet connectivity except for those at the bottom of the household income range. In broadband connectivity, gaps between metropolitan city and rural/remote areas were diminishing. However, those who were better off had broadband adoption rates consistently higher than those in the vulnerable groups. For mobile Internet access, steady increases across age and education groups were found, nevertheless, the gaps among these groups persisted.

Household Internet connection figures have increased significantly over the last decade in Hong Kong. About 70 percent of households had access to broadband connectivity. Personal Internet access rates also increased from 30 percent to 70 percent in the past decade. Consistently, the rate of having Internet access was slightly higher for males than their female counterparts. The divides between age groups were shrinking in general, although there was still a huge gap between the younger group and those aged 45 and over in 2009. A narrowing trend of Internet access was found between those who had graduated from senior high school and those who had college or higher degrees. However, the gap between the lowest and the highest education groups persisted, with an over 70 percent discrepancy. The slow increase of Internet access in the lowest income group led to a huge gap when compared to the highest income group in Hong Kong.

The China Internet Network Information Center (CNNIC) reported the number of Chinese Internet users had reached 457 million in 2010 and the Internet penetration rate was 34.3 percent. Almost all the Internet users had broadband access. At the end of 2010, China had 303 million users who used mobile phones to go online, which accounted for 66 percent of total Internet users. There was a slight gender difference in Internet access in the past few years. The upgrading trend of Internet access was observed for younger groups; however, the increasing rate of Internet access was sluggish for the older population groups, thus resulting in a huge difference compared to the top connected group and a widening trend of divide between these two groups. Internet access by different educational levels demonstrated a dramatic increase among those who had a college degree and a fast catch-up rate of high school graduates in Internet access. Yet the slow increase in the less educated population led to a persistent 80 percent gap of Internet access by educational level in the last few years. Despite the fast increase in the numbers of rural netizens, the urban/rural digital divide had widened: while 45 percent of the urban population had Internet access, only 15 percent of the rural population had used Internet services in 2009.

A cross-regional comparison of the first order divide

Table 9.1 shows the comparison of access divides in Taiwan, Hong Kong and China. First of all, the table indicates that the gender difference in Internet access was less significant in these regions. While the gender gap had disappeared in Taiwan, the proportions of female Internet users in Hong Kong and China were slightly less than their male counterparts. Age divides in Internet access in Taiwan and Hong Kong revealed an optimistic development for those aged under 40, yet the elder groups revealed persistent gaps when compared to the younger groups. Despite the impressive increase in numbers of Internet users in China, the age divide of access had widened, with those aged between 19 and 30 demonstrating a much higher increased rate of Internet access than the other groups. Although gradual increases within the less educated groups were found in Taiwan, the gaps in levels of Internet access across educational groups were persistent over time. A steady increase in secondary educational groups' Internet access led to a narrowing gap between this group and the higher educated group in Hong Kong, however, a huge gap between the higher educated and the less educated still remained. China revealed the same trend as Hong Kong did in the decline of the access gap between the secondary and post-secondary education groups. The secondary education group in China showed a significant improvement with a shrinking gap between them and the top group. Yet a persistent divide between the least educated group and the top one appeared in the past few years. The regional divide in Internet access in Taiwan demonstrated a similarity to the normalization model, in that all the remote and rural areas had increased connectivity and the gaps compared to the metropolitan city had narrowed over time. By contrast, the access divide had increased along the lines of geographic location in China, as the Internet access gap between the urban and rural areas had widened. The income divide in Internet access resembled the trends of age and education divides both in Taiwan and Hong Kong, in the manner that the gaps across income groups, except for those with the least affluent group, were diminishing.

Table 9.1 Summary of the first order divide in Taiwan, Hong Kong and China

		Taiwan	*Hong Kong*	*China*
Internet	Gender	High penetration Disappearing	High penetration Small gap persistent	Medium penetration Small gap persistent
	Age	Declining yet persistent in the older groups	Declining yet persistent in the older group	Widening
	Education	Huge gap persistent	Declining in secondary yet huge gap in the lowest group	Significantly declining in the high school group yet persistent in the less educated group
	Region	Declining	—	Widening
	Income	Declining yet huge gap persistent in the lowest group	Declining yet persistent in the lowest group	—
Household broadband	Region	Disappearing	—	—
	Income	Narrowing in the upper income groups, persistent in the lowest income groups	—	—
Mobile/ wireless	Gender	Small gap persistent	—	—
	Age	Persistent	—	—
	Education	Persistent	—	—

— Indicates data are unavailable.

The access to broadband services across different geographic regions in Taiwan showed a more optimistic development in that the regional gaps in household broadband access were diminishing. The income gaps in broadband connection were narrowing in the upper income groups, however, the gap persisted for the worst off group. The divides in mobile and wireless connection in Taiwan generally showed a declining trend. The gaps between age groups and educational levels were declining, yet the gaps still existed.

The second order divide: Digital usage

Recent research has shifted concerns from a simplistic conception of Internet access to a more complex approach to digital inequality as more people are using the Internet to communicate, search, entertain, and engage in online economic and political activities (DiMaggio *et al.*, 2001; Hargittai, 2002; van Dijk, 2005). A wider range of questions about the impact of digital access and use on social inequality was raised. In all, research on the digital divide has moved beyond physical access to pay closer attention to a multi-faceted concept of access. This second wave of research on the digital divide was called the "second-level digital divide" (Hargittai, 2002) or "usage divide" (van Dijk, 2005). By examining the variation of Internet use, the effects of the digital divide on educational attainment, earning, social participation and political engagement were addressed. Scholars focused on the usage gap in the digital divide conduct research reflecting their concerns of digital inequality across segments of the population depending on differences among several dimensions of Internet access and usage. The so called "the rich get richer" or the Matthew effect implies that in most spheres of societal participation and political engagement those already occupying the strongest positions tend to benefit more from access and usage of ICTs as potentially powerful tools than those occupying the weakest positions (van Dijk, 2005). If the effect were realized, then those who are already better off would gain more from the wide ranges of digital technologies used which would lead to a deepening inequality in society. Information technologies would then become one more resource for those who already have a large number of resources to amplify their social, economic and political advantages. In this section, trends of the usage divide in Taiwan and Hong Kong are delineated (see the figures in Appendix 9.2), followed by comparison of the usage divide in Taiwan and Hong Kong.[3]

Trends of digital usage

Searching for information has been the top reason for using Internet services in Taiwan. The second most common Internet activities were communication and online entertainment. The activity of online shopping has been increasing in usage since 2004. Online banking and online governmental services were used less than other activities in Taiwan. In Hong Kong, the main purpose of using Internet services has been searching for information and online communication since 2002. Clear gaps between using Internet services for these two top activities and using the Internet for entertainment and e-commerce purposes were shown. The less common activities were online shopping and banking. Usage of governmental services was generally low. In China, searching for information, online entertainment and instant communication were major Internet activities. Recent trends showed that searching for information was the highest priority of Internet usage. The need for online entertainment including music or video and online gaming has increased over the past few years. Instant communication has outnumbered email usage since 2007. The proportion of online users engaging in shopping reached one third of Internet users and slowly increased over time. This trend was followed by the usage of online banking in 2009.

A cross-regional comparison of the second order divide

The Internet offers a new range of usages to individuals; we adopt the classification of Internet usage suggested by the UK digital inclusion study (Helsper, 2008) to further compare the changes of these clusters of digital engagement across regions. The first cluster is basic users of the Internet who undertake practical activities such as information seeking, individual communication and online shopping. Intermediate users are those who use the Internet for participatory activities, including using government services and online financial services. Since Internet activity by socio-economic strata was only available in Taiwan and Hong Kong, Table 9.2 shows the trends of usage divides in these two regions.

For the basic Internet activities in Taiwan, the gender gap was shown to be either disappearing or diminishing; males had a slightly higher percentage in entertainment usage than females, while females had a slightly higher percentage in online shopping usage than their male counterparts. Age effects were generally declining in information searching, communication, and entertainment; nevertheless, the youngest group was far less engaged in information searching and the elder groups were less engaged in online communication and entertainment. The gaps between different age groups in online shopping activity persisted over time. The gaps between usage of basic activities among educational levels were either remaining or widening, except for online entertainment. In general, educational differences still matter in digital engagement. The effects of geographic location were gradually diminishing over time in usage of basic Internet activities. The trend of digital engagement in Hong Kong was similar to that of Taiwan. While the gender gap was disappearing, the educational effects on searching for information and

Table 9.2 Summary of the second order divide in Taiwan and Hong Kong

		Basic Internet activities			Online Shopping	Intermediate Internet activities	
		Information searching	Communication*	Entertainment		Online Banking	e-Government
Taiwan	Gender	Disappearing	Disappearing	Declining small gap (M>F)	Small gap persistent (F>M)	Disappearing	Disappearing
	Age	Declining except in the youngest	Declining yet gap persistent	Declining yet gap persistent	Persistent	Widening	Persistent
	Education	Persistent	Persistent, widening in the least educated	Declining	Widening	Widening	Persistent
	Region	Declining	Declining	Declining	Modest gap persistent	Persistent	Persistent
Hong Kong	Gender	Disappearing	Disappearing	Declining small gap (M>F)	Disappearing**	Disappearing	
	Age	Declining except the youngest	Widening	Widening	Persistent**	Persistent	
	Education	Persistent	Persistent	Declining	Widening**	Persistent	

*Communication in Taiwan is defined as instant communication; communication in Hong Kong is defined as communication with others.
**Indicates the activity of electronic commerce which includes online shopping and banking in Hong Kong.

communication were persistent. Moreover, age effects on online communication and entertainment suggested that the usage gaps in these two activities have widened among age groups. The trends of intermediate level digital engagement demonstrated that age, educational level, and geographic location continue to influence what people do online, although the effect of gender has become irrelevant. The usage gaps of intermediate Internet activities were either persistent or widening. These results also suggested that a greater number of socio-economic factors influence the use of intermediate applications than influence the use of the Internet for basic activities. Far from the optimistic prediction, those socially disadvantaged groups appear to be less included in the participatory use of the Internet that could affect their life chances most. On the contrary, those who are better off may benefit from the wider use of ICT technologies and re-enhance their social, economic and political advantages; digital divides thus lead to a deepening social inequality.

Discussion

The results of the cross-regional comparison of digital access suggested that the Internet access gap was narrowing in highly connected regions. However, after reaching the growing peak, the trend of the digital divide in these regions was parallel to the lines of social divides. Those who were most deprived socially, such as the elderly, less educated and the poor were also the least likely to be digitally connected. The persistent gaps in broadband and mobile access between high and low access populations suggested that low access groups were again lagging in adoption of new innovations. Moreover, for regions with rapid growth of digital access, the main policy should be to address the unequal rates of diffusion in the low socio-economic population. Without recognition of the unequal accessibility within the population, the gaps of digital access will widen and certain groups with social disadvantages will be at risk of exclusion from various aspects of the information society.

The gaps between figures for men and women in both basic and intermediate Internet usage have gradually improved. Regional gaps have declined in basic usage, but persisted in intermediate activities. Age gaps of online activity demonstrated different preferences between the young and the elderly. Education matters across all online usages and activities except for those recreational purposes. Less engagement in Internet activities might be due to a lack of training and direct hands-on experience. Along the lines of educational or ICT skills gaps, it is likely that Internet use will be stratified, with some using it as an entertainment device and some using it to seek and create new knowledge. Scholars have suggested the Internet will not create knowledge seekers out of those without the requisite background or skills (Warschauer, 2003). With more advanced activity that requires high levels of skill capacity, not surprisingly, the divides between people who have high and low educational levels were persistent or widening.

Furthermore, the number of barriers to digital engagement was higher for those intermediate activities than for basic uses of the Internet. A greater number of socio-economic factors, for example age, education and region, influenced the use of intermediate applications than influenced the use of the Internet for basic activities. This result indicated an intertwined link between digital engagement and social inclusion. Lack of usage of needed resources will make groups that are already socially disadvantaged fall further behind. On the contrary, individuals who already have valuable resources, including material wealth and skill assets, enjoy a privileged position to maintain their distinct advantages. Without proper intervention, the wider usage of ICTs may become a potent tool to deepen social divides and foster "the rich get richer" effect. These results suggest that exploring how people engage in ICT activities and the resultant impact on social exclusion is important in the current stage of digital divide scholarship.

A narrowing access divide in Taiwan can be attributed to the active government policy on bridging the digital divide. Several action plans have been launched since 2003, such as providing digital TV signals and reception devices in rural areas, connecting broadband networks to all villages, establishing digital opportunity centers in all counties, supporting small to medium enterprises to develop e-commerce, supporting digital opportunity centers in Asia-Pacific Economic Cooperation (APEC) economies and educating international trainers and professionals. While substantial growth of digital access in the past decade was found, persistent divides among the elderly, the least educated, and the poor in Internet, broadband and mobile access suggested technological and social disadvantages were inextricably linked. The growth of digital access did not automatically solve social problems. Overcoming barriers to access technologies in the socially disadvantaged groups requires active government intervention. A shrinking gap between rural and urban areas in Taiwan demonstrated a continued need for governmental policy to support socially excluded groups in preventing digital disengagement.

As a result of open competition in the telecommunications market, Hong Kong has shown that the pro-competition policy and pro-market approach has been very successful in facilitating high penetration of ICT development. Broadband Internet access in Hong Kong is among the highest broadband penetration rates, and the number of mobile service subscribers also represents one of the highest penetration rates in the world. However, the persistent gaps in Internet access among the elderly, less educated and economically disadvantaged demonstrated the need for governmental policy to advocate for digitally excluded populations. Those socially deprived are also the most at risk of lacking access to digital resources. They are the elderly, the less educated with limited skills and those with low socio-economic status. From the Marxist view of capital, those who are already disadvantaged in terms of social and economic resources are the most at risk of being excluded from the information society. The inequality will deepen as they are deprived of the digital resources and opportunities of engaging in online social, economic, and political activities. As technology continues to develop, those who are not included are at risk of being left further behind. Governments and other stakeholders need to focus on tackling digital exclusion among the socio-economically disadvantaged and bridging digital divides for these groups to access the digital resources they need.

China has experienced exponential Internet growth in the last decade. Despite the absolute number and percentage of Internet users having increased dramatically, Internet penetration in China remains relatively low when compared to the first tier digital nations. The slow increase in usage rates of the elderly has lead to a widening trend of an age divide. The trend shows a significant increase in the number of Internet users in rural areas, nevertheless, the increase rates are behind those in urban areas. The unequal distribution of Internet resources between segments of the population has profound impacts on the continuation of social inequality. While celebrating the huge growth of the Internet-using population in China, policy concerns should respond to the widening gaps of digital access and exclusion from digital engagement. The CNNIC pointed out that the rapidly growing numbers of rural netizens have become an important part of the new Internet population and most of this rural population with a poor educational background has been attracted to the Internet due to its recreational and entertainment functions (CNNIC, 2008). From the aspect of digital inclusion, the low use of online economic services and political functions let down the enabling power of the Internet to enhance digital engagement and social inclusion. In this regard, issues of wider uses of online functions and participatory activities in China, such as education, learning, job seeking, e-commerce and participating in public affairs should be addressed.

A relevant issue is Internet censorship. In China, only government-approved agencies and businesses are permitted to establish an Internet Interconnecting Network and to license the operation of Internet service providers at the next tier. All private Internet service providers are licensed through one of these backbone networks and are required to install filters to block undesirable content. In order not to risk having their licenses revoked, most of these companies complied with the self-censorship regulation in China (Liang and Lu, 2010; MacKinnon, 2008). Based on the CNNIC reports, a great loss of search engine usage was found in 2006. The downward trend in the usage of search engines might be a reflection of the broader censorship in China on the bulletin boards, blogs, and online news and information sites in the year of 2005. The usage of search engines and news browsing functions decreased almost 15 percent compared to the previous year. The number soon bounced back in 2007. This resilience might be due to a huge infusion of Internet population from the rural areas. Whether this downward trend of usage was due to measurement problems or a reflection of governmental regulation, long-term impacts of Internet censorship on social and political change in China deserve further investigation.

Currently, strategic responses to the digital divide by national, state, and local programs often focus on getting more equipment and connections, yet recent research has shown that it is insufficient to bridge the divide by only responding to physical access need. Digital access is essential, and interventions which provide access to the technology remain important aspects of increasing digital engagement. In addition, human resources, such as digital literacy, and social resources that engage in meaningful social practices are also important to realize the possibility of digital opportunity. From the Marxist perspective, this chapter contends that social inequality might accelerate in the information society for those privileged groups take uneven advantages and benefits from effective use of the Internet in the social, economic, and political spheres. The lack of effective digital skills and exclusion from the gains of the application of technology in the socially deprived groups as compared to their advantaged counterparts deepen social inequality in the information society.

Appendix 9.1 **Digital access in Taiwan, Hong Kong, and China**

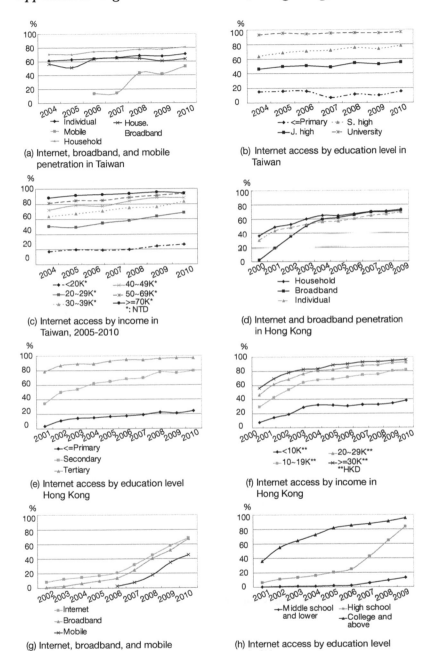

(a) Internet, broadband, and mobile penetration in Taiwan

(b) Internet access by education level in Taiwan

(c) Internet access by income in Taiwan, 2005-2010

(d) Internet and broadband penetration in Hong Kong

(e) Internet access by education level Hong Kong

(f) Internet access by income in Hong Kong

(g) Internet, broadband, and mobile penetration in China

(h) Internet access by education level in China

Sources:
(a)(b)(c) Individual/Household Digital Divide Survey in Taiwan, 2004-2010
(d)(e)(f) Thematic Household Survey 2000-2009, Census and tatistics Department of Hong Kong
(g)(h) Statistical Report on Internet Development in China, 2002-2010, CNNIC

Appendix 9.2 **Internet activities in Taiwan, Hong Kong, and China**

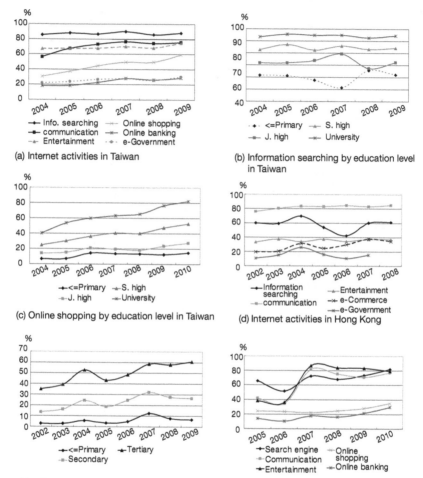

(a) Internet activities in Taiwan

(b) Information searching by education level in Taiwan

(c) Online shopping by education level in Taiwan

(d) Internet activities in Hong Kong

(e) e-Commerce by education level in Hong Kong

(f) Internet activities in China

Sources:
(a)(b)(c) Individual/Household Digital Divide Survey in Taiwan, 2004-2010
(d)(e) Thematic Household Survey 2000-2009, Census and tatistics Department of Hong Kong
(f) Statistical Report on Internet Development in China, 2002-2010, CNNIC. Note that there is no "information searching" category in the survey, use of "search engine" function is selected instead

References

Brotcorne, R., Damhuis, L., Laurent, V., Valenduc, G. and Vendramin, P. (2010). *The second order digital divide: Synthesis of the research report.* Foundation Travail-Universite (Namur). Retrieved from http://www.ftu-namur.org/fichiers/FTU-Second_order_digital_divide-Synthesis.pdf

Castells, M. (2000). *The rise of the network society,* 2nd edition London, UK: Blackwell.

Castells. M. (2001). *The Internet galaxy: Reflections on the Internet, business, and society.* New York: Oxford University Press.

China Internet Network Information Center (CNNIC) (2008). Statistical Survey Report on the Internet Development in China. Retrieved from http://www.apira.org/data/upload/pdf/Asia-Pacific/CNNIC/21streport-en.pdf

China Internet Network Information Center (CNNIC). (1997–2010). *Statistical report on Internet development in China.* Retrieved from http://www.cnnic.cn/research/bgxz/tjbg/

DiMaggio, P., Hargittai, E., Celeste, C. and Shafer, S. (2001). *From unequal access to differentiated use: A literature review and agenda for research on digital inequality.* Retrieved from http://www.eszter.com/research/pubs/dimaggio-etal-digital inequality.pdf

Hargittai, E. (2002). Second-level digital divide: differences in people's online skills. *First Monday,* 7(4), 1–19. Retrieved from http://chnm.gmu.edu/digitalhistory/links/pdf/introduction/0.26c.pdf

Helsper, E. (2008). *Digital inclusion: An analysis of social disadvantage and the information society.* London, UK: Department for Communities and Local Government.

International Telecommunications Union (ITU). (2010). *ICT data and statistics.* Retrieved from http://www.itu.int/ITU-D/ict/statistics/

International Telecommunications Union (ITU). (2011). *Measuring the information society.* Retrieved from http://www.itu.int/net/pressoffice/backgrounders/general/pdf/5.pdf

Liang, B. and Lu, H. (2010). Internet development, censorship, and cyber crimes in China. *Journal of Contemporary Criminal Justice,* 26(1), 103–120.

Lin, N. (2001). *Social capital: A theory of social structure and action.* New York: Cambridge University Press.

MacKinnon, R. (2008). Flatter world and thicker walls? Blogs, censorship and civic discourse in China. *Public Choice,* 134, 31–46.

National Telecommunications and Information Administration (NTIA). (1995). *Falling through the Net: A survey of the "Have Nots" in rural and urban America.* Washington, DC: US Department of Commerce.

Norris, P. (2001). *Digital divide: Civic engagement, information poverty, and the Internet worldwide.* New York, NY: Cambridge University Press.

Research, Development, and Evaluation Commission (RDEC). (2002–2010). *Individual/Household digital divide survey in Taiwan.* Yuan, Taiwan: Executive.

van Dijk, J.A.G.M. (2005). *The deepening divide: Inequality in the information society.* Thousand Oaks, CA, US: Sage.

Warschauer, M. (2003). *Technology and social inclusion: Rethinking the digital divide.* Cambridge, MA, US: MIT Press.

Witte, J.C. and Mannon, S.E. (2010). *The Internet and social inequalities.* New York: Routledge.

Notes

1 The Individual/Household Digital Divide Survey has been conducted annually by the Research, Development and Evaluation Commission (RDEC) (2002–2010), Executive Yuan in Taiwan since 2003. Take the 2010 survey, for example, carried out through phone interviews with those residents of Taiwan over the age of 12, with an effective sample size of 16,008 people.

2 The Statistical Report on Internet Development in China is conducted by the China Internet Network Information Center (CNNIC) (1997–2010). The first report appeared in 1997. Starting from 1998, the reports were issued twice a year. The twenty-sixth survey, for example, was conducted in 2010, with a total number of 30,000 residents at the age six or above interviewed by phone. Since these reports only show proportions of netizens, we used the total number of the population in each socio-economic category referenced by the National Bureau of Statistics of China to yield percentages of Internet access in each segment of the population. Usage of Internet services by Hong Kong residents has been researched annually by the Census and Statistics Department of Hong Kong since 2000 under its series of Thematic Household Surveys (THS). Some 10,000 persons aged ten and over in representative households were face-to-face interviewed in 2010. The reports of this survey are compiled in the Statistical Report on Internet Development in China.

3 Data of usage by socio-economic factors in China is not available in the CNNIC reports.

Section 4

Eastern Europe

10 The Internet and digital divide in South Eastern Europe

Connectivity does not end the digital divide, skills do[1]

Danica Radovanović
Belgrade Center for Digital Humanities

Introduction

The social paradigm of the information and communication technologies (ICTs) has fundamentally changed many aspects of everyday life but ICTs have also become an indispensable part of it. In this chapter, we take social theories developed by the classical sociologists like Weber (1924), Giddens (2006), and Meyrowitz (2008) and apply them to the issues of Internet inequality. Weber's stratification theory is grounded in the core perspective on inequality, and we examine how access to the Internet combines with variables such as class, status, education.

With this chapter, we are offering an understanding of social inequality in the information-driven networked society and we are focusing on South Eastern Europe (SEE) and on Serbia in particular. Serbia is an SEE country in transition, and the political, economic, and social turbulence of the 1990s have influenced its culture and ethical values, as well as the development of the ICTs and the creation of an online public sphere (Radovanović, 2010a, 2010b). The trends of Internet use in everyday life did not pass Serbia by. The socio-economic and moral crisis in Serbia has also reached the networked public and higher education.

It is not surprising that both the younger and the older generations in urban areas have embraced the new social media forms very quickly as an extension of their analog lives; but what about the necessity of new literacies in the twenty-first century? How should they acquire necessary skills that will enable them to use Internet services wisely and selectively, as well as to best utilize the collaboration practices in the academic environment?

We are all participating on a daily basis in a networked world and we are the creators of the content online, in the same hyper-connected world where the issues and patterns of social inclusion and exclusion need to be observed and addressed.

The goal of this chapter is to examine the paradox of how moving beyond digital divides in the context of the technological infrastructure would permit us to tackle other existing problems in order to explore the differences in how the online public in Serbia use the Internet, not just in their everyday lives, but also for learning, communication, and collaboration.

Some data in national and international reports on ICT use exists, but not on the subject of Internet use and the digital divide in higher education, and here we are trying to fill the gap in the existing reports and data, and present some empirical findings that cannot be found in these documents.

Finally, we indicate that there is a social stratification in regards to Internet use, social media, and collaboration in higher education in Serbia. The main empirical finding of the chapter has revealed the three main factors of the digital gap, the categories of community/sociality, participation and collaboration, as well as contradiction and its relation to the theoretical points of stratification. Crucially, motivated high status persons (professors at universities) are needed to advance digital literacy. Ironically, it is those who have less influence (junior faculty, graduate students, and undergraduate students) who are the savviest with Internet technology. The high status persons have less motivation. But how can we encourage the professors to adopt and use new ICTs? This is the underlying conundrum, and the results raise some important questions and shed light on current issues to be solved in the future.

Theoretical framework

Since we are examining stratification in the Internet from a socio-technological and educational perspective, we decided that the Weberian social stratification theory could be used as the theoretical approach for this chapter.

Many studies on inequalities focus mainly on differences in socio-economic backgrounds and in available resources, such as money or skills, or they focus on developing inequalities such as access to basic human resources including equipment, knowledge, or education. Those with more access to resources "use their relative advantage to increase the inequalities" (Meyrowitz, 2008, p.645).

Weber's principles (1924) of status and class present a good starting point for the Internet context of inequalities that are interconnected within online communities and the exploration of the social media as applied in educational communities. The access to produce information and knowledge, or create and distribute the content online in the information society, is stratified by socio-economic factors and skills or literacy abilities. We examine two groups within the higher education ecosystem in Serbia, in the context of status (or *Stände*) applying Weber's theory for analyzing Internet use.

In higher education, collaborative and communication processes determine and form the category of status or prestige one holds within one community. Conversely, outside academia, the possession of power is more interconnected with the technological and economic infrastructure that reflects the access to information, the Internet and computers (and other devices that connect online), as it refers more to material goods, social resources and the divide between the "haves" and the "have-nots" (Warschauer, 2003). For example, possession of information or knowledge can make one more powerful than others in society as one is in the dominant position and can control the access to information or media. These people are sometimes known as information gatekeepers. Social power in the Internet perspective denotes the existence of status groups that often show themselves in the form of communities sharing information and knowledge, social media content, or other benefits within likeminded groups online.

Internet access is a universal issue and of major concern to many policy makers and governments. Opening up the access to knowledge and its deployment in everyday work and education is crucial for producing results and fostering the competences of students, scholars, and knowledge workers. Access to information is the key to an individual's position in society; and still access is not everything, it is only the starting point in many countries and societies while the present power structures remain.

A communal action *Gemeinschaft*, according to Weber, is oriented to and fueled by an "emotional feeling of the actors that they belong together" (1924, p.150). Social networks and the networked sociality that people are gathered around online today on the Internet confirm this function within the *Stände*, i.e. defining one's status in the community. People are sharing in groups, gathered by some shared interest or purpose in a place with others of their choosing where they feel they can belong and validate each other.

On the other hand, on the issue of inequality, Giddens (2006) considers as fundamentally important that education plays a significant role in either strengthening or breaking down inequalities. Giddens argues the role of education is critical as he identifies a new divide emerging between those who have the opportunity to experience higher education and those who do not. He thinks it is important not to think of the education system as if it works in a vacuum – factors like changes in employment and the economy also figure.

Thus having defined theoretical perspectives from classical sociology that can help us understand and analyze the existence of a digital divide in contemporary societies, we are going to describe the specific case of such divides in Serbia in the rest of the chapter.

Methodology

Statistical data about the digital divide exists and many reports have considered who is and who is not online by gender, age, education, socio-economic status, or region. This brief review cannot be comprehensive about such broad topics, so we are focusing on higher education and the use of the Internet and social media with available data and research findings.

Most of the research on social inequalities with an Internet perspective to date in Serbia has stayed on the level of analyzing data from national and international statistical institutions, with the limitations of the study lacking theoretical background and exploratory research in specific environments. For example, no data was found in any report on Internet use and inequalities within higher education in Serbia. While information on Internet social media use in higher education has not been previously published and was not available in those reports for Serbia, we did locate individual Internet scholar research (Radovanović, 2010a, 2010b) that discussed social media and social network use among young adults in Serbia, and in higher education.

Data sources for the study, beside quantitative international indicators from the reports, represent statistical data analyzed from the secondary statistical sources. The Statistical Office of the Republic of Serbia (SORS) telephone survey presents a sample of n=2400 households in the territory of Serbia. SORS has been carrying out a panel study of Internet use in Serbia since 2006, using the Statistical Office of the European Commission (Eurostat)[2] methodology.

We also present data from the semi-structured in-depth interviews (n=32)[3] with higher education representatives from the region (North, Central, and South Serbia) with deeper insight into social media use and collaborative processes online. The study population was young adults – students (undergraduate and postgraduate) and teachers (professors and junior faculty) who gave extensive feedback in conversations both face-to-face and via telephone and Skype. Through exploratory and descriptive analysis of the content from the transcripts we came to interesting narratives expressed through offered input. Data from the interviews represents the respondents' opinions regarding the use of the Internet and social media to illustrate the divide in communication and collaborative processes in higher education, and social stratification between these status groups.

International and national data on ICT use in Serbia

The latest SORS report of Internet use in Serbia was published in September 2011 with data from surveys, providing a description of users as well as their socio-economic background. Internet usage is analyzed based on the penetration, type and frequency of Internet use, education and employment status. Internet penetration presents one of the key indicators related to widespread information society development. According to the Internet World Report statistics as of June 2011 (Internet World Stats, 2011), in Serbia there were 4,107,000 Internet users which represents a 56 percent Internet penetration, according to the ITU (International Telecommunications Union), and 2,866,200 Facebook users on June 2011, indicating a 39.2 percent penetration rate.

However, the SORS survey shows that social-economic factors are the main issue, and the correlation between the use of the Internet and the income of the user demonstrates a significant gap in usage rates depending on income level. Another evident divide is between rural and urban households with relation to ICT use, almost double in percentage for urban populations with 60.8 percent versus 39.7 percent for rural populations.

In Serbia 52.1 percent of households own a computer or Internet capable device, 50.6 percent of the users have a DSL connection, while 7.8 percent still use modems to get online, and 29.6 percent use cable Internet (SORS, 2011, p.18). The share of Internet users is linked to level of education: 73.8 percent of individuals with a university degree use the Internet, as compared to 57.4 percent of those with secondary school education and 17.7 percent of individuals with an educational level lower than secondary school.

There is only one information source in the SORS survey on social media usage among the population and it is based on the sole variable "types of Internet use." Respondents who used the Internet reported it was mostly for participation in social networks (69.8 percent). Also, 91.8 percent of the Internet population aged 16–24 has one or more accounts on Facebook and Twitter, which indicates that the most frequent users in Serbia are young adults, and most of their Internet time is spent on social networks. They use the Internet for education purposes as well, with 65.5 percent reporting that they search for information relating to education as well as browsing Wikipedia (45.5 percent).

In regards to e-learning and digital literacy, the survey (ibid., p.32) showed that only 5.6 percent of respondents had attended a course on using computers in the last three years. A surprising 79.7 percent of them said they had never attended any course. However, according to the UNDP Human Development Report (2010), the list of the Balkan countries by literacy rate places Serbia in sixty-fifth place (96.4 percent literacy rate). This report indicates that Serbia belongs to the high human development group, and as for education, it is interesting that there is no data on the adult literacy rate (Human Development Report, 2010, p.145).

With regard to the utilization of ICTs within education, computers and access to the Internet: 100 percent of primary and secondary schools have computer labs and 87 percent of schools have Internet access which is an average of 26 pupils per computer (eGovernance and ICT Usage Report for SEE, 2010, p.54). It is interesting that the curriculum for ICT skills and obtaining digital literacy is optional and that computer science is not a mandatory subject in primary schools, while in the secondary schools it is mandatory from the first or second grade, depending on the school's educational profile (ibid., p.57).

As for ICT use in higher education, there is no data available for very important indicators, such as the number of students per computer at a typical university, or the percentage of male and female student users or how often they use the Internet. It is unfortunate that this important information is not available officially and the lack of research and data should be addressed seriously by governments, higher education institutions and ministries. Moreover, the digital literacy among scholars and the monitoring of the intellectual potential in the ICTs should be improved through the further development of national academic networks, as well as the improvement of regional networks and educational interconnections.

Online collaboration and digital divide in higher education

> A good educational system should have three purposes: it should provide all who want to learn with access to available resources at any time in their lives, empower all who want to share what they know to find those who want to learn it from them; and, finally, furnish all who want to present an issue to the public with the opportunity to make their challenge known (Illich, 1971, p.75).

As Internet technologies are rapidly evolving, new digital divides on the Internet emerge. In this section we move the initial concept of digital divide toward the focus in its transition from a technological to a social context (Warschauer, 2002), and focus on social media use, digital literacy skills, and collaboration in higher education in Serbia. Weber's social stratification theory focuses on access to production rather than ownership of the capital of one's production. In doing so, access to production, in this context, is access to the Internet and e-resources in order to produce information or accomplish interaction. Those without access to the Internet cannot participate in collaboration, production, and education processes. Weber was right about social stratification given that the digital divide creates new boundaries. Besides basic social stratification from a lack of computers or Internet access, we can also consider a knowledge gap, and digital literacy skills. Having Internet access does not necessarily mean that one group will use it wisely or use its resources in a smart way. For example, if a group does not possess some amount of digital literacy skills, how would they know how to use browsers for research, or to edit a Wikipedia article?

In Serbia Internet access is not the major problem (Accessing and Disseminating Scientific Information in SEE, 2005, p.23). The challenges are different. For example, within the academic community, students and researchers complained that e-resources were not available, when in fact there are over 35,000 scientific journals available. We have the paradoxical situation of e-resources not been being used at a satisfactory level due to many factors and challenges. Among these challenges is a lack of awareness and promotion, digital illiteracy and other human and economic factors indicated by the knowledge gap.

Using Weber's concepts, we can relate to his principle of *Gemeinschaft* with collaborative networks of knowledge in education (Illich, 1971). They are communities in the sense that they differ from "societies" in which links between people are purely rational and extrinsically motivated. In a community, according to Weber, there is something more affective and personal which is an adequate context for online networks. If we look at the dynamics of online communities and social networks where communication and education processes are emerging, we find that people (re)connect, interact, "like" statuses, seek validation, and dozens of other things while constantly communicating and participating online. However, by participating and creating the online public sphere, they also learn, through the processes of socialization. They use e-resources for learning and education.

These social and communication practices – networking, collaboration, and interaction between groups who commonly use the Internet and social media in Serbia – are examined with regard to professors and students. In the Weberian stratification context we have two status groups from the academic community: they are stratified by the status of their respective roles. From the qualitative research data we analyzed, professors are more concerned with technological infrastructure, human relationships, Internet adoption and other problems while students are more concerned with the lack of professors' feedback via digital means and their willingness to adopt social media, illustrating the gap in the communication and collaborative practices between the two groups.

Here is what some respondents in the semi-structured interviews had to say:

> I think the lack of financial resources in academic and in individual frames is one of the key factors for the modest application of ICTs. Also important is the indifference of teachers (from primary school to university). One should not only observe the situation in Belgrade and other large cities (which is also not great), but also examine the situation inside Serbia (Nikola, professor).

DiMaggio and Hargittai (2001) point out that social inequalities influence digital literacy, engagement in social and educational life, and overall participation and collaboration in an online public sphere. We have marginalized groups who will not have access to the Internet and therefore are not going to be able to engage in this social life and those without the necessary networked literacy skills to navigate online. Professors concerned with equipment and implementation of software in teaching, think that "the Internet should be accessible to everyone and in every place at the universities, and that is not always the case, for now."

Besides the technological challenges, professors indicate other obstacles for collaboration and participation, including lack of motivation, problems with the staff in academia, interpersonal relations, and corruption in the academic community:

> The conditions are not the same in developed and underdeveloped cities. Schools are unequally equipped; teachers are unevenly trained and motivated. A lot depends on the Director/Dean of the institution (Marko, junior faculty).

> Unfortunately, in an environment where I work, there are personal and unscientific reasons. In my faculty, the Dean has created unhuman relationships, everything is subordinated to the whims of the Dean's Office, and the Ministry of Education does not care. Collaboration takes place in personal relationships (Vesna, Professor).

We also examined the possibilities of Internet usage and social media in the learning environment as a tool for collaboration and participation that encourages and fosters communication processes and decreases the widening gap. There were communication and collaboration issues detected among professors and students.

Respondents indicated that neither group was satisfied with the participation and communication levels of their colleagues.

> Professors are very inflexible on many issues. We study from the same books for ages and in my field of study things are changing every day. There are fewer practical examples than there should be. I think the key point is to convince the professors to do their job, and their work is "to promote and disseminate knowledge." The professor has to be a leader in that sense, the first one to have an account, to create a group that supports the dissemination of information and knowledge, and not to hide them from their students (Natasa, postgraduate student).

Despite not being satisfied, professors and students agree that it is possible to initiate and foster collaboration by the introduction of the Internet and social media services into classrooms and curricula. Professors believe that by the promotion of education platforms for collaboration and learning, along with the introduction of "distance learning" and formalization of the e-courses, the present levels of collaboration can improve.

When we talk about new literacy requirements (Haythornthwaite, 2007), we include competencies related to the set of skills required of an individual in order to perform tasks that include finding, processing, producing, and communicating information as well as fluency in online technologies, communication norms, application, and programming environments.

Students think that "professors must know how to use new platforms and be leaders in that, rather than waiting for the initiative from the students." In the first place students emphasize education and training as a major factor – for both status groups – in order to use these services and obtain the necessary set of skills:

> Education for professors to use social media (at the state universities) is needed as the initiative must come from them. Moreover, some of the tools should be accepted at the institutional level and all professors should be obliged to use them.

Also, students believe that collaboration is possible by enabling access to the Internet and the content. They report that the Internet in classrooms and "computers for each of them, for each student" is crucial. Accessibility of the resources is possible "by uploading more content on the web, where the information could be easily accessible, creating the networking capability for remote collaboration."

Some scholars do not think it is possible to initiate and foster collaboration by using Internet services and social media. Some professors have said that "it is too demanding, and students are changing." Others state: "the older generations of professors are still not educated and trained to communicate electronically, and are therefore not able to use this medium."

Professors have also expressed the following opinions and feelings: uncertainty ("I do not know how our students would accept new technologies"), doubt ("I'm not sure if they would be interested in this kind of collaboration"), and concern ("There is low awareness about the possibilities of implementing social media sites for collaboration"). Other professors also commented on the motivation of their colleagues ("willingness of both sides is needed to make a contact using this form of communication"), lack of initiative from both sides, then "insufficient education of colleagues" and "maybe even fear of the new," as important issues affecting the acceptance of new technologies to enhance collaboration and participation in the academic community.

When it comes to the potential improvements to be gained by the higher education community through ICT implementation that would facilitate and encourage collaboration, professors state that there should be initiatives within the faculty as well as "new and improved policies for ICT use in education," while, students consider "open and frequent communication between teachers and students" as a very important factor. Both groups agree on the need for promotion and organization of courses for students and teachers on digital literacy.

As regards the question referring to the limitations of the current education system, related to Internet use, respondents have indicated strongly that the lack of initiative in the faculty to implement these services and present them to students is a hindrance. Also, respondents (both professors and students) said that professors are not interested in participating and accepting the new software and web technologies. They "lean towards the older, traditional ways of communication and learning."

It seems that in the omnipresent social networking surroundings there is an unbalanced momentum between these status groups, where students are more prepared than professors to use Internet services and social media. On the other hand, it strongly depends on the willingness and the motivation of professors to adopt and adjust to new ways of interacting with students. Though there is a hope of junior faculty who have already embraced digital technologies, implementing them in the classroom, and communicating online with students. Not all universities are equipped but again the above statistics show that over 50 percent of the population is on the Internet and Facebook, and those are students, so maybe a solution is to look for the future collaborative practices among these two status groups via places where students spend most of their time – and those are online habitats.

Thus our main empirical finding has revealed factors of the digital divide in the academic community, related to the stratification theory and the Weberian concept of status (*Stände*) and social power between two groups. We now turn to the possible recommendations for solutions which might lessen the digital divides.

Conclusion and further recommendations

The results provided in the statistical and qualitative analyses above show relationships between socio-economic factors and Internet use. We presented some empirical data that cannot be found in the international and national reports to indicate the importance of collaborative and participatory possibilities for bridging the digital divide.

According to the results of this research, two status groups – professors and students – agree that the ministries are demonstrating a lack of initiatives for the implementation of ICTs and that they should encourage a change in the higher education system in Serbia. A lack of policy and action related to digital literacy could lead to even higher digital divides and inequalities among different social groups.

This chapter indicates that besides the unequal access to the Internet and computers, there is a social divide as regards Internet use, a lack of twenty-first century literacies, a knowledge gap, and communication and collaboration issues between the two status groups in the context of Weberian stratification theory.

The main empirical evidence has revealed the three main factors of the digital inequalities as a growing phenomenon in the academic community in Serbia. Those are the categories of community/sociality, participation and collaboration online, as well as the contradiction and its relation to the theoretical points of stratification. Crucially, high status persons (professors at universities) need to learn and adopt social media and new technologies in order to advance digital literacy. They need to implement and encourage the use of Internet services and web sites that would enable collaboration and communication amongst other colleagues and students. Ironically, it is those who have less influence, and social power according to Weber (junior faculty, graduate students, and undergraduate students), who would be savviest with ICTs. The high status persons have less motivation. How can we encourage the professors to adopt and use new ICTs? This is the underlying conundrum, and the results raise some important questions and shed light on current issues to be solved in the future.

Collaborative possibilities using the Internet and social media present one of the most engaging opportunities for overcoming inequalities in twenty-first century literacies and fostering better collaboration and participation in higher education environments.

National government institutions should play a key role in developing, implementing and promoting a consistent higher educational policy that would encourage a wider use of the Internet in higher education. Future research will show if new improved and implemented policies will facilitate bridging the social stratification online, in order to decrease the existing digital divides.

References

Accessing and Disseminating Scientific Information in South Eastern Europe (2005). UNESCO. Available online: http://unesdoc.unesco.org/images/0015/001532/153225e.pdf (accessed 11 October 2011)

DiMaggio, P. and Hargittai E. (2001). *Digital inequality: From unequal access to differentiated use: A literature review and agenda for research on digital inequality.* Available online: http://www.eszter.com/research/pubs/dimaggio-etal-digital inequality.pdf (accessed 19 January 2012).

eGovernance and ICT Usage Report for South East Europe, 2nd Edition (2010). Sarajevo: United Nations. Available online: http://www.undp.ba/upload/publications/eGovernance%20and%20ICT%20Usage%20Report%20for%20South%20East%20Europe%202.pdf (accessed 29 September 2011).

Giddens, A. (2006). *Sociology.* 5th Edition. London: Polity.

Haythornthwaite, C. (2007), Social facilitators and inhibitors to online fluency, HICSS, p.67a, *40th Annual Hawaii International Conference on System Sciences (HICSS '07)*. Available online: http://www.computer.org/csdl/proceedings/hicss/2007/2755/00/27550067a-abs.html (accessed 14 January 2012).

Human Development Report (2010). *The real wealth of nations: Pathways to human development.* 20th Anniversary Edition. New York: United Nations. Available online: http://hdr.undp.org/en/media/HDR_2010_EN_Complete_reprint.pdf (accessed 29 September 2011).

Illich, I. (1971). *Deschooling society.* New York, Harper & Row.

Internet World Stats. (2011). Available online: http://www.internetworldstats.com/europa2.htm#rs (accessed 10 October 2011).

Meyrowitz, J. (2008). Power, pleasure, patterns: Intersecting narratives of media influence. *Journal of Communication*, 58(4), 641–663.

Radovanović, D. (2010a). Интернет парадигма, структура и динамика онлајн друштвених мрежа: Фејсбук и млади у Србији (Internet paradigm, structure, and dynamics of online social networks: Facebook and young adults in Serbia). *Pancevacko citaliste*, 3(17), 20–26.

Radovanović, D. (2010b). Serbia: Better on Facebook than in the streets, In *Global voices online.* Available online: http://eprints.rclis.org/bitstream/10760/14941/1/Radovanovic_-_Better_on_Facebook_Than_in_the_Streets.pdf (accessed 26 October 2012).

Statistical Office of the Republic of Serbia (SORS). (2011). *The use of ICT in the Republic of Serbia*, 2011. Belgrade: Government of Serbia. Available online: http://webrzs.stat.gov.rs/WebSite/Public/PageView.aspx?pKey=206 (accessed 11 October 2011).

Warschauer, M. (2002). Reconceptualizing the digital divide. *First Monday*, 7(7), 2002. Available online: http://firstmonday.org/htbin/cgiwrap/bin/ojs/index.php/fm/article/view/967/888 (accessed 14 September 2011).

Warschauer, M. (2003). *Technology and social inclusion.* Cambridge, MA, US: MIT Press

Weber, M. (1924). Class, status and party. In H. Gerth and C.W. Mills (eds.) *Essays from Max Weber.* New York: Routledge and Kegan Paul.

Notes

1 The author acknowledges the assistance of Mr. Baudry Rocquin, D.Phil. in History, University of Oxford.
2 In Europe, Eurostat conducts surveys and publishes reports, including ones related to Internet use.
3 Respondents come from state and private faculties in the territory of the Republic of Serbia. The semi-structured interviews occurred in March 2011 and March 2012.

11 Closing the gap, are we there yet?

Reflections on the persistence of second-level digital divide among adolescents in Central and Eastern Europe[1]

Monica Barbovschi
Masaryk University

Bianca Balea
Babeș-Bolyai University

Introduction

In spite of the initial enthusiasm about the Internet's capacity to facilitate access to information and thus expand access to education, jobs and better healthcare, research showed, very early, that the new technology exacerbates inequality rather than ameliorates it (DiMaggio, 2001). It became increasingly obvious that access to the Internet is dependent on various characteristics such as socio-economic status, gender, race, age, and ethnicity, and these differences are likely to reinforce inequality in opportunities for economic mobility and social participation (DiMaggio *et al.*, 2004). Arguing that mere access is not enough to ensure equal take-up of opportunities, the theorists of the second-level digital divide (Hargittai, 2002) tried to move the debate onto factors of digital inequalities from a technological deterministic view of material access, to social and cultural factors that shape patterns of use (Selwyn, 2004). In addition, the conflict perspective of digital inequalities states that without the development of Internet competencies, as a particular set of skills, access to the Internet may in fact foster enduring social inequalities (Witte and Mannon, 2010).

In line with the "emerging digital differentiation" (Peter and Valkenburg, 2006), we expected the patterns of digital inequality to be no less relevant for children than they are for adults and that socio-economical and digital inequalities among adults (parents) would reinforce/perpetuate digital inequalities among children. As in the case of adult users, significant differences can be found in the way children access and use the Internet, as indicated by research that has tried to debunk the myth of the monolithic image of the techno-savvy child (Livingstone *et al.*, 2005). Demographic variables, breadth and depth of Internet use were expected to play a role in accounting for differences in children's digital skills. In addition, parental socio-economic status and demographic variables, along with variables of parental Internet access and use were expected to influence children's Internet access and use, as well as their digital skills.

The EU Kids Online data confirms that within the 25 European countries, children differ in their level of digital skills, regardless of whether it is measured by self-reporting, the range of online activities or the beliefs in their Internet abilities, which points towards a second-level digital divide (Hasebrink *et al.*, 2011: 30). Moreover, children in Romania and Bulgaria (both countries with low GDP and recent introduction of broadband) report both the highest levels of Internet use and a very low range of online activities and digital skills as reported in Lobe *et al.* (2011), which might be an indicator of digital inequalities. These countries seemed to be perfect examples of second-level digital divide, where access is available, usage is high, but the differences in opportunities taken online, digital skills and, consequently, benefits are still widespread. For comparison purposes Poland was chosen as a country with high use, while Hungary was chosen as one of the countries with low Internet use among children. At country levels, GDP per capita and broadband penetration had no influence on children's Internet use (Lobe *et al.*, 2011), therefore, we looked at the individual level in order to account for the differences. However, the number of education years was a relevant national indicator. The fact that data from all four of these countries demonstrated cases of "digital natives," with children's Internet use surpassing that of their parents, was also noteworthy.

Building on the data from the EU Kids Online II project (2009–2011), the chapter explores the difference in access, use and skills among adolescents (aged 11 to 16) in four Central and Eastern European (CEE) countries, namely Bulgaria, Hungary, Poland and Romania, under the assumption that these differences might still be attributed to socio-economical inequalities (Witte and Mannon, 2010).

Literature review

Two dominant perspectives have emerged in the attempt to understand the connection between social categories and digital inequalities: enthusiasts of the digital revolution, who prophesized a relationship between the increase in level of access and a decrease of the digital gaps (Howard *et al.*, 2001; Norris, 2001) and pessimists, who foresaw deeper divides appearing (van Dijk, 1999; van Dijk, 2005; DiMaggio, 2001; Hargittai, 2002; Katz and Rice, 2002; Wellman and Chen, 2005).

According to the latter, the differences in the way we use the Internet go much deeper. Hargittai and Zillien (2009) highlight that individuals cultivate different forms of Internet practice depending on their socio-economic background. Individuals with high status are much more likely to engage in capital-enhancing activities[2] online and subsequently, to reap more benefits from their time spent online than users from lower socio-economic backgrounds. Scholars like DiMaggio (2001; DiMaggio *et al.*, 2004), Hargittai (2010) and Zillien (Hargittai and Zillien, 2009), Wellman and Chen (2005), and van Dijk (2005) have advanced original theoretical models for the studying of digital divides which include differences in equipment, autonomy of use, social support, skill, and the purposes for which one is using the Internet (DiMaggio *et al.*, 2004; Hassani, 2006 as cited by Hargittai and Hinnant, 2008).

Another model advanced by van Dijk (2005) takes into account a number of personal and positional categorical inequalities in society, the distribution of resources[3] relevant to this type of inequality, a number of types of access to ICTs and a number of fields of participation in society. The relationship between these factors can be summarized as follows: personal and positional categorical inequalities in society produce an unequal distribution of resources, which leads to an unequal access to digital technologies, causing unequal participation in society, which reinforces categorical inequalities, and unequal distribution of resources. In other words, as one gap closes, another one opens, pointing towards a rather dystopian view of social inequalities.

Adolescents and the digital divide

Most studies have shown that traditional measures of inequality – age, gender, socio-economic status (SES) – influence access, use and online skills. However, few have been preoccupied with the differences in digital access, use and skills among children and adolescents. These few studies (e.g. Livingstone *et al.*, 2005; Livingstone and Helsper, 2007), however, suggest that demographic factors directly influence young people's experience of both online opportunities and risks. Older children, it seems, both take up more opportunities (educational, civic, communicative, creative, etc. [see Livingstone *et al.*, 2005]) and encounter more risk. Also, there is evidence that those from higher SES homes not only have better Internet access, but also take up a greater range of opportunities online (Kaiser Family Foundation, 2005; Livingstone and Helsper, 2007). According to Livingstone and Helsper's study (2007), SES has no direct influence on either opportunities or risks, but only influences access, resulting in inequalities that have indirect but significant consequences. The policy implications were intriguing; while middle-class parents often provide better access for their children, for those middle- and working-class children with equivalent access, there are few or no direct effects of SES on use, literacy or opportunities. Enhancing quality of access (i.e. more sites of access, more private use) for less privileged teenagers could, therefore, reduce the digital divide among young people (Livingstone and Helsper, 2010).

In addition, a "rich get richer" model of online communication (Kraut *et al.*, 2002; McKenna *et al.*, 2002) can envision the development of skills as a consequence of a more intense communication pattern. In their study on Dutch adolescents aged 13 to 18, Peter and Valkenburg (2006) pitted the perspective of a disappearing digital divide against the perspective of an emerging digital differentiation and found support for the latter. They advanced the prediction that teenagers with more socio-economic, cognitive and cultural resources will use the Internet more as an information and social medium, while less advantaged adolescents will mostly use the Internet as an entertainment medium. This appears to be the case for Romanian and Hungarian teenagers in the EU Kids Online study, since they engage mostly in entertainment activities rather than in creative, advanced uses (Hasebrink *et al.*, 2011).

Moreover, since educational background is related to the integration of digital technologies in the daily lives of individuals (Bonfadelli, 2002; Korupp and Szydlik, 2005), we can expect that the educational level of parents has an influence on how their children make use of these digital technologies.

Drawing from the same perspective, we would expect to see some relationship between types of Internet use and class position/class background (Witte and Mannon, 2010: 84), since "conflict" theorists argue that class inequality is reproduced across generations. Another interesting concept, "the sedimentation of racial inequality" (Oliver and Shapiro, 1995), offers a similar understanding of the perpetuation of digital inequalities from one generation to another. This chapter aims to contribute to our understanding of the phenomenon of digital "stratification" and inter-generational digital inequalities, in a region where these differences are expected to matter most.

The EU Kids Online project (2009–2011) has showed, beyond any doubt, that most children are fully online at an increasingly earlier age. The findings presented in Livingstone *et al.* (2011); Lobe *et al.* (2011); and Hasebrink *et al.* (2011) offer detailed accounts on patterns of access, use and skills among children aged 9 to 16 across Europe. Half of European children use the Internet from a private room at home and older children spend nearly two hours online every day (Livingstone *et al.*, 2011). Among the findings that are relevant for this chapter are: private use is strongly differentiated by age and the education of the household; more various and sophisticated access and use is differentiated by SES and education; children are further differentiated in terms of breadth of online activities, which points towards a "ladder of opportunities" influenced by age, gender (boys conduct more online activites) and parental education. Digital literacy skills and safety skills also differ by age, gender (boys declare more) and parental education (Hasebrink *et al.*, 2011: 22–23, 27).

Among the four countries investigated, the differences are strongly marked: in terms of locations of use and devices for accessing the Internet, all reported below average figures (Lobe *et al.*, 2011: 23). Bulgarian children have the highest number of average skills (4.7) and highest number of reported activities (7.8), followed by Poland with 4.5 and 7.1 respectively, then Hungary and Romania (both scoring 3.4 average skills, and 7.5 and 7.3, on online activities respectively). The European averages were 4.2 for skills and 7.2 for activities (Lobe *et al.*, 2011: 26). If we look in the ladder of opportunities at "advanced and creative uses," Poland and Romania have the lowest levels among all European countries (15 and 14 percent), while Bulgaria and Hungary have quite high levels, (27 and 33) compared to the 23 percent European average.

Our research questions, inspired by the ideas advanced by Livingstone and Helsper (2007), are related to the three perspectives taken into consideration: children's emerging digital differentiation, the conflict perspective and the inter-generational transfer of digital inequalities:

1   Is there a digital divide among adolescents in CEE countries? If so, what role do age, gender and type of Internet use play in the digital skills of adolescents?
2   Does the parental digital divide perpetuate the digital divide among children?
3   Does the parental background perpetuate the digital divide among children?

Our analytical model

Four major types of variables were employed to explain differences in digital skills and confidence in Internet use for children in Hungary, Romania, Poland and Bulgaria. A first set of parental background variables was included in order to establish a "class positioning" or parental background. Second, another set, related to parental Internet use and level of support for various online activities of the child, was included. The child demographics were also taken into account and last, variables related to children's access and use were introduced. Also noteworthy, the two types of dependent variables, confidence in one's Internet abilities and digital skills (or competencies) of children are all interdependent with children's online activities.

The digital skills of children included in the questionnaire can be divided into what van Dijk and Hacker (2003) call instrumental and informational skills (for detailed description, see Hasebrink *et al.*, 2011).

While we can assume that more activities lead both to more confidence and more skills, building up more skills and more confidence also works as a facilitator for taking up more activities (opportunities) online. Therefore a causal link is difficult to pinpoint. Based on these assumptions and on previous literature, we propose the following analytical model, with all four sets of predictors having direct and indirect influences on the dependent variables (Figure 11.1).

Concretely, the analysis was driven by the testing of the following hypotheses:

H1. In line with the "emerging digital differentiation" and the "rich get richer" model, we expect inequalities in confidence and skills among adolescents, even if they all have access to the Internet. Specifically, we expect that differences in private use, number of years online and range of activities undertaken online will account for differences in confidence and skills.

H2. In line with the conflict perspective, we expect that differences in socio-economic status/educational background will account for differences in the range of activities undertaken online and range of digital skills developed by adolescents.

H3. According to a model of "inter-generational digital transfer", we expect that parental usage influences the children's digital outcomes (confidence and skills).

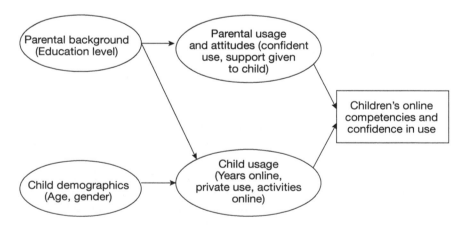

Figure 11.1 Analytical model for children's digital competencies and confidence in own Internet use in Bulgaria, Hungary, Poland and Romania.

Method

The EU Kids Online project collected data from a random stratified survey sample of 1000 children and one of their parents in each participating country. For the purpose of our study, only responses from children 11 to 16 years old in the four countries were taken into account (N=3154). The sample includes 48 percent girls and 52 percent boys with an average age of 13 years (*SD*=1.7). Our analyses included two types of dependent variables: children's confidence in their use of the Internet (child confident use, or children's belief in their Internet abilities, in Hasebrink *et al.*, 2011) and their digital competencies or skills (online competencies).

The variables used in our analyses were grouped in four categories: independent parent related; intermediate parent related; independent child related; and intermediate child related (Table 11.1).

Correlations among all variables entered in the analytical model revealed systematic relations between demographic variables of parent and child, parent's Internet use, child's Internet access and use, and finally, the child's online activities and competencies.

However, in order to account for causal effects between variables, a path analysis was conducted with AMOS. In order to control multicollinearity problems,[4] we decided to include the highest level of education in the household instead of SES (since SES was derived from the education and occupation of the household main wage earner), even if the same relations were observed when using SES. Following the previous literature and based on the correlation indicators, some relationships were hypothesized (such as the link between use and confidence in personal use, or use and skills); also, following the logic of second-level digital divide and inter-generational digital transfer, we expected significant relationships between parent-related variables and intermediate children-related variables, on one hand, and the dependent variables, on the other hand.

Analyses and results

The correlations indicators suggest that older teenagers and boys have more years online than girls, engage in more online activities, are more confident and report more online competencies. Children from more privileged backgrounds receive more support from their parents, are more confident in their usage, are online longer, experience greater private use, and also display more digital skills than the less privileged children. But it is not only demographics variables that create differential usage. There are significant correlations between intermediate variables as well. More time spent online and the possibility to use the Internet in a private manner can also affect the way children use the Internet.

Table 11.1 Descriptive statistics of variables employed

Variable type		Mean	Standard Deviation	Description
Independent parent related	Education level	4.2	1.2	Highest education level completed by the head of the household.
Independent child related	Age	13.4	1.72	Scale variable, 11–16 years old.
	Gender	—	0.5	Dummy, Female=0.
Intermediate parent related	Parent confident use	0.7	0.4	Dummy, Confident=1.
	Parental support	5.7	3.2	Range 0 to 11, calculated from "Yes" responses to the question "Which of the following things, if any, do you sometimes do with your child?" Eleven activities listed, such as talking to the child about what he or she does on the internet. Full list in Hasebrink *et al.* (2011).
Intermediate child related	Years online	3.9	2.07	Number of years online, scale variable, Highest=13.
	Private use	0.6	0.4	Private use from the bedroom and/or mobile. Dummy variable, Yes=1.
	Online Activities	7.3	3.3	Scale variable, the number out of 16 possible activities, such as using the internet for schoolwork or visiting a chat room.
Dependent variables	Child confident use	0.8	0.3	"I know lots of things about using the internet." Dummy variable, True=1.
	Digital competencies	3.9	2.6	Scale variable, the number out of 8 in total.

Figure 11.2 presents the causal paths between our variables, for all four countries, with the significant path (beta) coefficients.

In the European dataset, activities, skills and children's belief in their Internet abilities are all positively associated (Hasebrink *et al.*, 2011: 30). This remained true, unsurprisingly, in our general model and at country levels as well: children with higher activity on the Internet become more confident and more skilled.

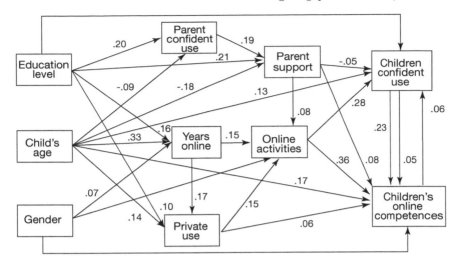

Figure 11.2 Path model for children's digital competencies (skills) and confidence in own Internet use in Bulgaria, Hungary, Poland and Romania

Source: EU Kids Online dataset, own Path analyses; Base: all children 11–16 in Bulgaria, Hungary, Romania and Poland who use the Internet; all path coefficients significant at p < .01 and p < .05 levels. The model fit was considered acceptable based on the following indicators for complex models: RMSEA values=.046 (with a confidence interval .812) and a CFI value=.970. The value of chi-square ($\chi 2$ (16) = 121.7 significant at p < .01) isn't relevant since chi-square values are known to be very sensitive to large sample sizes (Kline, 2005). The model is confirmed for each individual country.

First, as predicted in our first hypothesis, the analysis revealed a differential usage pattern for the children 11 to 16 years old who use the Internet. Both parent and child-related variables have significant influence on children's digital outcomes. Moreover, parents with higher educational backgrounds are more confident in their use and provide more support for their children, which in turn increases their online competencies. However, older children have less confident parents and receive less support from their families, which is to be expected with the increasing autonomy of adolescents and their gaining more confidence in using the Internet. Conversely, the more the parents know about and use the Internet, the less children report confidence in their own use.

Regarding child-related variables, boys display more Internet self-confidence than girls, regardless of parental background or Internet usage. Moreover, older children and boys are more experienced than younger children and girls, are online longer and are engaging in more online activities, also becoming more confident and skilled. In terms of the "rich get richer" paradigm, our analysis sustains that more privileged children are using the Internet for a longer time and more privately, which helps them rally more online activities and also develop more confidence and more skills. This might be a late effect of the first-level digital divide, with parents in more privileged positions having been able to offer earlier Internet access to their children.

Parents from higher SES households are also more active in terms of giving advice about use and safety (since they are more likely to be users themselves and more technically competent, according to Hasebrink *et al.*, 2011: 12). In our analyses, parents' education is a predictor for their confidence in Internet use as well as for the amount of support given, which, in turn, work as predictors for their children's Internet competencies.

Country-specific results

As in the general model for all four countries, in the case of Romanian teenagers ($\chi2(16)$=42.46, *CFI*=.97, *RMSEA*=0.047), age holds a direct relation with all dependent and independent variables, while gender has a slight influence on children's years online (boys generally having more than girls). The influence of parental support is higher for Romanian teenagers when it comes to their online competencies, but has no influence on children's confident use. Educational level remains a strong predictor for intermediate variables, with more influence on parental support and online experience (years online), which becomes a stronger predictor for the number of activities that children are conducting online. Apparently the digital gap between children, based on their background, is increasing: on the one hand, the chances that less privileged children access the Internet earlier are decreasing, as is the range of online activities they embrace, this results in them being less skilled and less confident than the privileged children. On the other hand, Romanian teenagers rely more on parental support than other children, which provides evidence for an inter-generational transfer, which might not always carry the best outcomes for children (fewer skills to pass on to their children, less effective mediation, etc.).

In the Bulgarian model ($\chi2(16)$=40.41, *CFI*=.974, *RMSEA*=0.031), as in the case of the general model, age and child usage variables have significant correlations with all dependent variables. Parental educational background remains a strong predictor for the child-related variables, thus confirming the second-level digital divide (with differences in access and use accounting for differences in activities and skills). However, parental usage variables have no significant influence on child's digital outcomes, indicating the lack of support for an inter-generational digital transfer.

As in the case of Bulgarian adolescents, the educational background of Hungarian parents has an indirect impact on the digital skills and confidence of Hungarian adolescents ($\chi2(16)$=31.72, *CFI*=.976, *RMSEA*=0.036). However, parental usage seems to have a slight impact on children's digital outcomes. The case of the Hungarian digital divide is more a case of second-level digital divide rather than a case of inter-generational digital transfer, with differences in access and use (determined also by socio-economical background) accounting for differences in skills. Child-related variables (demographics and usage being the ones that hold the most important effect), support an "emerging differentiation" pattern of the divide.

Finally, the Polish model ($\chi2(16)$=32.73, *CFI*=.978, *RMSEA*=0.036) shows support for the "emerging differentiation" paradigm, for the inter-generational transfer and for the second-level digital divide. Poland was the only case where parental usage variables had a substantial impact on both of the children's digital outcomes.

Discussion

The population that the EU Kids Online project surveyed was children 9–16 who use the Internet across Europe therefore the discussion around this data has to be already situated in the framework of "second-level digital divide." The present chapter aimed to offer a comprehensive explanatory framework for the patterns of digital inequalities among adolescents (aged 11 to 16) in four CEE countries, namely Bulgaria, Hungary, Poland and Romania. Taking into account different theoretical approaches, we pitted several models against each other, in order to make sense of the second-level digital divide(s) among the teenagers in our sample. Simultaneously, we examined the plausibility of a model of emerging differentiation, with a specific variant of the "rich get richer" hypothesis (with differences in access and use accounting for differences in activities, skills and confidence), of the conflict perspective (differences in socio-economical background determining differences in activities, skills and confidence) and finally, a model of inter-generational digital transfer, where parental digital literacy and competence influence their children's own skills and confidence in Internet use.

Consistent with previous evidence, we found that older children and those coming from households with higher educational backgrounds enjoy better access (more private use, both at home and mobile) and longer use (more years online, longer time spent online). Gender did not hold a particularly strong effect, although, as in previous findings, boys tend, to some degree, to use the Internet longer (for more years, also more throughout a day) or to develop more confidence in using the Internet. Due to the connection between educational background and domestication of digital technologies (Bonfadelli, 2002; Korupp and Szydlik, 2005), we expected a connection between parental education and children's Internet use. In all four cases, the socio-economical background (here, the education of the household) held significant influences on children's digital outcomes (competencies, confidence). As we found, Internet inequalities are mapped into existing inequalities and further amplify these inequalities in some cases, indicating support for the conflict paradigm (Witte and Mannon, 2010).

The data from all countries demonstrated child-specific differentiations, with variables of background and usage having a strong impact on the digital outcomes, offering support for the emerging differentiation model and the "rich get richer" paradigm (years online for Romania and Bulgaria, and private use for Poland and Hungary).

Finally, the model of inter-generational digital transfer was moderately supported only for Romanian and Polish teenagers.

In terms of policy recommendations, Romanian and Polish children could benefit more from the opportunities the Internet has to offer if given stronger parental guidance and support. As long as the parents remain digitally illiterate, there is little they can offer to their children in order to ensure the maximization of "digital benefits." In addition, the strong link between children's usage, activities, competencies and confidence in own Internet skills, evidenced also by Hasebrink *et al.* (2011), indicates that policy interventions (from politicians, teachers, educational providers, industry, e-safety networks, etc.) should be directed towards developing more digital competencies in children and teenagers, thus creating a "virtuous circle" (more competencies, resulting in more activities, leading to more confidence, allowing more opportunities). Finally, as confirmed by previous studies (Livingstone and Helsper, 2010), increasing quality of access (more private use, more points of access) would contribute to closing the gap between the level of Internet opportunities accessed by children. We are not there yet, but hopefully we are slowly getting closer.

The limitations of our analyses touch different levels, two of them being more salient for the scope and purpose of this book. First, the data collected in the EU Kids Online project allows analyses mostly at a level of second-level digital divide, since the survey population was children aged 9–16 who use the Internet. Another limitation sprang from our theoretical framework: although we tried to compare different theoretical models, deciding *a priori* which theories to include is an intrinsic flaw of "quantitative sociological thinking." For example, our model did not include variables related to the mediation of children's Internet use by peers or teachers. In spite of these, we hope that our chapter has offered a substantial contribution in providing a nuanced understanding of the digital differences among teenagers in CEE countries. Much remains to be explored and constantly updated due to the changing nature of the digital landscape.

References

Bonfadelli, H. (2002). The Internet and knowledge gaps. A theoretical and empirical investigation. *European Journal of Communication*, 17, 65–84.

DiMaggio, P. (2001). Social implications of the Internet. *Annual Review of Sociology,* *27,* 307–336.

DiMaggio, P., Hargittai, E., Celeste, C. and Shafer, S. (2004). *Digital Inequality: From unequal access to differentiated use.* New York: Russell Sage.

Hargittai, E. (2002). Second-level digital divide: Differences in people's online skills. *First Monday,* 7(4). Retrieved 25 October 2011 from http://www.uic.edu/htbin/cgiwrap/bin/ojs/index.php/fm/article/view/942/864.

Hargittai, E. (2010). Digital na(t)ives? Variation in Internet skills and uses among members of the Net generation. *Sociological Inquiry, 80* (1), 92–113.

Hargittai, E. and Hinnant, A. (2008). Digital inequality: Differences in young adults' use of the Internet. *Communication Research, 35* (5), 602–621.

Hargittai, E. and Zillien, N. (2009). Digital distinction: Status-specific types of Internet usage. *Social Science Quarterly, 90*(2), 274–291.

Hasebrink, U., Görzig, A., Haddon, L., Kalmus, V. and Livingstone, S. (2011). *Patterns of risk and safety online. In-depth analyses from the EU Kids Online survey of 9–16 year olds and their parents in 25 countries.* London: EU Kids Online.

Howard, P., Rainie, L. and Jones, S. (2001). Days and nights on the Internet: The impact of a diffusing technology. *American Behavioral Scientist, 45* (3), 383–404.

Kaiser Family Foundation (2005). *Generation M: Media in the lives of 8–18 year-olds.* Released at a forum on 9 March 2005 in Washington DC. Available online: http://www.kff.org/entmedia/upload/generation-m-media-in-the-lives-of-8-18-year-olds-report.pdf

Katz, J. E. and Rice, R. E. (2002). *Social consequences of Internet use: Access, involvement and interaction.* Cambridge, MA, US: MIT Press.

Kline, R. B. (2005). *Principles and practice of structural equation modeling,* 2nd Edition. New York: Guilford Press.

Korupp, S. E. and Szydlik, M. (2005). Causes and trends of the digital divide. *European Sociological Review, 21,* 409–422.

Kraut, R., Kiesler, S., Boneva, B., Cummings, J., Helgeson, V. and Crawford, A. (2002). Internet paradox revisited. *Journal of Social Issues,* 58, 49–74.

Livingstone, S. and Helsper, E. (2007). Gradations in digital inclusion: Children, young people and the digital divide. *New Media & Society,* 9, 671–696.

Livingstone, S. and Helsper, E. (2010). Balancing opportunities and risks in teenagers' use of the Internet: The role of online skills and family context. *New Media and Society,12*(2), 309–329.

Livingstone, S., Bober, M. and Helsper, E. (2005). *Internet literacy among children and young people.* Findings from the UK Children Go Online project. London: London School of Economics and Political Science. Retrieved 25 October 2011 from http://www.children-go-online.net.

Livingstone, S., Haddon, L., Görzig, A. and Ólafsson, K. (2011). *Risks and safety on the Internet: The perspective of European children. Full findings.* London: EU Kids Online.

Lobe, B., Livingstone, S., Ólafsson, K. and Vodeb, H. (2011). *Cross-national comparison of risks and safety on the Internet: Initial analysis from the EU Kids Online survey of European children.* London: EU Kids Online.

McKenna, K. Y. A., Green, A. S. and Gleason, M. E. J. (2002). Relationship formation on the Internet: What's the big attraction? *Journal of Social Issues,* 58, 9–31.

Norris, P. (2001). *Digital divide: Civic engagement, information poverty, and the Internet worldwide.* Cambridge, UK: Cambridge University Press.

Oliver, M. and Shapiro, T. M. (1995). *Black wealth/white wealth: A new perspective on racial inequality*. New York: Routledge.

Peter, J. and Valkenburg, P. M. (2006). Adolescents' Internet use: Testing the "disappearing digital divide" versus the "emerging digital differentiation" approach. *Poetics*, 34, *293–305*.

Selwyn, N. (2004). Technology and social inclusion. *British Journal of Educational Technology*, 35(1), 127–127.

Van Dijk, J. (1999). *The network society: Social aspects of new media*. London: Sage.

Van Dijk, J. (2005). *The deepening divide*. London: Sage.

Van Dijk, J. and Hacker, K. (2003). The digital divide as a complex and dynamic phenomenon. *The Information Society*. 19, 315–326.

Wellman, B. and Chen, W. (2005). Minding the cyber-gap. The Internet and social inequality. In M. Romero and E. Margolis (Eds.). *Blackwell companion to social inequalities*. Oxford, UK: Blackwell.

Witte, J. and Mannon, S. 2010. *The Internet and social inequalities*. New York: Routledge.

Notes

1   This chapter is based on the data collected by the EU Kids Online II project, funded by the EC Safer Internet Programme, http://ec.europa.eu/information_society/activities/sip/ from 2009–2011 (contract SIP-KEP-321803). For detailed reports, consult www.eukidsonline.net.

2   DiMaggio and Hargittai name capital-enhancing activities as those activities that may lead to more informed political participation, help with one's career advancement, or consultation of information about financial and health services. They argue that not all online activities are equally important to enhancing one's human, financial, and social capital (Hargittai and Hinnant, 2008; DiMaggio *et al.*, 2004).

3   These are resources linked to different kinds of access to digital technology that van Dijk (2005: 20) discusses: temporal resources, material resources, mental resources, social resources, and cultural resources.

4   All VIF and toleration coefficients were at acceptable levels.

12 Behind the slogan of "e-State"

Digital stratification in Estonia[1]

Veronika Kalmus
Kairi Talves
Pille Pruulmann-Vengerfeldt
University of Tartu

Introduction

The post-socialist transition in Estonia is often viewed as a particular case among Central and East European countries. Specifically, the economic reforms in Estonia have been most radical, particularly with regard to highly liberal transformation policies, sometimes highlighted as the key component of the success of the Estonian case. Moreover, societal changes mixed with political aspirations and radical reforms enjoyed high legitimacy, largely due to the still-perceived "Russian threat" and narratives about the first period of independence (1918–1940) as the "good old days" (Vihalemm and Kalmus, 2009), enabling the presentation of the transition as a "return to Europe" or even as a "return to normality" (Helemäe and Saar, 2011). However, Lauristin and Vihalemm (2009) emphasize that the economy-centered transition culture has taken the perspectives of the most successful social actors and framed these as self-evident aims for the whole society, thus legitimizing the political approaches that prioritize the economic dimensions of the reform and devalue their social implications. Closely related to the economy-dominated paradigm, technological change has also been a crucial component of Estonian transition. "Internetization" has become one of the central symbols of the rapidly changing society, leading to a widely held perception of Estonia as a leading e-state (Runnel *et al.*, 2009).

Witte and Mannon stress the need for understanding "how the Internet is mapped onto existing social inequalities" and "the ways in which digital technology feeds off the social context wherein inequality plays a starring role" (Witte and Mannon, 2010, p. 51). In this chapter, we aim to analyze digital stratification in Estonia with the focus on different aspects of access to and use of the Internet. We place our analysis in the context of social stratification in Estonia to see whether the hopes prevailing in the information society policies about ICTs closing the gaps between different social groups can be confirmed.

Partially due to the 50-year-long Soviet regime, which almost totally eradicated class-based social differentiation, the class structure in Estonia is vague, unsettled and blended with different markers of social status. Therefore, our starting point for exploring (digital) stratification in Estonia is a cultural perspective, which turns "attention to the multi-dimensional nature of inequality" and "raises the issue of lifestyle and consumption, which become critical angles to evaluate the impact of new forms of information and communication technology" (Witte and Mannon, 2010, p. 86).

Stratification in Estonia

Max Weber has drawn a distinction between "class" and "status", arguing that classes are groups of people who, from the standpoint of specific interests, have the same economic position. Positively and negatively privileged status groups are formed on the basis of claiming social esteem or lack of it, which is typically practiced as well as expressed through a specific style of life. Status may rest on class position; however, it is not solely determined by it. Money and entrepreneurial position are not in themselves status qualifications, although they may lead to them, and the lack of property is not in itself a status disqualification, although this may be a reason for it (Weber, 1978 [1922], p. 306).

Similarly, Pierre Bourdieu accepts economic capital as the main principle of domination in capitalist society, but observes that the efficacy of economic capital as a principle of stratification is constantly challenged by fractions of the dominant class (e.g. artists, professionals and academics) who are relatively poor in economic capital, but who by nature of their social role, are rich in cultural and/or other forms of capital, striving to enhance their specific form of capital as a rivaling principle. Bourdieu, thus, extends the concept of capital with multiple forms of capitals, which are increasingly becoming a new basis of social stratification. He argues that members of the class share the same objective structures, which give them the same objective meanings of collective practices. These common practices include similarities in lifestyle or certain "taste" that is reflected in "habitus" (Bourdieu, 1984 [1979], p. 311). In contemporary societies where ICTs are becoming increasingly important in almost all spheres of life, differences in capitals, taste, and habitus manifest more and more in distinctive consumption patterns, self-expression, and cultural practices that are based upon unequal access to ICT products and digital services.

Patterns of social and digital stratification in Estonia need to be seen in the context of yet unsettled and somewhat paradoxical differentiation of classes and status groups, resulting from rapid changes in the political and economic order in the past century. After the collapse of the Soviet Union in 1991, emerging stratification manifested in significant income differences. Processes of privatization and liberalization of the market resulted in a remarkable gap between different classes with regard to quantitative (e.g. Gini index) and qualitative (e.g. lack of social coherence) measures. Emerging economic inequality led to a discourse about "two Estonias" where the "winners" of the transformation enjoyed the benefits of the growing economy and the "losers" were lagging behind (Lauristin, 2003). Additionally, such division clearly reflected the mind-set and value system of the society, which highlighted economic means as the measure of success and emphasized individuals' responsibility in social mobility.

Although stratification is still largely explained by the economic aspect, studies have indicated the diversification of stratification and emergence of the gaps between class-based and status-based social esteem (Lindeman, 2011). Perceived social status is more clearly shaped not just by labor market success as measured by income, but is also dependent on demographic predictors such as age, gender, and ethnicity. Increased risks and vulnerability to transformation were shifted towards more disadvantaged social groups. For example, it is argued that Estonia experienced a change from a "gerontocratic" to a "youth-oriented" society (Tallo and Terk, 1998). Studies of perceived social status (e.g. Lindeman, 2011) indeed have shown significant differences from Western countries with Estonian young people estimating their social position to be higher, compared to other age groups, regardless of education and income. The oldest age group that mostly includes pensioners has the lowest perceived social status. Such differences may seem surprising, taking account of the fact that the youth unemployment rate in Estonia is one of the highest in Europe. The paradox can be explained by considering that status-based stratification is related to lifestyle and social practices. Studies of consumption and media use in Estonia (Lauristin, 2004) demonstrated that perceived social status was strongly influenced by the level of adaptation to the standards of the emerging consumer and information society. Consumerist orientation and digital skills as new success markers were most rapidly adopted by younger generations, while more inert elderly people experienced a decline in social status and even marginalization.

Status-based stratification is also influenced by complex and multi-dimensional inequalities between men and women. On the one hand, women have, on average, higher education levels than men, and they enjoy equal participation in jobs. On the other hand, gender segregation on the labor market, a high gender pay gap, and unbalanced gender roles in the domestic sphere (Vainu *et al.*, 2010) are still marking the reproduction of traditional patriarchal structures and gender stereotypes in the society.

After 1991, Russians and other ethnic minorities faced a double challenge of self-determination: in terms of post-socialist transition and the restored Estonian nation-state (Vihalemm and Kalmus, 2009). The new situation set the Russian-speaking community into a marginalized position, characterized by objective indicators such as higher unemployment rates and job insecurity, as well as subjective feelings of inequality and exclusion, and non-activism in politics.

Education and employment status are also important resources for sensing oneself higher in the social hierarchy. Compared to people with higher levels of education, those with lower levels of education are more likely to give a lower estimation of their social status. People who are employed are more likely to estimate their social position significantly higher than the unemployed or retired people, even when income is controlled for (Lindeman, 2011).

To sum up, the most privileged group in Estonia regarding both the class and status characteristics is young, employed ethnic Estonians with high education and income levels (Lindeman, 2011). In the following analysis, we explore whether this pattern also holds with regard to digital stratification.

From digital divide to digital stratification

The term "digital divide" was coined to indicate the gap between "haves" and "have-nots," resulting directly from lack of access or related skills to use ICTs in order to maximally gain in terms of information, various types of capital, and other socially desirable benefits. Lack of access will result in "digibetism" (that is, lack of digital literacy), which in turn will lead to societies divided between the information rich and the information poor (Carpentier, 2003).

Access-related questions dominated in digital divide research in the 1990s. In the next decade, the focus shifted to more diverse and rich descriptions of various shades of inequalities related to the new information and communication technologies. For example, Jan van Dijk (2006) has drawn attention to skills, knowledge, and motivation as important aspects of creating digital stratification. Furthermore, the digital divides are no longer seen as a problem of an individual but rather as resulting from contextual and social resources (Tsatsou *et al.*, 2009). Deepening digital divides, in turn, reproduce and aggravate social stratification, thus effectively hindering information society developments, especially in the context where both public and private sphere services are increasingly becoming available exclusively online. Hence, the digital divides are both seen as a symptom and a cause of broader economic inequality and social exclusion (Parayil, 2005).

In proceeding to analyze digital stratification in Estonia from the cultural perspective, we view digital inequality as multi-dimensional, that is, as being related to class position and status differences (Witte and Mannon, 2010). On top of that, we assume that differences in Internet use are conditioned by a number of other factors such as individuals' lifespan, their social roles and duties, and social capital and integration in the society. These factors vary greatly depending on demographic characteristics that are, together with indicators of social class and status, the focus of our chapter.

Our analysis is based on data from the third wave of the survey Me. The World. The Media, conducted in October 2008. The survey covered the Estonian population aged 15 to 74 years, with a total sample size of 1,507 respondents. A proportional model of the general population (by areas and urban/rural division) and multi-step probability random sampling (realized through primary random sampling of settlements with a proportional likelihood related to the size of the settlement, followed by random sampling of households and individuals) was used. In addition, a quota was applied to include a proportional number of representatives of the ethnic majority and the minority, differentiated according to the preferred language of the survey interview (Estonian or Russian, respectively). A face-to-face interviewing method was used.

In our analysis, we employ three demographic characteristics: gender, age, and ethnicity. For the latter, we use the preferred language of the survey interview (Estonian for the ethnic majority, and Russian for the minority). In addition, we make use of two indicators of social class – level of education and income per family member – and an indicator of social status. The latter was conceptualized in the study as social representation of stratification, and operationalized as respondents' self-evaluated position on the imagined social ladder, visually presented in the questionnaire in the form of a stairway, rising from step one to step ten (cf. Lauristin, 2004). The resulting variable was shortened to a five-point scale, ranging from 1 – low stratum to 5 – high stratum. This indicator of social status, approximating to normal distribution, was not dependent on gender. Ethnic Estonians estimated their status somewhat higher ($M = 3.25$; $SD = 1.30$) than the Russian-speaking minority did ($M = 3.09$; $SD = 1.33$; $p < 0.05$). As expected, perceived social status was negatively correlated with age ($r = -.25$; $p < 0.001$). Furthermore, status was positively correlated with the number of years in education ($r = 0.24$; $p < 0.001$), but even more strongly with income per family member ($r = 0.33$; $p < 0.001$). This suggests that in Estonia, as a transition society, economic success still tends to dominate over educational and cultural factors in the formation of social representation of stratification, confirming the findings of the first wave of the Me. The World. The Media survey in 2002 (Lauristin, 2004).

To find out patterns of digital inequality, we first introduce a basic division of Internet users and non-users. Altogether 73 percent of the respondents were Internet users at the time of the survey. Figure 12.1 shows statistically significant differences based on language, age, education, income and social status. Thus, the divides in access and basic usage of the

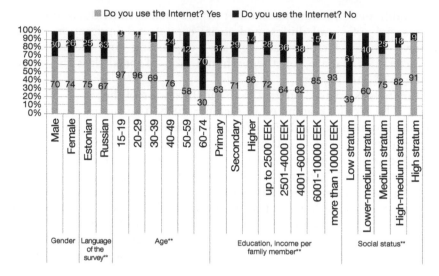

Figure 12.1 Internet users and non-users in Estonia (N = 1,507).
Note: ** p < 0.01.

Internet mirror quite adequately the patterns of social stratification described above. Compared to the results of the 2002 survey data (Runnel and Pruulmann-Vengerfeldt, 2004), according to which significantly more men were using the Internet, we can say that the gender gap in access has closed. The divides based on language, age and education have remained the same. The relationship with income was linear in 2002 with fewer Internet users among the low-income groups but showed a non-linear curve in 2008 with somewhat more Internet users in the two lower and the two higher income groups compared to the middle-income group. This may be explained by the fact that families with children tend to have lower income per family member, while being avid Internet users.

Inequalities in Internet use

In the following analysis we focus on socio-demographic differences in the intensity and versatility of Internet use. We employ the sub-sample of Internet users of the 2008 wave of the Me. The World. The Media survey. As 369 respondents answered that they had never used the Internet, and 38 respondents did not answer the question, 1,100 participants remained in this analysis with mean age of 38.29 years (*SD* = 14.76). Of the remaining sample, 55 percent were females; 70 percent of the respondents completed the questionnaire in Estonian and 30 percent in Russian, respectively.

For the indicator of the intensity of Internet use we employ an index of the frequency of Internet use, measured with three items: How frequently do you use the Internet (1) at work or school, (2) at home, and (3) elsewhere (Internet cafés, public Wi-Fi hotspots, at friends' places, etc.). The respondents were asked to answer each question on a five-point scale, ranging from 0 – not at all to 4 – almost every day. The maximum value of the index is, thus, 12.

To compare the versatility of Internet use, extending to different spheres of life, we make use of an empirically robust and theoretically easily interpretable classification of online activities, drawn upon the same database in a previous analysis (see Kalmus *et al.*, 2011). Based on factor analysis of 30 online activities, the previous study proposed a simple and stable two-factor structure. The first factor, labeled as "social media and entertainment related Internet use" (hereafter, SME), contains variables such as searching for and managing information regarding friends and acquaintances on social networking portals; searching for entertainment; participating in forums, blogs, surveys, and writing comments; communicating with friends and acquaintances; and sharing music, films, and programs, and is indicative of personal need for entertainment, fun, self-expression, and maintaining social relations. The second factor, labeled as "work and information related Internet use" (hereafter WI), includes activities such as searching for information about public institutions, ministries, courts, etc.; using e-services (tax board, forms, citizens' portal, etc.); work-related communication with clients and colleagues; searching for practical information (weather, timetables, etc.); within-organization communication (intranet, lists, etc.); searching for information and tips on relationships, family, children, child-rearing, health and other aspects of personal life, and refers to people's motives to use the Internet for practical and work-, role- or institution-driven purposes. It can be suggested that these factors and, accordingly, two underlying motives for Internet use, correspond to two aspects of an information environment – a personal/relational aspect and an institutional aspect – delineated by Lievrouw (2001) in her insightful theoretical essay.

Table 12.1 presents the mean values of the index of Internet use frequency and the mean factor scores of two factors of online activities among gender and ethnic groups. The difference between men and women in the intensity of Internet use was not statistically significant. An interesting polarization between males and females, however, appeared with regard to the types of online activities: women scored significantly higher than men on WI, whereas men used the Internet more than women for SME. These gender differences might be explained by the so-called second shift (Hochschild and Machung, 1989): the gender regime, while favoring women's active participation in the labor market, simultaneously associates home-making and child-rearing mostly with females. This implicates that women have less spare time compared to men. Recent studies indicate that this phenomenon is particularly prominent in

Estonia: according to the 2010 Time Use Survey, women, on top of their daily paid labor, spend on average 4.1 hours a day on household duties, compared to men's 2.6 hours. At the same time, women have on average 5.3 hours a day as leisure time, while men have 6.1 hours (Tasuja, 2011). Thus, the overwhelming importance of institutional duties, including gendered role division in families, probably motivates women to use their time online for practical and work-related purposes, while hindering them from pursuing those motives for Internet use that are related to their agency and personal needs. Similar explanations to gender inequalities in Internet use have also been proposed by other authors (e.g. Hargittai and Shafer, 2006; Dutton *et al.*, 2009).

The difference between the ethnic majority and the minority with regard to Internet use frequency was not significant (Table 12.1). Those who completed the questionnaire in Estonian used the Internet significantly more for WI, that is, the institutional aspect of the information environment, than those who responded to the survey in Russian. Members of the ethnic minority, however, scored significantly higher on more personal uses of the Internet (SME) than Estonian-speakers did. These findings may be indicative of a weaker vertical integration of the minority group in the Estonian society, that is, their looser ties with state institutions (Ehin, 2009), and lower use of national online and offline news media (Vihalemm, 2008). Still, the findings point at the potential for horizontal integration of the ethnic minorities through social networking sites (SNS) and interpersonal online communication.

Table 12.2 displays Pearson's correlations between the characteristics of Internet use, age and indicators of social class and status. Age was strongly

Table 12.1 Characteristics of Internet use by gender and language (N = 1,100)

	Frequency of Internet use		Work and information related Internet use (WI)		Social media and entertainment related Internet use (SME)	
	Mean	*SD*	*Mean*	*SD*	*Mean*	*SD*
Males	6.32	2.97	−0.15**	0.98	0.13**	1.01
Females	6.02	2.90	0.12**	1.00	−0.10**	0.98
Estonian speakers	6.26	2.89	0.09**	1.01	−0.04*	0.99
Russian speakers	5.91	3.02	−0.22**	0.94	0.10*	1.02

Note: * $p < 0.05$; ** $p < 0.001$.

Table 12.2 Correlations between the characteristics of Internet use, age and indicators of social class and status

	Frequency of Internet use	Work and information related Internet use (WI)	Social media and entertainment related Internet use (SME)
Age	−0.41***	0.01	−0.62***
Education (in years)	0.16***	0.36***	−0.19***
Income	0.17***	0.17***	−0.09**
Perceived social status	0.28***	0.19***	0.08*

Note: $*p < 0.05$; $**p < 0.01$; $***p < 0.001$.

and negatively correlated with the frequency of Internet use and SME, while the correlation between age and WI was near zero.

Figure 12.2 shows the mean levels of the two types of Internet use in age and gender groups. WI trajectory across the lifespan is better described as curvilinear, with this motive for Internet use being relatively low among the youngest and the oldest age group, and reaching its highest level around 30 to 44 years of age. This suggests that the importance of the institutional aspect of an information environment is related to one's lifespan and social roles, implicating that older age groups are still more deprived of the opportunity of interacting with societal institutions via new media.

SME was highest among the youngest age group, decreasing steadily throughout the lifespan. Our results, in line with the findings of other studies (e.g. Dutton *et al.*, 2009), thus, suggest that young people's motives for using the Internet indeed largely derive from their agency, free will, and interest in interactive opportunities offered by the new media.

Interestingly, differences between males and females are non-existent among 15 to 19 year olds, and become particularly notable between the ages of 30 and 54. These dynamics of gender differences lend support to the above-proposed explanation that the double workload, most acute at the age of parenting, leads women to use their time online for practical and work-related purposes, while limiting entertainment-oriented uses.

The intensity of Internet use was significantly positively correlated with the indicators of social class, that is, education and income, as well as with perceived social status (Table 12.2). Similarly, correlations between WI and all three indicators of social class and status turned out to be positive, being especially strong with regard to the level of education. Interestingly, the indicators of social class were negatively correlated with the personal aspect of Internet use (SME), while perceived social status, on the contrary, turned out to be weakly, but still significantly, positively correlated with

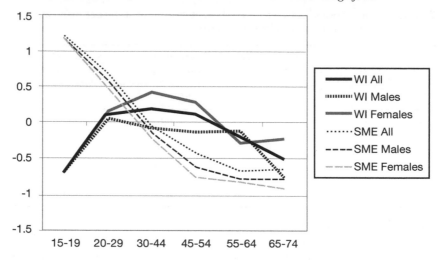

Figure 12.2 The motives for Internet use in age and gender groups (N = 989).

Note: The difference between age groups in WI and SME scores was statistically significant in the whole sample and among both gender groups at p < 0.001.

SME. These correlation patterns demonstrate, in line with the cultural perspective presented in Witte and Mannon (2010), that the association between Internet use and social status is independent of the effects of class differences. It is possible that better-off and, in particular, better-educated users are driven by pragmatic motivation as they might benefit from WI related activities much more compared to SME related use in their pursuit to maintain the position of advantage (cf. Zillien and Hargittai, 2009). Accordingly, they may prioritize work and information related activities over more entertainment-oriented uses in allocating their scarce time resources. Scoring higher on *both* types of online activities as well as on the overall intensity of Internet use seems to be, somewhat differently, the function of higher social status and the corresponding values, habitus and lifestyle.

To find out to what extent the three characteristics of Internet use are predicted by demographic variables versus the indicators of social class and status we conducted a series of linear regression analyses (Table 12.3). Starting from the intensity of Internet use we can observe that younger age was the strongest predictor of Internet use frequency, followed by higher education levels, status and income. The ethnic majority status was a weak but significant predictor in the two regression models. Altogether, the indicators of social class and status increased the explained variance by 12 percent.

Due to the curvilinear relationship between WI and age, the age-squared variable was added to the regression models predicting work and information related Internet use. Higher education levels turned out to be the strongest predictor of WI, with the ethnic majority status, being a female, higher social status, higher income and the age variables all significantly contributing to predicting this type of Internet use. Similarly, to the case of Internet use frequency, adding the indicators of social class and status considerably enhanced the model, increasing the explained variance by 13 percent.

Finally, SME was, by far, most strongly predicted by younger, followed by being a male, lower level of education, higher social status and, in one of the models, weakly but significantly by the ethnic minority status. Differently from the cases of Internet use frequency and WI, adding the indicators of social class and status did not enhance the model remarkably, suggesting that the more personal and agency-related aspect of Internet use is, predominantly, the function of inter-generational differences.

From our analytical perspective, it is important to note that perceived social status was the only variable that was significantly positively correlated with all aspects of Internet use, that is, with the intensive as well as extensive nature of online activities. This can be seen as a particularity

Table 12.3 Linear regression analysis exploring how demographic variables and indicators of social class and status predict the characteristics of Internet use

	Frequency of Internet use		Work and information related Internet use (WI)		Social media and entertainment related Internet use (SME)	
	Model 1	Model 2	Model 1	Model 2	Model 1	Model 2
Gender	0.03	0.01	−0.12***	−0.11***	0.09***	0.08**
Language	0.07*	0.07*	0.15***	0.16***	−0.04	−0.05*
Age	−0.41***	−0.45***	1.34***	0.90***	−0.61***	−0.60***
Age squared	—	—	−1.36***	−0.98***	—	—
Education (in years)	—	0.19***	—	0.32***	—	−0.08**
Income	—	0.12***	—	0.07*	—	−0.01
Perceived social status	—	0.17***	—	0.09**	—	0.06*
R^2	0.17	0.29	0.10	0.23	0.39	0.41

Notes:
Language of the survey (1 = Estonian; 0 = Russian); gender (1 = male; 0 = female).
*$p < 0.05$; **$p < 0.01$; ***$p < 0.001$.

of a rapidly informatizing transition society where higher perceived social status not only fosters and urges individuals to advance the intensity and scope of their online activities, but is also influenced by successful and swift adaptation to social and technological changes (cf. Lauristin, 2004).

Conclusions

Our analysis indicated that the socio-demographic differences in access to and use of the Internet largely correspond to the patterns of social stratification in Estonia. With regard to access and use frequency, more advantaged social groups (younger generations, well-educated and well-off people, those with higher social status, and, to some extent, the ethnic majority) have maintained their lead in adaptation to social transition. In terms of Internet uses, a clear differentiation has emerged, with females, the ethnic majority, middle-aged people, and better-educated and better-off people leaning towards the institutional aspect of an information environment, and males, the ethnic minority, the youngest generations, and people with lower education levels and income preferring the personal/relational uses. Somewhat differently from American society where the well-off and well-educated succeeded in the intensive as well as extensive nature of Internet use (Witte and Mannon, 2010), social status rather than social class predicted both the intensity and versatility of Internet use in Estonia. We may conclude that in a rapidly changing society where the class structure is still unsettled, a set of different resources such as economic and cultural capital, digital literacy and sufficient leisure time are needed to flourish in all aspects of the emerging information society, which, in turn, contributes to advancing one's capitals and the perceived social status.

References

Bourdieu, P. (1984 [1979]). *Distinction: A social critique of the judgment of taste.* Cambridge, MA, US: Harvard University Press.

Carpentier, N. (2003). Access and participation in the discourse of the digital divide: The European perspective at/on the WSIS. In J. Servaes (ed.) *The European information society: A reality check.* Bristol, UK: Intellect, 99–120.

Dutton, W.H., Helsper, E.J. and Gerber, M.M. (2009). *Oxford Internet Survey 2009 report: The Internet in Britain.* Oxford, UK: Oxford Internet Institute, University of Oxford. Online. Available HTTP: http://microsites.oii.ox.ac.uk/oxis/publications (accessed 21 February 2011).

Ehin, P. (2009). Political support and political participation: comparison of Estonians and non-Estonians. In M. Lauristin (ed.) *Estonian human development report 2008.* Tallinn, Estonia: Estonian Cooperation Assembly. Online. Available HTTP: http://www.kogu.ee/public/EIA2008_eng.pdf (accessed 9 April 2011).

Hargittai, E. and Shafer, S. (2006). Differences in actual and perceived online skills: The role of gender. *Social Science Quarterly,* 87, 432–48.

Helemäe, J. and Saar, E. (2011). An introduction to post-socialist transition in Estonia. In E. Saar (ed.) *Towards a normal stratification order.* Frankfurt am Main: Peter Lang, 13–33.

Hochschild, A. and Machung, A. (1989). *The second shift: Working parents and the revolution at home.* New York: Viking Penguin.

Kalmus, V., Realo, A. and Siibak, A. (2011). Motives for Internet use and their relationships with personality traits and socio-demographic factors. *Trames,* 15(65/60), 385–403.

Lauristin, M. (2003). Social contradictions shadowing Estonia's "success story." *Demokratizatsiya,* 11, 601–16.

Lauristin, M. (2004). Eesti ühiskonna kihistumine [The stratification of Estonian society]. In V. Kalmus, M. Lauristin, P. Pruulmann-Vengerfeldt (eds). *Eesti elavik 21. sajandi algul: ülevaade uurimuse Mina. Maailm. Meedia tulemustest [Estonian life-world in the beginning of the 21st century: Overview of the results of the survey Me. The World. The Media].* Tartu, Estonia: Tartu University Press, 251–85.

Lauristin, M. and Vihalemm, P. (2009). The political agenda during different periods of Estonian transformation: External and internal factors. *Journal of Baltic Studies,* 40, 1–28.

Lievrouw, L.A. (2001). New media and the "pluralization of life-worlds": A role for information in social differentiation. *New Media & Society,* 3, 7–28.

Lindeman, K. (2011). The changing perception of social position. In E. Saar (ed.) *Towards a normal stratification order* (481–500). Frankfurt am Main: Peter Lang.

Parayil, G. (2005). Digital divide and increasing returns: Contradictions of informational capitalism. *The Information Society,* 21, 41–51.

Runnel, P. and Pruulmann-Vengerfeldt, P. (2004). Mobiilid, arvutid, Internetid: Eesti infoühiskonna künnisel [Mobiles, computers, Internets: Estonia on the verge of the information society]. In V. Kalmus, M. Lauristin, P. Pruulmann-Vengerfeldt (eds). *Eesti elavik 21. sajandi algul: ülevaade uurimuse Mina. Maailm. Meedia tulemustest [Estonian life-world in the beginning of the 21st century: Overview of the results of the survey Me. The World. The Media].* Tartu, Estonia: Tartu University Press, 147–62.

Runnel, P., Pruulmann-Vengerfeldt, P. and Reinsalu, K. (2009). The Estonian tiger leap from post-communism to the information society: From policy to practice. *Journal of Baltic Studies,* 40, 29–51.

Tallo, A. and Terk, E. (1998). The generations in Estonia's transition period. In E. Terk (ed.) *Estonian human development report.* Tallinn, Estonia: UNDP, 14–16.

Tasuja, M. (2011). Gender differences in time use. In K. Põder (ed.) *Man's home is the world, woman's world is her home?* Tallinn, Estonia: Statistics Estonia. Online. Available HTTP: http://www.stat.ee/publication-download-pdf?publication_id=25640 (accessed 18 November 2011).

Tsatsou, P., Pruulmann-Vengerfeldt, P. and Murru, M.F. (2009). Digital divides. In S. Livingstone and L. Haddon (eds) *Kids Online: Opportunities and Risks for Children.* Bristol, UK: Polity Press, 107–19.

Vainu, V., Järviste, L. and Biin, H. (2010). *Soolise võrdõiguslikkuse monitooring 2009. Uuringuraport. [Gender equality monitoring 2009. Research report.]* Tallinn, Estonia: Ministry of Social Affairs. Online. Available HTTP: http://www.sm.ee/fileadmin/meedia/Dokumendid/V2ljaanded/Toimetised/2010/toimetised_20101.pdf (accessed 21 February 2011).

van Dijk, J. (2006). Digital divide research, achievements and shortcomings. *Poetics,* 34, 221–35.

Vihalemm, P. (2008). The infosphere and media use of Estonian Russians. In M. Lauristin (ed.) *Estonian Human Development Report 2007.* Tallinn, Estonia: Estonian Cooperation Assembly.

Vihalemm, T. and Kalmus, V. (2009). Cultural differentiation of the Russian minority. *Journal of Baltic Studies,* 40, 95–119.

Weber, M. (1978 [1922]). *Economy and society: An outline of interpretative sociology.* Berkley, CA, US: University of California Press.

Witte, J.C. and Mannon, S.E. (2010). *The Internet and social inequalities.* London: Routledge.

Zillien, N. and Hargittai, E. (2009). Digital distinction: Status-specific types of Internet usage. *Social Science Quarterly,* 90, 274–91.

Note

1 The writing of this chapter was supported by grants from the Estonian Research Agency (ETF8527 and SF0180017s07).

Section 5
The Middle East region

13 Digitally divided we stand

The contribution of digital media to the Arab Spring

David M. Faris
Roosevelt University

Introduction

On a bright summer night in July 2011, Egyptian digital activists gathered in Tahrir Square to discuss police abuse and torture, and ongoing failure of the military regime that succeeded Hosni Mubarak to reform the country's corrupt Ministry of Interior. The "Twitterati," as these elite, Cairo-based activists were derisively known, were not sitting alone in their apartments tweeting, texting and posting on Facebook, but rather engaged in an attempt to include their non-wired citizens in a dialogue about important national issues. Two or three hundred Egyptians sat in solidarity at the far edge of the square, with the burned-out husk of the recently-deposed National Democratic Party headquarters in the background, and communicated not just with the microphone but also with the non-verbal hand-signals that would become famous in the United States when employed later that summer by Occupy Wall Street protestors. These events had become known as "Tweet Nadwas" – hash-tagged, ad-hoc conferences about the significant challenges facing the Egyptian revolution and the dangers of losing the energy and exuberance of Tahrir Square to the forces of what had become known as the "counter-revolution." Sitting in the crowd were the familiar faces of Egypt's decade-long digital counter-public, but also a cross-section of less privileged Egyptians, who were sharing the square in an attempt to realize justice for the revolution's "martyrs" – those who lost their lives in Cairo, Suez and other parts of Egypt during the 18 days of the uprising in January and February of 2011 against one of the longest-tenured authoritarian regimes in the world.

The well-known role of digital activists in the Egyptian uprising in particular, and the Arab Spring in general, raises important questions about digital access and fluency in the developing world, and about the relationship between elites and non-elites on the Internet. Egypt is both a relatively poor and unequal society, with the benefits of Mubarak-era neoliberal reforms distributed quite unevenly. On the one hand, largely urban business elites and upper middle class Egyptians have captured the very real growth of the past 20 years, and are connected to global capital flows and trends. It is these groups who have seen their access to broadband Internet and wireless networks grow substantially since the turn of the century, while digital infrastructure in the rest of the country lags seriously behind. Is Egypt's (and the region's) digital divide merely reinforcing extant social inequalities, or are digital tools increasing access to information and economic opportunities for regional citizens who might otherwise be left behind? These important questions will be examined through the lens of classic sociological theories about inequality and class.

The digital divide and social science traditions

In Witte and Mannon's *The Internet and Social Inequalities* (2010), the authors analyze the "digital divide" through the lens of three major sociological traditions: the material, cultural and functional perspectives. For the functionalist perspective, Witte and Mannon ask, "Does it matter that many individuals do not use the Internet on a daily basis if, in the end, society benefits from information and innovations provided by the Internet?" Functionalism in fact became one of the defining foundations of contemporary political science (Sil, 2000, p. 355), as "modernization theory" – the idea that through increasing specialization, urbanization, and technological advancement, all societies were on a common trajectory from traditional to modern. The explosion of Internet penetration into less developed countries would fit squarely into the tradition's focus on the number of telephone lines and television sets as proxies for the "modern." While the materialist tradition would decry the inequalities wrought by and reinforced by the unequal spread of digital technologies, the functionalist paradigm would see in them merely a reaffirmation of the division of labor. Not everyone can be an expert in digital technologies, nor each individual an activist. And society as a whole might benefit from their efforts, even if they do not quite share in them equally. For Durkheim, the division of labor allows the "cohesion of societies," and thus "must possess a moral character" (Durkheim, 1984, pp. 23–24). Therefore, while allowing that the benefits of digital technologies have been unequally shared, in both the developed and developing worlds, can we make a case for their essential utility for social solidarity and cohesion?

Without offering an unconditional "no" to this question, this essay will adopt the functionalist perspective for analyzing the broad contributions of the Internet to societies in the Middle East. In other words, even while acknowledging the unequal impact of digital tools on different social classes in countries like Egypt and Tunisia (Fahmy and Rifaat, 2010) (which do matter, of course), I will argue that the Internet has brought benefits that both justify some of the optimism surrounding these technologies, and offer hope that some of those benefits might ultimately redound to the benefit of less privileged classes and groups. Insofar as they have contributed to a political shake-up across the region, that promises to empower citizens to make political and economic choices about their own lives, rather than submitting to the whims of authoritarian rulers, digital inequalities can be at least temporarily justified.

The spread of the Internet has been beneficial for the Middle East in a multitude of ways. First, there are, in fact, many ways that visitors to the region can see some of the benefits brought by the increasing penetration of broadband access. From e-government initiatives that put crucial information for citizens online, to the proliferation of food-ordering Web sites that connect individuals with food vendors that they might not have ordinarily encountered nor had immediate access to, the Internet has almost certainly contributed to both economic growth and general transparency. In Cairo, for instance, you can now order food from nearly any restaurant in the city through a site called Otlob and have it delivered to your doorstep. Restaurants whose markets might once have barely extended beyond a three-block radius can now count half of sprawling Cairo as their customer bases. Anyone who has actually been to Cairo and tried to decipher its labyrinthine street grid should understand what an accomplishment this truly is. And while reaping the economic gains of these innovations is more difficult the further down the economic food chain you move, it is also true that even working class Egyptians might make occasional use of such services through Internet cafes or the common broadband connections in apartment buildings. This is a clear example of a broad social benefit that can be justified morally despite the fact that its benefits are not shared equally.

States in the Middle East have long posed increased access to information technology as one of the keys to building more prosperous global economies. In 1999, the government of Hosni Mubarak unveiled a major initiative to enhance Egypt's digital infrastructure, forming a cabinet ministry called the Ministry of Communication and Information Technology (Wheeler, 2003, p. 631). That initiative has paid dividends, as rates of Internet access have risen rapidly in the past ten years, a pattern that has been clear across the region, as governments scrambled to catch up to other countries. Countries are also scrambling to claim a share of the market for digital platforms and applications. In fact, while rates of access have started to level off in many parts of the world, the Middle East is still witnessing explosive growth due to its initial lag in widespread adoption of the technologies. It is not just broadband – across the region digital mobile networks have grown at astonishing rates, and many individuals who can afford to do so now access the Internet primarily through their mobile phones. This has, of course, only reinforced the divide between elites with the income to spend on such devices, and the masses, who still access the Internet communally, sporadically in Internet cafes, or through poor-performing home access points.

But the Middle East is not an ordinary region – as of December 2010, it was characterized by pervasive authoritarianism, and had seemed to completely avoid the movement toward electoral democracy witnessed in East Asia, Latin American and Africa during the 1980s, 1990s, and 2000s (Bellin, 2004; Posusney, 2004). Regimes had, in fact, seemingly mastered techniques of controlled openings and liberalization for the purpose of self-preservation rather than democratization. Prior to the uprising in Tunisia that swept away longtime dictator Zine El-Abadine Ben Ali, the region was characterized with few exceptions by countries with robust repressive apparatuses, minimal civil and political rights, and economies distorted in various ways by bloated bureaucracies, kleptocratic ruling families, and domination by small cliques of financiers and in some cases, military elites who captured most of the rents from liberalization for themselves and a small coterie of clients. Media environments were dominated more or less extensively by state-owned or state-affiliated newspapers, television stations and radio outlets, with only satellite TV stations like Al-Jazeera and Al-Arabiyya relieving the tedium, and even then, both stations were owned and operated out of states that were among the most regressive in the region. The Internet, beginning around the turn of this century, offered dissidents in nearly all of the authoritarian countries of the region, an alternate platform for expressing and organizing dissent. The question for our purposes, is whether the use of the Internet as an alternate public sphere and organizing platform reinforced existing gender, religious and class hierarchies, or whether it in some way subverted them. As I will argue below, it is clear in the cases of Egypt and Tunisia that the digital divide is the result, rather than the cause of, social inequalities, and that activists have used the medium to pursue a clear set of social and political goals from which no one can be reasonably excluded.

The digital divide and the Middle East

The term "digital divide" was used by Pippa Norris (2002) to describe disparities in access to the Internet across social classes worldwide. Early boosters of the Internet believed that digital tools might mitigate extant social inequalities by providing marginalized groups with access to information and tools of organization that might bypass barriers created by social class. Norris argued, on the other hand, that the Internet "reflects and thereby reinforces" political realities and social inequalities, instead of undermining or changing them (Norris, 2002). Norris's book was a useful corrective to more optimistic accounts of the Internet and social change, and sparked a debate about the potentialities of digital tools and ways to increase access and equality on the Internet. Arguments based on Norris's concept of the digital divide have in fact been quite prominent in general skepticism about the Internet's potential to transform developing societies, and as such are particularly relevant to discussions of the Internet in the Middle East.

The most recent data suggests that region-wide, women constitute only one-third of all Facebook users, a finding that respondents attribute to general regional cultural constraints (Arab Social Media Report, 2012). This finding tracks generally with the lower general levels of female literacy across the region, and thus it is not surprising to find this divide recapitulated in the digital realm. Despite these constraints, however, women have played a significant role in the digital dissent that has swept the region over the past ten years, and a number of young Arab women played prominent roles in national dramas beginning in December 2010. Radsch argues that Arab women were relatively equal participants in blogging (though equal participation does not of course mean equal influence), but clearly the gender divide in digital access has prevented such equality from reaching the more recently-developed social media sphere (Radsch, 2012, p. 7). Etling, Faris and Palfrey, on the other hand, found that only 34 percent of Arab blogs were written by women (2009, p. 36). Women who have become successful activists, though, have tended to come from the upper levels of regional class hierarchies.

Modes of inequality

The growth of broadband in places like Egypt, Yemen, and Syria slowed throughout the 2000s, partly for economic and partly for geopolitical reasons. In Egypt, while there were a number of vendors for broadband service, for most of this period it remained prohibitively expensive for average Egyptians. In cities like Cairo, the need for Internet access was filled by two competing and stratified institutions. On the one hand, the country witnessed the proliferation of Western-style cafes with names like Cilantro, Joffrey's, and Costa Coffee – in some cases these restaurants were international ventures of companies like Coffee Bean & Tea Leaf. Stepping off the hot, dusty streets of Cairo into one of these cafes is tantamount to entering an alternate universe, where trendy and well-dressed Cairenes sip expensive lattes and pick at Western-style sandwiches and paninis that cost more than the daily salary of many other citizens. de Koning argues that these cafes, indeed, became sites for the production and display of wealth and status for upper middle class Cairenes (de Koning, 2006). For years these cafes provided Internet access free of cost, but in 2008 and 2009 they started charging for that as well, whether hourly, or by purchasing cards with scratch-off codes that allowed for a certain time period of access. But of course, most of the people who could afford the expensive sandwiches and drinks in such cafes probably had Internet connections at home or work as well.

At the same time, there developed another business model of Internet cafes – places that did not serve up anything but access to the Web, and for a small fraction of the cost of access at Cilantro. These cafes are often located off side streets and down a set of stairs, where the proprietors usher you to a seat and hand you a time card that keeps track of how long you spend surfing the Internet. While this access is still pricey by the standards of ordinary Egyptians, even working class individuals are able to afford a few hours a week if they so desire. This is to say nothing of common practices such as the residents of apartment buildings sharing a single broadband connection (known as "thief nets"), or of a single mobile phone providing the point of Internet access for multiple friends or family members. While the official Internet penetration rate in Egypt stood at 26 percent in 2011, the actual rate of effective access might be quite a bit higher. But it forces us to ask whether disparities in digital access time and quality might lead to inequalities in how the Internet is harnessed for social and economic empowerment. In other words, it is quite likely that the elite Egyptian with unlimited broadband can do more with his or her access than a working class Egyptian who can get online for three or four hours a week.

Access and revolution

While general research has yet to be conducted on the demographics of protestors during the Arab Spring more broadly, there is some data on Internet usage and access in the Egyptian events. These access disparities can be seen in the latest research on the Egyptian uprising, demonstrating that it was in fact wealthier Egyptians who heard about the January 25 demonstrations on the Internet, through online social networks, and who were overwhelmingly more likely to show up on the first day to protest. Tufekci and Wilson's data also show that 77 percent of the respondents who participated in the protests had Internet at home, a rate that far eclipses that of ordinary Egyptians (Tufekci and Wilson, 2012, p. 369). The proportion of survey respondents who also reported using Facebook to discuss the protests was 51 percent, as opposed to just 13 percent for Twitter (p. 370). What this suggests is that it was precisely wealthier, more connected Egyptians who hatched the plans for protest and executed them, but that it was only when the non-wired citizens joined in on the protests that they were actually able to affect large-scale change in the country. This process of elite-led diffusion in the context of persistent social stratification reinforces the central argument of this article, that elite digital activists enabled broad-based and important change in spite of the digital divide.

What was the relationship between access and uprising across the region? Diving into the data, it becomes difficult to assert any clear relationship between rates of Internet access and the onset of revolutionary uprisings. What seems clear is that some of the most-connected states, including the UAE, Saudi Arabia, and Qatar, saw minimal mobilization, or at least mobilization that did not lead to the kind of political upheaval witnessed in more low-connectivity states like Egypt, Libya and Syria. In fact it is the four states with the lowest levels of Internet access in the entire region – Egypt, Yemen, Libya, and Syria – which have so far witnessed the most dramatic political uprisings, all of which were backed by robust Internet-based mobilization campaigns. In the case of Egypt, the time, date and initial mobilizing strategies were all conducted on Facebook, making it perhaps the first mobilization that truly deserves the term "social media revolution." The starkness of this contrast should lead us to conclude that something beyond simple "access" to the Internet is required to spark dissent in authoritarian countries. Indeed, it is not access itself, but, to borrow Witte and Mannon's terminology, "use" of the Internet that can best predict under what circumstances an authoritarian regime is likely to have to contend with an uprising (2010, p. 44).

One aspect of the digital divide in the Middle East that is most salient is the population bulge dynamics that inhere across many of the states in the region. Many regional states have populations that are disproportionally young, from Iran to Egypt. It is also unquestionably true that these youth populations are much more likely than their elders not only to have Internet access, but to be fluent in how to most efficiently use the tools at their disposal. As the Open Net Initiative notes, "Demographic factors are also expected to contribute to the growth of Internet population" (Open Net Initiative, 2009). Therefore even as rates of access across the region continue to lag behind their counterparts in Western Europe and Asia, increases in Internet access will be captured disproportionately by the young. The salience of youth access to digital media was highlighted during the Arab Spring, as Egyptian and Tunisian youth activists used their preferred social media platforms to organize the initial protests (as in Egypt) or to coordinate and amplify ongoing protests after they had begun, as in Tunisia (Faris, 2012).

It is not just any young people, however, who are most likely to have a dramatic impact on the politics of regional states. It is unquestionably college-educated, middle and upper middle class youth who have seized the mantle of digital organizing across the region. Matthew Hindman argued that far from empowering marginalized groups in the United States, the Internet merely transferred power to a new networked elite, largely comprised of privileged, Ivy-League educated white men (Hindman, 2008). Rather than leveling the playing field between different groups and classes in American society, the Internet instead reinforced existing class, gender, and racial hierarchies. Looking at the most popular and influential blogs in the American "blogosphere," Hindman concluded that, if anything, minority representation was worse online than it was offline. If we expect the digital divide to mirror, if not exacerbate, a country's general inequality, it should be no surprise that the US has a substantial gap in this regard. Table 13.1 provides the relevant Gini

Table 13.1 Comparative measures for selected Middle Eastern countries

	Gini Coefficient	Internet Access* %	Literacy** %
United States	45.0	78.3	99.0
Egypt	34.4	26.4	66.4
Libya	N/A	5.9	97.7
Qatar	41.1 (2007)	66.5	N/A
Saudi Arabia	N/A	43.6	86.1
Tunisia	40.0	36.3	88.9
United Arab Emirates	N/A	69.0	90.0
Yemen	N/A	10.8	62.4
Syria	N/A	19.8	87.9

Notes: * Source: Internet World Stats. http://www.internetworldstats.com/ (accessed May 30, 2012); ** Source: United Nations Development Program, 2011.

coefficients for the countries under consideration in this essay. The United States is provided for comparison. Because of the relative newness of the Gini measurements, it is impossible at present to determine whether increased Internet access has had a measurable effect on inequality in general.

Interestingly, the regional countries that have data available on this question are all substantially less unequal than the United States. It should also be noted that equality does not necessarily translate to prosperity. While the world's most equal country, Sweden, also happens to be quite prosperous, very poor countries like Afghanistan and Ethiopia have lower levels of inequality than, for instance, the EU countries as a whole (Gini Index, 2011).

Models of dissent

What seems clear is that there is no linear relationship in the Middle East between general levels of Internet penetration, and the use of such technologies by dissident entrepreneurs. It is more appropriate to consider the different models of digital activism that were deployed across the Middle East during the Arab Spring, and to understand the ways in which those models are influenced by architectures of state control and surveillance. In a small number of countries like Egypt and Bahrain, state authorities opted not to tightly filter and censor the Internet. From the dawn of Egyptian digital activism around the turn of the century, dissidents found few obstacles between themselves and their ability to create or access content on the Internet. This seemingly open road contrasted sharply with the media environment, which even after the liberalization of press laws in 2004, remained dominated by state TV and state-owned or affiliated newspapers. The lack of access to traditional channels of expression and dissent led many dissidents to use the new tools of Web 2.0 – at the time primarily off-the-shelf blogging technology through Blogger – as platforms for writing and thinking about ways to challenge the state. For Egyptians, this led to a small but robust and tightly-linked network of about 1,000 activists, many based in Cairo and Alexandria, who coordinated both with the protest movement Kefaya, and with the new independent newspapers, to get their message out to the broader, non-wired population. While many members of this community were harassed, arrested, and blacklisted by traditional media organizations, the state made little to no effort to actually block or take down their content. In time, this allowed dissidents to build a campaign of dissent around a small number of widely shared goals – goals that transcended other divisions (largely between secularists and Islamists) that have come to define post-revolutionary Egypt. Dissidents sought an end to the Mubarak dictatorship, a lifting of the emergency law that had governed Egypt since the 1981 assassination of President Anwar El-Sadat, an end to practices of torture and indefinite detention, and a shifting of Egypt's foreign policy away from a blind subservience to US and Israeli interests. In other words, in the open Internet environment of pre-2011 Egypt, digital activists were both thought leaders as well as coordinators of protest (Khamis and Vaugh, 2011; Faris, 2013; Radsch, 2012; Lynch, 2012). Likewise, while Bahrain's uprising was ultimately crushed, its robust blogging community is widely seen as having been at the forefront of dissent and organizing during the 2000s (Schleusener, 2007).

Other states, however, including Syria, Tunisia, and Saudi Arabia, opted for the "China model" of a closed Internet, governed by intrusive state filtering and censorship. This strategy, while it successfully drove digital activism to the margins, and forced many dissidents to do their writing and thinking abroad, clearly gave many regimes a false sense of confidence in their own ability to continue governing. Whereas in Egypt, dissent was increasingly open over the past decade, in Tunisia the first inklings of broad dissatisfaction really only became apparent in 2010, when digital activists began holding small rallies to protest state corruption and abuse of power. In the case of both Syria and Tunisia, the state's decision not to block seemingly innocuous sites like Facebook led activists to use the group-forming and sharing capabilities of these platforms to amplify and coordinate large-scale protests whose causes could not necessarily be found in digital activism itself (Khamis and Vaugh, 2011). The number of individuals involved in digital activism inside Tunisia was quite limited. As the journalist and activist Afef Abrougui noted, "the number who were active was limited, people were careful."[1] But once the floodgates of protest had opened, Tunisians took full advantage of social media to get the word out about protests, share images and videos of what was happening in the streets, and to build linkages with activists outside the country. Activists consider the contribution of these technologies to the success of the Tunisian revolution to be quite significant. Across the region, digital tools played an important role in coordinating and amplifying dissent. In Syria, where protests most unexpectedly erupted in March 2011, Facebook and Twitter were critical organizing nodes for the Friday protests that eventually threatened the authoritarian regime of Bashar Al-Asad (Blanford, 2011).

Conclusion

Egyptian and Tunisian digital activists have made persistent attempts to undermine repressive and corrupt state structures that are deeply implicated in social inequality. Their success in supporting and amplifying movements to change those structures thus gives those activists, as Durkheim would argue, a positive moral dimension that a narrow focus on the digital divide would obscure. In other words, even if access to digital technologies is unequal, elites have used their privileged access to fight for a series of changes that they believe will redound to the broad benefit of society. This is particularly true because the Middle East is a region still characterized, even after the Arab Spring, by non-democratic or proto-democratic governments that have proven unequal to the task of broad economic development with prosperity shared by all citizens. In most cases, it seems clear that the benefits of digital diffusion have been captured by classes and population segments who already occupy a privileged position in these societies. Despite the claims of digital enthusiasts, it is not clear that the astronomical increase in rates of digital penetration in the 2000s has had any discernible effect on extant social inequalities in the states of the Middle East. In poorer countries like Egypt, Syria, and Algeria, a great deal of economic activity remains beyond the reach of the state, and thus largely outside of state-planned projects for digitally enhanced economic development. However, from a functionalist perspective, it is clearly possible to see the contribution of social media to economic change and political development. Access to alternate forms of digital media has proven critical to the formation of what I have called "social media networks" – loosely linked, non-hierarchical networks of activists and dissidents that cross class, religious and national boundaries across the region (Faris, 2013). These Social Media Networks were critical actors in a drama that unfolded over the course of the past decade in Egypt, Tunisia, Bahrain, and elsewhere: the collation and organization of dissent in closed societies. While states adopted different policies toward digital activism – with Tunisia extensively filtering and blocking political Web sites, and Egypt merely harassing practitioners – the activists themselves were able to adapt to these differing architectures of control to exert significant influence on public debate, and to use the evolving ecosystem of social media platforms to continue organizing protests and rallies that contested the arbitrary nature of state power in these societies. Those architectures of control, and the legal frameworks that govern access to the Internet, will remain both a topic of extensive debate in the coming years, and will affect the ability of activists to use digital tools for the common good (MacKinnon, 2012).

In sorting through the ultimate effects of digital media, it remains true that those best positioned to capture the benefits of new media technologies will be the immediate beneficiaries. As Ronald Deibert argued 15 years ago, "the properties of a communications environment— the unique ways in which information can be stored, transmitted, and distributed in that environment—'favor' the interests of some social forces and ideas over others" (1997, p. 30). For the past ten years, digital media in the Middle East has benefitted social forces and contributed to the progressive ideas of elite, networked dissidents – middle class and upper middle class activists who have been able to harness the power of digital technologies for the purpose of undermining and challenging what had seemed to be hegemonic state power. That means, of course, that many people have been excluded from this nascent public sphere, and that concerns about poverty and equality have not typically received the same level of attention by these activists as issues about torture, corruption and arbitrary state power. In many ways this allows us to confirm materialist assumptions about the disparate impact and use of these technologies (as well as culturalist understandings about the particular ways that women are excluded from power and society in the Middle East), and to understand that simple diffusion of Internet access and wireless technologies will not, in and of themselves, undermine entrenched gender hierarchies or class relations. Digital media both reflect and reinforce certain inequalities, but at the same time, they offer elites the opportunity to subvert dominant paradigms and discourses, and to organize dissent even under stifling conditions of authoritarianism. And we should not be surprised if, at some point in the future, these tools are married to a project of class and gender equality that includes not just the Twitterati but also people who have thus far been excluded from the general march of progress.

References

The Arab Social Media Report. (2012). Dubai, United Arab Emirates: Dubai School of Government.

Bellin, E. (2004). The robustness of authoritarianism in the Middle East: Exceptionalism in comparative perspective. *Comparative Politics, 36* (2), 139–157.

Blanford, N. (2011). On Facebook and Twitter, spreading revolution in Syria. *Christian Science Monitor,* April 8, 2011.

Deibert, R. J. (1997). *Parchment, printing and hypermedia: Communication in world order transformation.* New York: Columbia University Press.

de Koning, A. (2006). Café latte and Caesar salad: Cosmopolitan belonging in Cairo's coffee shops. In D. Singerman and P. Amar (eds.), *Cairo cosmopolitan: Politics, culture and urban space in the new globalized Middle East.* Cairo, Egypt: American University in Cairo Press.

Durkheim, E. (1984). *The Division of Labour in Society.* New York: Palgrave, 23–24.

Etling, B., Faris, R. and Palfrey, J. (2009). Mapping the Arab blogosphere: Politics, culture and dissent. Berkman Center Research Publication, 2009–06, 1–62.

Fahmy, E. I. and Rifaat, N. M. (2010). Middle East information literacy awareness and indigenous Arabic content challenges. *International Information & Library Review, 42* (2), 111–123.

Faris, D. (2012). Beyond social media revolutions: The Arab Spring and the networked revolt. *Politique etrangere 77,* (1), 99–109.

Faris, D. (2013). *Dissent and revolution in a digital age: Social media, blogging and activism in Egypt.* London: I.B. Tauris & Co.

Gini Index. (2011). *World Bank development indicators,* 2011. Retrieved from http://data.worldbank.org/indicator/SI.POV.GINI (accessed May 30, 2012).

Hindman, M. (2008). *The myth of digital democracy.* Princeton, NJ, US: Princeton University Press.

Khamis, S. and Vaugh, K. (2011). Cyberactivism in the Egyptian revolution: How civic engagement and citizen journalism tilted the balance. *Arab Media and Society, 14* (3).

Lynch, M. (2012). *The Arab uprising: The unfinished revolutions of the new Middle East.* New York: PublicAffairs.

MacKinnon, R. (2012). *Consent of the networked: The worldwide struggle for Internet freedom.* New York: Basic Books.

Norris, P. (2002). *Digital divide: Civic engagement, information poverty and the Internet worldwide.* Cambridge, UK: Cambridge University Press.

Open Net Initiative. (2009). Internet filtering in the Middle East and North Africa. Retrieved from http://opennet.net/research/regions/mena (accessed May 30, 2012).

Posusney, M. P. (2004). Authoritarianism: Middle East lessons for comparative theory. *Comparative Politics, 36*(2), 127–138.

Radsch, C. (2012). *Unveiling the revolutionaries: Cyberactivism and the role of women in the Arab uprisings.* Houston, TX, US: James A. Baker III Institute for Public Policy, Rice University.

Schleusener, L. (2007). From blog to street: The Bahraini public sphere in transition. *Arab Media and Society, 1* (1).

Sil, R. (2000). The foundations of eclecticism: The epistemological status of agency, culture and structure in social theory. *Journal of Theoretical Politics, 12*(3), 353–387.

Tufekci, Z. and Wilson, C. (2012). Social media and the decision to participate in political protest: Observations from Tahrir Square. *Journal of Communication, 62,* 363–379.

Wheeler, D. (2003). Egypt: Building an information society for international development. *Review of African Political Economy, 98,* 627–642.

Witte, J. C. and Mannon, S. E. (2010). *The Internet and social inequalities.* New York: Routledge.

Note

1   Interview with Afef Abrougui, Tunis, Tunisia, July 27, 2011.

14 Explaining digital inequalities in Israel

Juxtaposing the conflict and cultural perspectives

Gustavo Mesch
Ilan Talmud
Tanya Kolobov[1]
University of Haifa

There are many scholarly concerns that the Internet, rather than reducing existing inequalities, is actually exacerbating them (DiMaggio *et al.*, 2001; van Dijk, 2005). "Digital inequality" refers to the uneven access to and use of information and communication technology (ICT) (Anderson *et al.*, 1995). With the advent of the World Wide Web, early studies of "digital inequality" focused on understanding the factors associated with physical access to the Internet at home, at work and in other settings (Hargittai, 2007). As Internet access has become more universal in Western societies, studies have focused on more subtle indices of use, including the quality of access, the context and intensity of use, types of use, and users' computer skills (van Dijk, 2005; Hargittai, 2007).

Ethnicity is an important dimension of both social and digital inequality in multi-ethnic societies. Studies on the digital divide have shown that ethnic minority groups are less likely to access and use the Internet (Dupagne and Swalden, 2005; Fairlie, 2007; Mesch and Talmud, 2011). Various factors have been identified as the antecedents of these inequalities, most notably: income, educational level, occupational standing, and attitudes toward technology (Witte and Mannon, 2010; Mesch and Talmud, 2011). Thus, ethnic disparities in ICT access may reflect social-structural disadvantages and cultural differences. The purpose of this study is to investigate the sources of gaps in access to and use of the Internet among ethnic groups in Israel. The study focuses in particular on the differential contribution of ethnicity, human capital, occupational structure and attitudes to ICT accessibility and use.

The context: Israel as a deeply divided society

Israel is a multi-ethnic society. Approximately 79 percent of the population is Jewish, and the remainder is Arab. Jewish immigrants have come to

Israel in a sequence of waves. As a result, the Jewish population consists of various groups from different backgrounds (Lewin-Epstein and Semyonov, 1993). The establishment of the Jewish state in 1948 and the Arab-Israeli wars that followed left the Arab minority subordinated to the Jewish majority, and in an inferior position in the Israeli economy and labor market. The Arab minority is disadvantaged in its educational level and socio-economic status (Okun and Friedlander, 2005). The result is that while Jews are overrepresented in higher status occupations, and are more likely employed in professional, scientific, and managerial positions, Arabs are overrepresented in skilled and unskilled manual occupations (Kraus and Yonay, 2000). This disparity accounts in part for the income differences between Jews and Arabs (Lewin-Epstein and Semyonov, 1993). Residential segregation also plays a role in the digital divide in Israel. Most of the Arab population lives in peripheral areas of the country and in small localities in which they are the vast majority of the population. Partly because of state policies, Arab communities are allocated fewer resources and have a less well developed infrastructure (Mesch *et al.*, 1998; Smooha, 2002).

Another important group in the Israeli population is immigrants from the former Soviet Union (FSU). Immigration to Israel took place in two waves. The first was between 1968 and 1979, when 150,000 Jews arrived in Israel. The second large wave of immigration began after 1989, shortly after the dissolution of the Soviet Union. Since then, an estimated one million immigrants from the FSU have arrived in Israel, becoming 15 percent of the total population and 20 percent of the Jewish population. Some sociologists have concluded that because of their high degree of residential and social segregation, and high level of language and culture conservation, the FSU immigrants have become a new ethnic group (Al-Haj, 2004).

Thus, the multi-ethnic nature of Israeli society, and the high level of residential and social segregation of Arabs and immigrants makes Israel a perfect setting for conducting this study on social position and the pattern of access to and use of computer mediated communication.

Internet technology in Israel

In Israel, the proportion of users of computers from any place (home, work, elsewhere) increased from 47 percent of the population in 2002 to 58 percent in 2006. In 2006, 63 percent of the Jewish population reported having access to the Internet, but only 35 percent of the Arab population had such access (Central Bureau of Statistics, 2008a, 2008b). A recent survey found that while 77.3 percent of the Jewish population reported they had used the Internet in the last 24 hours, only 61.9 percent of the Arabs had done so. On average, Internet users are online 16 hours a week. Cell phone access to the Internet is limited but expanding. According to the same survey, while 28 percent of Israeli Jews had mobile access, only 20 percent of the Arab population reported using a mobile device to access the Internet (Amichai-Hamburger, 2011). Studies also reported differences in ethnic groups with regard to how they use the Internet. Israeli Arabs are more likely to use the Internet to access health information and online news, while Israeli Jews are more likely to use the Internet for communication, financial and consumption purposes (Amichai-Hamburger, 2011; Mesch, Mano and Tsamir, 2011; Mesch and Talmud, 2011).

The sociological literature uses various perspectives for explaining digital inequalities. Following the work of Witte and Mannon (2010), we will adopt the cultural and conflict perspectives with a focus on ethno-national inequalities.

Inequality from a conflict perspective

According to the conflict perspective, Internet literacy is tightly linked with the division of power in society. Such literacy is a contextual set of skills and knowledge whose possession is mainly used to maintain class advantage and class boundaries. In fact, knowledge and skills are examples of effective exclusionary practices of the ruling groups. Even with the advent of universal education, knowledge and skills are not distributed equally in society. The unequal distribution of funding to schools, a curriculum that appeals to the values of the upper and middle class, and conditions of poverty imply that large segments of the population are denied particular forms of knowledge and skills.

Internet access may have a similar effect, reproducing social divisions even while we celebrate the equalizing potential of ICT (Witte and Mannon, 2010). Without the development of actual Internet competencies, access to the Internet may in fact veil enduring social inequalities. In their study on the US, Witte and Mannon (2010) found that, without controlling for measures of class (education and income), race had a statistically significant association with going online the previous day. Blacks and Asian Americans were less likely to go online. However, when measures of social class were included, the effects of race became statistically non-significant. This result provides support for the conflict perspective by showing that the negative effects of race and ethnicity on Internet use are the result of social class.

We believe that an alternative reason for this effect is that in multicultural societies, over and above other socio-economic factors, ethnicity and occupational structure often overlap. Members of majority groups are overrepresented in professional, scientific and managerial occupations, and minorities are overrepresented in blue-collar and low skilled occupations. Occupation is an important variable in explaining the rate of adoption of technology as well as the effects of computers and the Internet on income level (Reese, 1988; Brynin, 2006; DiMaggio and

Bonikowski, 2008). In addition to using ICT in the workplace, white-collar workers are more likely to understand the potential uses and applications of ICT. Therefore, they develop positive attitudes about these technologies and through them help workmates solve technical problems (Reese, 1988). In Israel, ethnic minorities are more likely to belong to economically disadvantaged social groups who have blue-collar jobs. Therefore, they are generally not exposed to ICT at work, do not have the social support necessary to learn about using the Internet, and often cannot afford a computer at home, or the necessary Internet connection hardware. This argument suggests the reproduction of digital inequality through the replication of existing inequalities in access to the occupational structure and to ICT (Mesch and Talmud, 2011).

Following the arguments of the conflict perspective, we expect that ethnic differences in the use of computers at work and access to the Internet will be partially explained by the individual's ethnic background and occupational class. More importantly, though Israel is characterized by status group politics where ethnic background plays an increasing role (Arian and Talmud, 1991; Smooha, 2002; Al-Haj, 2004) we expect that the individual's occupation serves as a structural container of attitudes, literacy, and skills, and thereby would contribute in explaining the observed variation in digital divide, over and above the pronounced effect of income and education.

Inequality from a cultural perspective

The cultural perspective focuses on the multi-dimensional nature of inequality. As presented by Witte and Mannon (2010), the cultural perspective has its roots in the work of Max Weber's distinction between class and status. The latter reflects stratification according to lifestyle and consumption. Specifically, restrictions on social interactions set high-status group members apart from non-members: stratifying society along social lines. According to this view, status stratification rests on social prestige, rather than on mere economic assets. Once established, distinctions in status are converted into particular lifestyles and approaches to conducting one's life. Distinctions in status are important because they define the lens that people use to create their worldview. From the cultural perspective, even class is not simply a structural position relative to markets, but a shared perspective that defines and enables patterns of social interaction among individuals with a common social background. Thus, according to this perspective, social status is associated with the lifestyles, values, and attitudes that are characteristic of each class position in the stratification system.

Members of each class have a body of tacit knowledge including attitudes, habits, and a deep understanding of "information orders" (Ryan, 2006). Such knowledge is not easily attained, but it constitutes the cultural (or symbolic) capital by which social actors deploy their "habitus" (shared or taken-for granted mental models or "doxa") of the world (Bourdieu, 1984; Calhoun *et al.*, 1993). According to this view, attitudes toward technology and digital competency are key factors in mastering the digital field and benefitting from the advantages of ICT use (Calhoun *et al.*, 1993).

At the very core of a group's habitus (doxa) are the building blocks of lifestyle and consumption. The habitus provides a unique environment for evaluating the social role of information and communication technologies. From the cultural perspective, social prestige and the inter-generational transmission of lifestyles are important for the shared understanding of social inequality. The focus of this perspective is on the relationship between occupational prestige and Internet use. Witte and Mannon (2010) considered the extent to which the Internet may be viewed as a feature of middle class or upper middle class lifestyle, and as a cultural boundary marking the class divide. In this study, we look at central factors that play an especially important role in distinguishing one's status position, and hence, one's lifestyles choices: occupational prestige and attitudes toward Internet use.

According to the cultural perspective, to the extent that the Internet is associated with prestige and status, individuals in high prestige occupations and individuals from prestigious families should be more likely to use the Internet on a daily basis. These effects should be independent of class differences, understood here as income and education. In addition, if status implies consumption and lifestyle, then we should see a positive association between occupational prestige and the use of the Internet across a variety of domains, in consumption as well as in production, and for purposes of communication as well as information.

Attitudes toward technology reflect a worldview (or habitus) associated with social status. Theoretical models of technology adoption have suggested that attitudes toward technology play an important role in accessing and using information and communication technologies (Rogers and Kincaid, 1981; Porter and Donthu, 2006). More specifically, the technology acceptance model (TAM) suggests that perceived attributes of the technology such as perceptions about the benefits of the technology and its ease of use influence attitudes toward and use of the technology (Porter and Donthu, 2006). The central assumptions of the model are that the adoption and use of ICTs are associated with positive attitudes that it turn are associated with a greater likelihood of access to ICT. In a similar vein, Internet anxiety, such as expressing negative feelings and attitudes about ICT and its effect on society, are negatively associated with the likelihood of access and the frequency of ICT use (Meuter *et al.*, 2003). Negative attitudes toward computers and the Internet were found more frequently in low income and minority groups (Jackson *et al.*, 2001).

Certainly, attitudes are related to social status. Social groups vary in their attitudes toward technology, according to their position in society (Jackson *et al.*, 2001; Porter and Donthu, 2006). More specifically, disadvantaged minorities may hold negative attitudes toward technology as a reflection of their disadvantaged social position. Supporting this argument, a study that investigated the effect of socio-demographic characteristics on the adoption of the Internet found that age, education and income were associated differently with attitudes and beliefs about the Internet, and that beliefs mediated respondents' attitudes to, and ultimately use of, the Internet (Porter and Donthu, 2006). In addition, due to their disadvantaged position in society, ethnic minorities are less likely to be exposed to new technologies such as the Internet. A lack of exposure to technology influences one's self-concept (Reese, 1988; Dupagne and Swalden, 2005). Jackson *et al.* (2001) argued that minorities often internalize the stereotypes conveyed by the majority. According to this viewpoint, a social stereotype linking minority status with poor performance in technological domains may cause group members to avoid engaging with that domain. Jackson *et al.* (2001) found that minority groups are less likely to use ICTs because of a higher level of negative attitudes toward ICT. In that sense, their lack of exposure may lead to anxiety about, and fear and mistrust of, ICTs, causing them, in turn, to avoid their use. The argument of the cultural perspective implies that occupational prestige and attitudes toward ICT will be positively associated with access to and variations in ICT use. Individuals in high prestige occupations and individuals from prestigious families should be more likely to hold positive attitudes toward ICT and use it on a daily basis. These effects should be independent of class differences, understood here as income and education.

Additional variables

There are additional variables that may be associated with access to and use of ICT. Many studies have found a negative relationship between age and Internet use (e.g., Kraut *et al.*, 1998), with younger people being more likely to go online (Rogers and Kincaid, 1981). ICT literacy, meaning the degree of software competence, and the ability to use the Web are clearly conversely related to age (Hargittai, 2007; Gilleard and Higgs, 2008). Several other studies also found gaps between men and women in Internet use (DiMaggio *et al.*, 2001; 2004), claiming that male dominance in the quantity and quality of usage reflects cultural stereotypes in Western society. While in the past, several studies revealed a direct relationship between gender and Internet access and ICT use, the gender gap in ICT access appears to be disappearing. Nevertheless, a gender gap clearly remains, at least in terms of the Internet user's type of activity if not duration of use (van Dijk, 2005).

Data

The data for this study were gathered during the months of April–May 2009, and are part of a larger longitudinal study on the association between Internet use and social capital. The Statistical Unit at the University of Haifa created a sampling frame, containing a random sample of the population of the State of Israel. The sampling frame included the various groups that comprise the Israeli population. The unit contacted 2,792 households and conducted telephone interviews in Hebrew, Russian, and Arabic. Of those contacted, 620 refused to be interviewed, 306 found it difficult to understand the questionnaire and 100 did not complete the interview. Overall, 1,792 valid questionnaires were obtained, and the analysis is based on them.

When investigating the role of income, education, occupational prestige and ethnicity on Internet use, a complex relationship between the independent variables can be expected. In deeply divided societies, ethnicity is likely to be highly correlated with education, income, and occupation. Thus, multicollinearity might be problematic in the multivariate analysis. We inspected the correlation matrix of all the independent variables, and did not find any bivariate correlation higher than 0.40. The highest values were between occupational prestige and income, and between education and occupational prestige (p=0.36). Other correlations were much lower. In addition, we conducted an exploratory factor analysis to investigate whether education, income and occupational prestige were part of single underlying latent variable. The analysis resulted in three independent factors. We concluded, accordingly, that statistical multicollinearity did not seem to be a problem that either harmed the estimates' precision or limited the validity of the analysis.

Results

Table 14.1 presents data about physical access to ICT by ethnic group, and indicates the existence of statistically significant differences in computer use at home, at work and Internet use. Israeli Jews report the greatest use, followed by immigrants from the FSU. Israeli Arabs are the least frequent users in every category. Such findings confirm the existence of digital inequality among social groups.

After documenting the differences in ICT use, the next task was to investigate whether the conflict and cultural perspective can account for these differences. In this next step, we conducted a logistic regression analysis predicting Internet use. Model 1 includes only the variables derived from the conflict perspective – education and income. Model 2 adds the variables from the cultural perspective – occupational prestige and attitudes toward the Internet.

Table 14.1 Descriptive statistics of computer use and Internet use by social group

Variables	Population Group			F	Total %
	Jews – Non-immigrants %	*Jews – Immigrants from the FSU %*	*Arabs %*		
Computer use at home	80.3	74.9	70.0	8.6**a	77.8
Computer use at work	57.7	41.0	32.3	39.7**b	51.3
Computer use anywhere	84.3	76.4	72.2	14.51**c	81.3
Internet use	73.9	71.3	63.6	6.9**d	71.8
N	1270	195	327		

* $p < 0.05$, ** $p < 0.01$
a Difference between: Jews – Non-immigrants and Arabs
b Difference between: Jews – Non-immigrants and Jews – Immigrants from the FSU, Jews
   – Non-immigrants and Arabs
c Difference between: Jews – Non-immigrants and Jews – Immigrants from the FSU, Jews
   – Non-immigrants and Arabs
d Difference between: Jews – Non-immigrants and Arabs

The results of the first model do not provide empirical support for the conflict perspective. The effects of income and virtually all of the occupational categories are statistically non-significant. The only effect that is statistically significant – providing partial support for the conflict perspective – is the positive effect of education. However, the most impressively salient outcome is that even when occupation, income, and education (as well as other variables) are controlled, the effect of ethnicity persists. Thus, ethnicity has a direct net effect on Internet use, over and above other indicators of social hierarchy. In other words, social class alone does not explain why Israeli Arabs are less likely to use the Internet.

The second model introduces measures derived from the cultural perspective – occupational prestige and attitudes toward technology. The effect of these variables is statistically significant. Most importantly, when these variables are introduced, the effect of ethnicity becomes statistically non-significant, indicating that ethnic differences in Internet use in Israeli society appear not to be related to income and occupational differences between groups. Instead, these differences seem to arise from different cultural orientations rooted in the status hierarchy, and associated with hierarchically conceived lifestyles and occupational prestige. Furthermore,

Table 14.2 Logistic regression, predicting Internet use at home according to class variables (education, income) and cultural variables (occupational prestige, attitudes towards technology)

	Model 1			Model 2		
	B	SE	Odds	B	SE	Odds
Age	−0.02	0.007	0.97**	−0.02	0.008	0.97**
Marital Status (1=married)	−0.45	0.22	0.63*	−0.24	0.23	0.78
Gender (1=male)	0.37	0.21	1.45	0.03	0.22	1.03
Education	0.19	0.04	1.21**	0.14	0.04	1.15**
Income (log)	0.68	0.35	1.97	0.76	0.39	2.15
High grade professionals						
Low grade professionals	0.42	0.33	1.51	0.52	0.35	1.69
Routine non-manual laborers	1.077	0.42	2.93*	0.97	0.45	2.64*
Small employers and self employed	0.50	0.46	1.65	0.43	0.49	1.54
Technicians and workers[3]	0.73	0.47	2.08	0.73	0.51	2.08
Occupational prestige				0.02	0.008	1.02**
Immigrants from the FSU	0.64	0.36	1.89	0.60	0.39	1.82
Israeli Arabs	−0.60	0.25	0.54**	−0.43	0.26	0.64
Attitudes				−0.98	0.10	0.37**
Constant	−0.88	1.20	0.41	−0.01	1.28	0.98
Naglerke Pseudo R-square	0.18			0.32		

*$p < 0.05$, ** $p < 0.01$
Note: High grade professionals is the dummy category of comparison.

the introduction of the cultural variables substantially increases the explained variance of the model from 0.14 to 0.32 ($p < 0.001$).

The cultural perspective assumes that status is a central cause of social hierarchy, and a reflection of social inequality. Occupations differ from one another not just in terms of their salaries, but also in terms of the lifestyles and mental models they bring in their wake (Bourdieu, 1984; Calhoun *et al.*, 1993). Hence, occupational prestige is ultimately a determinant of Internet use.

In the next model, we examined this hypothesis further by conducting a multivariate regression, predicting negative attitudes toward the Internet. In this analysis we expected to find that to the extent to which the predictions of the cultural perspective hold, occupational prestige and ethnicity would each have an independent effect on attitudes toward the Internet.

Table 14.3 presents the results, indicating that both perspectives play a role in explaining negative attitudes toward the Internet. Education and income have an independent (net) negative effect on attitudes toward the Internet. The findings show that the higher the level of education and the higher the amount of reported income, the less negative the attitudes toward the Internet. Occupation is not associated with attitudes toward the Internet. However, as expected by the cultural approach, occupational prestige and ethnicity are significantly associated (in the expected direction) with attitudes toward the Internet. In other words, the higher the occupational standing, the lower the level of negative attitudes toward the Internet. Finally, Israeli Arabs and immigrants from the FSU express more negative attitudes toward the Internet than Israeli Jews.

An additional hypothesis, derived from the basic assumptions of the cultural perspective, is that Internet use represents variations in the lifestyle of various status groups in the population. According to this perspective, different groups will use the Internet differently. We tested this hypothesis by conducting a multivariate analysis, predicting five different types of Internet use from the indicators of social class, and from

Table 14.3 OLS regression, predicting attitudes toward the Internet

	B	SE	β
Age	0.004	0.002	0.055
Marital Status (1=married)	0.24	0.06	0.11**
Gender (1=male)	−0.32	0.06	−0.17**
Education	−0.05	0.01	−0.16**
Income (log)	−0.13	0.11	−0.03
High grade professionals	—	—	—
Low grade professionals	0.03	0.09	0.01
Routine non-manual laborers	−0.28	0.12	−0.12*
Small employers and self employed	−0.16	0.14	−0.05
Technicians and workers	−0.13	0.13	−0.05
Occupational prestige	−0.008	0.002	−0.17**
Immigrants from the FSU	−0.20	0.09	−0.06*
Israeli Arabs	−0.20	0.09	−0.06*
Constant	0.98	0.25**	—
Adj. R-square	0.10	—	—

*p < 0.05, ** p < 0.01
Note: High grade professionals is the dummy category of comparison.

the variables associated with status and ethnicity. Table 14.4 presents the results. One very salient outcome is that both education and occupational prestige are positively associated with most of the examined activities. Education is positively associated with user-generated activities (using a social networking site, etc.), with financial activities (checking and conducting banking activities online), and with searching for information and communicating using e-mail. Occupational prestige is positively associated with four out of the five activities (including creating a homepage, banking online, and online information searching and communication). This finding provides more support for the cultural perspective. More to the point, immigrants from the FSU are more likely to be involved in Internet activities that deal with production (creating a Web site) and information searching than native-born Israeli Jews. Similarly, Israeli Arabs are more likely to be involved in information searching only. By contrast, Israeli Jews are more likely to be involved in the construction of user-generated content such as social networking, online banking, and communication, and less likely to be involved in information searching.

Discussion

The purpose of this study was to apply the conflict and cultural sociological perspectives to the study of digital inequality in Israel. We focused on the explanation of ethno-national variations in access, attitudes, and types of use. In this study, we showed that occupational categories explain variations in the use of computers at work, as well as differences in Internet access, over and above the effect of income and education. We also showed that ethnicity explains differences in the use of computers at work and access to the Internet, which are also partially explained by one's occupational class.

We found repeated and systematic evidence that one's place in the social hierarchy, particularly cultural factors that reflect habitus or vertically situated lifestyles and mental models, predict Internet access and use, and attitudes toward ICT. These practices of virtual reality are embedded in other kinds of practices common to Israeli society, which are typically attributable to other indicators of social prestige and ethnicity as well.

Our findings tend to support the cultural perspective for explaining inequalities in the use of digital technology. Despite the existence of ethnic differences in the level of schooling and income between Arabs, Jews from the FSU and native-born Israeli Jews, we found that the main inequality in access was between Israeli Jews and Israeli Arabs. Furthermore, this inequality was explained by variations in occupational prestige and attitudes toward technology. However, the picture we portray here is complex. On one hand, Israeli Arabs have a significantly more

Table 14.4 OLS regression, predicting conducting Internet activities

	Create a home page			Create an SNS site			Check bank account			Search for information			E-mail		
	B	SE	β	B	SE	β	B	SE	β	B	SE	β	B	SE	β
Age	−0.01	0.005	−0.12**	−0.04	0.006	−0.19**	−0.01	0.004	−0.13**	−0.008	0.003	−0.09**	−0.009	0.004	−0.07*
Marital Status (1=married)	−0.02	0.13	−0.005	−0.47	0.15	−0.10**	0.02	0.11	0.007	−0.18	0.08	−0.07*	−0.03	0.10	−0.01
Gender (1=male)	0.24	0.12	0.07*	0.46	0.14	0.11**	0.28	0.10	0.09**	−0.08	0.08	−0.03	−0.02	0.10	−0.008
Education	0.03	0.02	0.06	0.06	0.02	0.08**	0.05	0.01	0.10**	0.04	0.01	0.11**	0.07	0.01	0.15**
Income (log)	0.08	0.23	0.01	0.70	0.27	0.08**	0.23	0.19	0.04	−0.09	0.15	−0.02	0.35	0.19	0.06*
High grade professionals	—	—	—	—	—	—	—	—	—	—	—	—	—	—	—
Low grade professionals	0.22	0.19	0.05	−0.05	0.22	−0.01	0.29	0.16	0.07	0.07	0.12	0.02	0.13	0.15	0.03
Routine non-manual laborers	0.39	0.25	0.10	0.38	0.29	0.07	0.67	0.21	0.19**	0.07	0.16	0.03	0.74	0.20	0.21**
Small employers and self employed	0.30	0.28	0.04	0.19	0.33	0.02	0.42	0.24	0.07	0.16	0.18	0.04	0.60	0.23	0.10**
Technicians and workers	0.44	0.27	0.09	0.42	0.31	0.07	0.26	0.23	0.06	0.13	0.17	0.04	0.47	0.22	0.12*
Occupational prestige	0.01	0.005	0.12*	0.003	0.006	0.03	0.01	0.004	0.15**	0.008	0.003	0.14**	0.02	0.004	0.33**
Immigrants from the FSU	0.47	0.19	0.08**	−0.25	0.22	−0.03**	−0.01	0.16	−0.003	0.33	0.12	0.08**	−0.11	0.15	−0.02
Israeli Arabs	0.11	0.18	0.02	−0.88	0.21	−0.13**	−1.01	0.15	−0.22**	0.27	0.11	0.08**	−0.61	0.14	−0.13**
Constant	1.46	0.71*		0.476	0.82**		2.74	0.60**		1.84	0.46**		−0.13	0.58	
Adj. R-square	0.02			0.12			0.08			0.04			0.11		

* $p < 0.05$, ** $p < 0.01$
Note: High grade professionals is the dummy category of comparison.

negative attitude toward ICTs, net of the pronounced effects of income and education. Nevertheless, their lower rate of digital access is mainly due to their disadvantaged social status. In this sense, ameliorating the economic inequality between ethnic groups is likely to reduce the digital divide between Israeli Jews and Israeli Arabs. Future research should expand the exploration of the conflict and cultural perspectives in a more refined way.

The study has various limitations. As we noted, over time there has been a reduction in the differences in access to ICT. This reduction and the extent to which it affects more affluent sub-groups of Arabs could not be investigated here as we relied on a cross-sectional data set. Furthermore, future longitudinal studies should focus not only on the determinants of social inequality, but also on its consequences in terms of the attainment of status and the acquisition of social capital.

References

Al-Haj, M. (2004). *Ethnic formation in a deeply divided society: The case of the 1990s immigrants from the former Soviet Union in Israel.* Leiden, Netherlands: Brill Academic Publishers.

Amichai-Hamburger, Y. (2011). *Survey on Internet use in Israel.* Unpublished research report. Downloaded on 11.20.2011 from http://data.isoc.org.il/data/109

Anderson, R.H., Bikson, T.K., Law, S.A. and Mitchell, B.M. (1995). *Universal access to e-mail: Feasibility and societal implications.* Santa Monica, CA, US: RAND.

Arian, A. and I. Talmud, (1991). Economic control and electoral politics. In Frances Piven Fox (ed.), *Popular power post-industrial societies.* New York: Oxford University Press, 169–189.

Bourdieu, P. (1984). *Distinction.* UK: Routledge.

Brynin, M. (2006). Gender, technology and jobs. *British Journal of Sociology,* 57(3), 437–453.

Calhoun, C., Lipuma, E. and Postone, M. (1993). *Pierre Bourdieu: Critical perspectives.* Chicago, US: University of Chicago Press.

Central Bureau of Statistics. (2008a). *Technology use among Israelis over 20 years old.* Jerusalem: Israeli Government.

Central Bureau of Statistics. (2008b). *Employed persons and employees by occupation and population group.* Jerusalem: Israeli Government.

DiMaggio, P. and Bonikowski, B. (2008). Make money surfing the Web? The impact of Internet use on the earnings of U.S. workers. *American Sociological Review,* 73, 227–250.

DiMaggio, P., Hargittai, E., Celeste, C. and Shafer, S. (2004). Digital inequality: From unequal access to differentiated use. In K. Neckerman (ed.), *Social inequality.* New York: Russell Sage Foundation, 355–400.

DiMaggio, P., Hargittai, E., Neuman, W.R. and Robinson, J.P. (2001). Social implication of the Internet. *Annual Review of Sociology,* 27, 307–336.

Dupagne, M. and Swalden, M.B. (2005). Communication technology adoption and ethnicity. *Howard Journal of Communication,* 16, 21–32.

Fairlie, R.W. (2007). Explaining differences in access to home computers and the Internet: A comparison of Latino groups to other ethnic and racial groups. *Electronic Commerce Research, 7,* 265–291.

Gilleard, C. and Higgs, P. (2008). International use and the digital divide in the English longitudinal study of ageing. *European Journal of Ageing,* 5, 233–239.

Hargittai, E. (2007). A framework for studying differences in people's digital media uses. In N. Kutscher and Hans-Uwe (eds), *Cyberworld unlimited.* Wiesbaden, Germany: VS Verlag für Sozialwissenschaften.

Jackson, L.A., Ervin, K.S., Gardner, P.D. and Schmitt, N. (2001). The racial digital divide: Motivational, affective and cognitive correlates of Internet use. *Journal of Applied Social Psychology,* 31(10), 2019–2046.

Kraus, V. and Yonay, Y. (2000). The power and limits of ethnonationalism: Palestinians and Eastern Jews in Israel. *British Journal of Sociology,* 51, 525–551.

Kraut, R., Patterson, M., Lundmark, V., Kiesler, S., Mukopadhyay, T. and Scherlis, W. (1998). Internet paradox: A social technology that reduces social involvement and psychological well-being? *American Psychologist,* 53, 1017–1031.

Lewin-Epstein, N. and Semyonov, M. (1993). *The Arab minority in Israel's economy: Patterns of ethnic inequality.* Boulder, CO, US: Westview Press.

Mesch, G. and Talmud, I. (2010). *Wired youth: The social world of adolescence in the information age.* Oxford, UK: Routledge.

Mesch, G.S. and Talmud, I. (2011). Ethnic differences in Internet access: The role of occupation and exposure. *Information, Communication and Society,* 14, 445–472.

Mesch, G.S., Gustavo, S. and Talmud, I. (1998). The influence of community characteristics on police performance in a deeply divided society: The case of Israel. *Sociological Focus* 31(3), 223–248.

Mesch, G., Mano, R. and Tsamir, Y. (2011). Access and use of health information in Israel. Research Report. Tel Aviv: Maccabi Medical Services Foundation.

Meuter, M.L., Ostrom, A., Bitner, M.J. and Roundtree, R. (2003). The influence of technology anxiety on consumer use and experiences with self-service technologies. *Journal of Business Research,* 56 (11), 899–906.

Okun, B.S. and Friedlander, D. (2005). Educational stratification among Arabs and Jews in Israel: Historical disadvantage, discrimination and opportunity. *Population Studies, 59,* 163–180.

Porter, C. and Donthu, N. (2006). Using the Technology Acceptance Model to explain how attitudes determine Internet usage: The role of perceived access barriers and demographics. *Journal of Business Research,* 9, 999–1007.

Reese, S. (1988). New communication technologies and the information worker: The influence of occupation. *Journal of Communication,* 38 (2), 59–70.

Rogers, E.M. and Kincaid, D.L. (1981). *Communication networks: Toward a new paradigm for research.* New York: Free Press.

Ryan, D. (2006). Getting the word out: Notes on the social organization of notification. *Sociological Theory,* 24(3), 228–254.

Smooha, S. (2002). The model of ethnic democracy: Israel as a Jewish and democratic state. *Nations and Nationalism,* 8(4), 475–503.

van Dijk, J.A.G.M. (2005). *The deepening divide.* London: Sage Publications.

Witte, J.C. and Mannon, S.E. (2010). *The Internet and social inequalities.* London: Routledge.

Note

1 All of the authors have contributed equally to the writing of this chapter. The research was supported by a grant from the Israel Science Foundation (#1014/08). Direct all correspondence to Gustavo S. Mesch, Department of Sociology and Anthropology, University of Haifa, Israel. E-mail: Gustavo@soc. haifa.ac.il

15 An analysis of the second-level digital divide in Iran

A case study of University of Tehran undergraduate students

Hamid Abdollahyan
University of Tehran

Mehdi Semati
Northern Illinois University

Mohammad Ahmadi
University of Tehran

Introduction

This chapter offers a descriptive analysis of second-level digital divide in Iran with a special reference to the case of second-level digital divide among University of Tehran students. After explaining the problematic of the paper, we will introduce second-level digital divide as a conceptual framework that can explain and address second-level digital divide as a larger problematic within Iranian society. Then we will offer the methodology of this research that is in line with our conceptual framework. Finally, we will present an analysis on the empirical data that was collected through a survey study of undergraduate students of the University of Tehran.

Problematic of research

Along with the development of the Internet and its use since the early 1990s there was an increasing interest among scholars in researching inequalities in Internet use by focusing mainly on the distinction between information haves and have-nots (Sassi, 2005; Yu, 2006; Crenshaw and Robison, 2006; Livingstone and Helsper, 2007). Various scholars later conceptualized this distinction as digital divide, which produced numerous books and papers on the topic of digital divide. From the early years of the twenty-first century, however, a new turn began to take shape regarding the study of inequalities caused by the development of new media technologies (e.g., Abdollahyan and Ahmadi, 2011).

The main idea supporting these new studies revolved around the fact that mere access to the Internet does not mean there is a uniform use of the Internet, and mere use of the Internet does not mean every user equally enjoys the opportunities available to them. Among the new concepts there was also the "second-level digital divide," which referred to the inequalities of Internet use among the users. Each research project pointed out a different type of inequality among the users, including inequality of usage based on age (Bonfadelli, 2002), gender (DiMaggio *et al.*, 2001; Herring, 2001), economic and social status (Wilson *et al.*, 2003; van Dijk, 2005) and education (Hargittai and Walejko, 2008; Hargittai, 2002) to name a few.

Generally speaking, however, there was a consensus among scholars (e.g., Hargittai, 2002) to distinguish three levels of digital divide. First there is a divide that is mostly noticeable between the poor and the rich nations; then there is the second divide that exists between the poor and the rich within the same society; finally, there is the third type of inequality that exists between the skilled and the new users. Here, we study various elements of the second-level digital divide within an educational setting (the University of Tehran). When we started this research our main objective was to identify differences of skills among undergraduate students at the University of Tehran. Here we offer an argument that concerns a different digital divide. We argue that in order to get education and an occupation and to live in knowledge societies,[1] the mere abilities to read, write and do simple arithmetic (i.e., traditional literacy) are not enough and students need to acquire new set of skills. Moreover, new media and the technological boom in recent decades have made dramatic changes in the ways people interact with one another, work together and so on. As van Dijk (2006a, p. 243) puts it, new media are trend amplifiers and in this case they produce a wider skill divide among the Internet users than ever before. We believe the second-level digital divide would provide a satisfactory and plausible concept that can explain the skills gap between various groups of users in Iran (see also Abdollahyan and Ahmadi, 2011).

Differences in skills can cause formation of new inequalities in the new media world (Gui and Argentin, 2011). Therefore, access to the Internet is not the only matter of concern in understanding the world of the Internet. Rather, the differences in digital skills are a primary aspect of the second-level digital divide (Hargittai, 2002; van Deursen and van Dijk, 2010).

However, the question is why differences in skills are an issue. As Hargittai (2004) emphasizes, even if higher access rates are achieved in developing countries, large portions of certain populations would still not be able to benefit from this medium. Accordingly, drawing the attention of scholars and governments to such problems would help address the issue. And, considering that Internet use in Iran is comparatively high (46.9 percent penetration, according to Internet World Stats, 2011), the following observations indicate that the second-level digital divide is an issue in Iran and needs to be addressed.

The first observation concerns the changing patterns of Internet access in Iran. Internet access is equally distributed across various groups.[2] The second observation refers to the gap between the Internet use and the new skills needed for knowledge-based societies. In Iran, this gap becomes more evident when one is involved in participatory observation of Internet use. In addition, in the early years of the invention of the Internet the digital divide was the main issue of concern, today there are more concerns expressed about the ways people practically use the Internet (Gilster, 1997; Hargittai, 2002, 2005, 2009; Eshet, 2002; Eshet and Aviram, 2006; Eshet-Alkalai, 2004; Eshet-Alkalai, and Chajut, 2009; Eshet-Alkali and Amichai-Hamburger, 2004; Perez Tornero, 2004a, 2004b; Tyner, 1998; New Media Consortium, 2005; Jenkins *et al.*, 2006; Dobson and Willinsky, 2009; Livingstone and Helsper, 2010). In other words, the digital divide has expanded to include the issue of utilization. Accordingly, the most important issue of today is not whether there is access, or lack thereof, to new media technologies. Rather, the major concern is recognizing the fact that there is a divide between information haves and have-nots as a result of lack of skills.

Some scholars (e.g., Norris, 2001) maintain that digital divide in Internet use is not a new divide and it only mirrors existing inequalities in use of communication technologies. In other words, such a divide is an extension of the existing divides. Nevertheless, the increasing rate of Internet use in Iran requires research and policies to go hand-in-hand in order to offer plans for decreasing this divide and its socio-cultural and economic consequences. In addressing such an objective, we first conceptualize the second-level digital divide, and then report on our empirical study to highlight the implications of this divide.

Conceptual framework

This study approaches the second-level digital divide in Iran through a communication and sociological perspective. At the communication level, it can be argued that the new studies on literacy and on studies related to the effects of media literacy and media education now focus on addressing the required skills and abilities to use new media technologies (Livingstone and Helsper, 2010; Tyner, 1998; Warnick, 2002). Here we emphasize the "differential possession of digital skills" (van Deursen and van Dijk, 2010). Accordingly, we review some of the major works that seek an explanation for new divides in knowledge societies.

Tsatsou (2011) categorizes four groups of digital divide studies: 1) techno-centric, 2) economy-driven, 3) socio-cultural, and 4) policy motivated. Van Dijk (2006b) refers to five different types of inequalities: 1) technological inequality, which conceptualizes it in relation to technological opportunities, 2) immaterial inequality, which is related to life chances and freedom, 3) material inequality that involves various forms of capital including economic, social, cultural capital, 4) social inequality, which includes positions, power and participation, and finally; 5) educational inequality, which is related to capabilities and skills. Van Deursen and van Dijk (2010) proposed a range of Internet skills including operational Internet skills, formal Internet skills, information Internet skills and strategic Internet skills. Van Dijk and Hacker (2003) also distinguish between four types of access: 1) mental access, 2) material access, 3) skills access, and; 4) usage access. Selwyn (2004) distinguishes between access to ICT, use of ICT and meaningful use of ICT. He defines digital divide as "a hierarchy of access to various forms of technology in various contexts resulting in differing levels of engagement and consequences." Hargittai (2004) introduces multiple dimensions in digital divide that include technological access, autonomy, social support, skill and types of uses.

At the sociological level, we maintain that social capital is a more important factor in Iran as a stratifying factor, although economic factors play a role. This is the case because education has become widely available in Iran, as the government has pursued a policy of education for the masses for the past three decades (see Semati, 2008). The growing number of educational institutions, including universities, most of them subsidized public universities available to individuals across different strata in Iranian society, has entailed a growing population of pupils and university students with access to the Internet either at the institutional sites or via personal computers (ibid., 2008). Accordingly, we suggest that access to educational settings and computers (i.e., being a student) is a key factor in digital divide. A Weberian approach that emphasizes factors in stratification beyond the economic factors is an appropriate framework.

Both from a communication perspective and a sociological one, we can conclude that second-level digital divide is a skill-based divide and can cause inequality of literacy in Iran, which in turn can cause other inequalities across various groups. That is the reason we have chosen the University of Tehran as a case in which digital divide can be studied and used to think about the future and the divide in the larger context of the Iranian society.

Methodology

This study falls into the category of user-oriented studies (Pinto and Sales, 2007). We conducted a survey to identify various digital skills among undergraduate students from the University of Tehran. To design the questionnaire we used Jolls and Thoman's model of media literacy process skills (2004; 2008). They present a set of five process skills that are necessary to be able to live, study and work in a world saturated with (old and new) media. Their definition concerns media literacy process skills and includes the abilities to "access, analyze, evaluate, create and participate".

We used self-assessment through questionnaire (Hargittai, 2002; 2005), which is a suitable approach for large sampling. Based on Jolls and Thoman's (2004; 2008) definitions of media literacy process skills and our understanding of digital skills according to the needs of Iranian students we defined five process skills as follows:

1   Accessing ability, which refers to users' ability to access information and digital resources;
2   Analyzing ability, which refers to users' ability to analyze the messages and information students receive;
3   Evaluating ability, which refers to users' ability to judge and evaluate the credibility of information;
4   Creating ability, which refers to users' ability to produce new contents and not merely be consumers (becoming "prosumers");
5   Participating ability, which refers to users' ability to publish digital contents and interact with other users.

In order to define these skills we focused on basic computer and web operating skills. Based on each skill, we defined a set of sub-skills that could measure University of Tehran undergraduate students' digital abilities. We considered the educational and professional necessities of university students in Iran as various elements of the measurement and placed them in the questionnaire. We put an emphasis on information-retrieving skills rather than communicative skills. Moreover, we considered Web 2.0 related skills as being critical for students.

Operationalization and structure of the questionnaire

In order to examine the hypothesis and measure various levels of skills and other variables we organized the questionnaire in such a way to include the following items. A set of questions was considered to obtain general personal information. These consisted of questions regarding the samples' gender, field of study, age, the starting date of university education, and places of access to computers and the Internet. We also used scales such as five-point self-reported ratings to measure the familiarity of the samples with the following digital skills items: basic knowledge of the English language for using computers, file compression, reboot, preference settings, back up, modem, "save as", Microsoft Word, Microsoft PowerPoint, Microsoft Access, Microsoft Excel, JFV, PDF, JPG, refresh/reload, add to favorites/bookmarking, spam, BCC in email, Boolean operators (or, and), ISP, HTML, server, firewall, .gov, .org, the Internet country code top-level domain, .ac ("academic") second-level domain, the Internet ads, cookie, mirror websites, e-zine, database, open access journals, XML, Unicode, shareware, filtering software, wiki, feed, RSS, blogging, podcasts and Proxypod.[3] We also used questions to measure the time samples spent on the web daily and years using the Internet. In order to measure the digital skills of self-efficacy,[4] we used the following question: "Regarding your familiarity with computers and the Internet, how do you evaluate your abilities?" (This was a five-point scale consisting of a) not at all skilled, b) not very skilled, c) fairly skilled, d) skilled; and, f) very skilled).

Sampling

For this study we used proportionate stratified sampling techniques (see Ruane, 2005, pp. 114–115). We first acquired the total number of undergraduate students (N=17,310) from the university's Center for Statistics and Informatics. Then we classified students based on their majors and disciplinary affiliation. Eventually, we selected sample elements in proportion to their actual numbers in the overall population of undergraduate students. Based on this technique we arrived at a total sample of 376 students.

Analysis and findings[5]

Descriptive data analysis

In our data analysis we used both descriptive and inferential statistics. At the descriptive level, we offer an analysis of the demographic information of the research sample. According to our data, 42.5 percent of the samples were male and 57.5 percent were female students. The data showed that 70 percent of the respondents were between 20 and 22 years old, 18 percent were 18 and 19 years old and about 12 percent were 22 years and older. The data also indicates that 18.1 percent of the respondents were first year students, 26.9 percent were second year, 23.1 percent in third year and 31.9 percent were fourth year BA students.

One important variable, however, is Internet use. According to the research data, 74.2 percent of the respondents used the Internet in only one place (mainly at home, school or the work place). While 24.7 percent of the respondents used the Internet in two places, only a small percentage (1.1 percent) used the Internet in three places. This means students at the University of Tehran are dependent upon the university's Internet facilities.

On average, more than half of the respondents (56.6 percent) use the Internet for up to one hour per day. Those who used the Internet for two to three hours a day made up 31.4 percent of the users. About 12 percent use it for more than three hours a day. We used daily usage to gauge the weight of the Internet use and our data indicates that about half of the respondents have been working with the Internet for four to seven years. About 25 percent started to work with the Internet seven to thirteen years ago and less than 25 percent of the students started to work with the Internet from three years to one year ago. This descriptive data indicates that undergraduate students on average are professional users as over 75 percent of them have been familiar with the Internet for between four and 13 years.

Table 15.1 Distribution of frequencies based on daily Internet use

Daily use	Sex		Total	%
	Female	Male		
1 hour and less	123	90	213	56.6
2–3 hours	71	47	118	31.4
4–5 hours	17	21	38	10.1
6–7 hours	4	0	4	1.1
8–9 hours	1	1	2	0.5
10 hours and more	1	0	1	0.3
Total	217	159	376	100.0

Table 15.2 Distribution of frequencies based on Internet usage history

Usage history	Sex		Total	%
	Female	Male		
One year and less	12	10	22	5.9
2–3 years	27	20	47	12.5
4–5 years	59	51	110	29.3
6–7 years	59	38	97	25.9
8–9 years	40	27	67	17.9
10–11 years	18	11	29	7.7
12–13 years	1	2	3	0.8
Total	216	159	375	100.0

One of the female respondents did not answer this question.

Inferential data analysis

We calculated 41 digital skill-related items to form a "digital skills" variable. Our data revealed that 62.2 percent of the respondents marked "not at all skilled" or "not very skilled". The percentage who reported that they are "fairly skilled" was 18.9. Also, 18.9 percent marked "skilled" or "very skilled".

We also tested the possible causal relationship between various variables and discovered that there is an association between the sex of the respondents and their familiarity with digital skills, since the result of

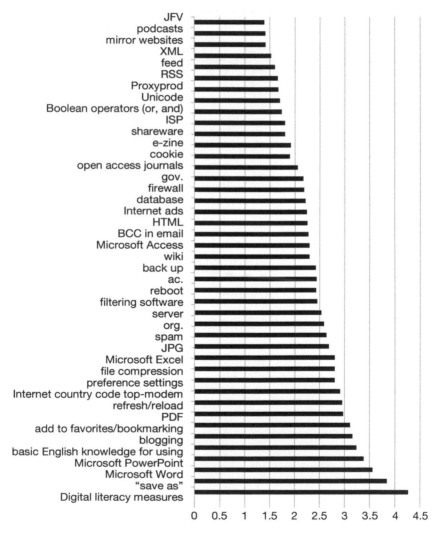

Figure 15.1 Means of digital skills items

Cramer's V test amounted to 0.16, indicating a positive association between the two variables. We used 41 variables as indicators for measuring the samples' level of familiarity. According to the Lambda results of the 41 variables, it can be concluded that male students are slightly more familiar with digital skills than female students are.

The data also indicates that there is a positive correlation between age and familiarity with digital skills (R=245; E=0.01). This means that older students report more familiarity with digital skills than younger ones. Probably because more time spent at the university contributes to having more opportunities for gaining new skills and having access to broadband Internet facilities.

It can also be argued that based on the date of entering university, the fourth and third year students indicated more familiarity with digital skills than the second and first year students did. In addition, there is a positive correlation between the length of the students' study time and their familiarity with digital skills (Kendall's tau-c=0.2). The data also indicates that there is a positive, though weak correlation (r=0.22) between owning a PC or a Notebook and an increase or a decrease in digital abilities. There is also a weak but positive correlation between places of access and familiarity with digital skills. This means the students who have used the Internet in two or three places (home, university, dormitory, work place, etc.) are more familiar with the digital skills than others (see also Livingstone and Helsper, 2010).

The data also revealed that there is a very strong and positive correlation between time spent on the web daily and years of using the Internet on one hand, and digital skills on the other. That means the students with more daily usage time were more likely to report a higher level of familiarity with digital skills than others (r=0.47). Moreover, students who started to use the Internet earlier are more familiar with digital skills (r=0.47).

Further measures of self-efficacy show a strong correlation with real skills of students (Kendall's tau-b = 0.53). This means the students who report higher digital skills in their five-point scale self-efficacy question are also more familiar with the digital skills than those who had a lower level of digital skills.

Analytical findings

We offer the following nine measures for predicting university students' digital skills along with some results coming from application of such measures:

1 Gender: male students reported more familiarity with the digital skills than female students did;
2 Age: older students reported more familiarity with the digital skills, although this might not be true beyond an educational setting;

3   Years of studying and living on campus: fourth and third year students reported more familiarity with digital skills;
4   Owning a laptop or a desktop computer;
5   Number of places of access: the higher the number of places of access available to a student, the more effectively he/she is able to use computers and the Internet;
6   Time spent on the Internet daily: users with higher daily usage tend to report more familiarity with digital skills;
7   Years using the Internet: students who started using the Internet earlier than their cohorts tend to report more familiarity with digital skills;
8   Digital skills self-efficacy: respondents who evaluate their digital skills as "skilled" and "very skilled" are more familiar with digital skills;
9   The set of the digital skills measures: the set of 41 digital skills measures, introduced and tested in this study give us the ability to predict digital skills of university students.

Generally speaking, our measurement indicates that the second-level digital divide is noticeable among undergraduate students of the University of Tehran and among various age and gender groups. The findings also indicate that the pattern of Internet use (years using the Internet) and the amount of daily use of the Internet, and the possession of a laptop or a desktop determine the factors affecting the second-level digital divide.

Conclusion

The research findings contribute to our understanding about the mechanism of educational inequality in the University of Tehran. For example, it is safe to claim here that a difference of skills among students has caused an educational inequality as the prime source of inequality among students. Differences in skills are important because, as Friemel and Signer (2010) put it, such differences would produce non-egalitarian use of the Internet applications and content, something that bring us to a Weberian type of social stratification across Internet users in Iran.

Although it is generally taken for granted that younger Internet users are very skilled, our study shows this is not necessarily true. With respect to educational systems' approaches toward new media technologies, in many countries including Iran, funding and planning are more focused on equipping educational institutions with new devices rather than helping students develop a new approach toward new media technologies.

In terms of the techniques that we employed to produce such a conclusion, it should be noted that the measures that we introduced and tested in this study are developed in an educational environment. Using such measurements for other socio-cultural environments, age groups or for specific professional purposes would require some modifications.

Also, there might be questions regarding censorship and how it could have affected the research results. It should be noted here that our research was conducted in an academic environment. Generally speaking, censorship could deepen digital divide because more skilled users can overcome censorship attempts (anti-filtering software, for example). Less skilled users lack such abilities and that can affect their access and Internet usage and produce more stratification. It should also be added that we have observed that almost all known social networking and micro blogging websites are subject to government blocking regulations in Iran. Nevertheless, some 66.5 percent of the respondents reported they were familiar with Internet forums and some 64.4 percent of them claimed to have had access to social networking websites. We should add that our own personal observations indicate that a large number of university students are regarded as Facebook users although it is hard to provide reliable statistics for that claim.

We are certainly aware that some of the inequalities we report in our work follow similar patterns in other parts of the world. Issues such as gender gap (DiMaggio *et al.*, 2001; Herring, 2001), number of places of access (Livingstone and Helsper, 2010), time spent on Internet and years using the Internet (Hargittai, 2002, 2005) are among a few that seem to be similar to what is addressed here. Nevertheless, this shows that, although Internet penetration rate in Iran is lower than some advanced societies, similar patterns in Internet usage exist. We also tried to make sense of it and show how it might affect future generations in Iran.

Finally, there are some limitations to this study especially where units of observations are concerned. We still need more studies on a national level to measure digital divide in Iran in order to be able to make a conclusion about Iran. We are aware that although access rates are growing in Iran, a broadband divide is developing and this is where new measures are needed to determine the dimensions of second-level digital divide.

References

Abdollahyan, H. and Ahmadi, M. (2011). A survey analysis of digital literacy among undergraduate students of the University of Tehran. *Amity Journal of Media and Communication*, 1(1)m, 1–6.

Bandura, A. (1994). Self-efficacy. In V.S. Ramachaudran (ed.), *Encyclopedia of human behavior (Vol. 4, pp. 71–81)*, New York: Academic Press. Available from: http://www.des.emory.edu/mfp/BanEncy.html (retrieved 15 April 2010).

Bandura, A. and Locke, E.A. (2003). Negative self-efficacy and goal effects revisited. *Journal of Applied Psychology*, 88(1), 87–99.

Bandura, A., Barbaranelli, C., Caprara, G.V. and Pastorelli, C. (2001). Self-efficacy beliefs as shapers of children's aspirations and career trajectories. *Child Development*, 72(1), 187–206.

Bandura, A. (1977). Self-efficacy: Toward a unifying theory of behavioral change, *Psychological Review*, 84(2), 191–215.

Bonfadelli, H. (2002). The Internet and knowledge gaps: A theoretical and empirical investigation. *European Journal of Communication*, 17(1), 65–84.

Crenshaw, E.M. and Robison K.K. (2006). Globalization and the digital divide: The roles of structural conduciveness and global connection in the Internet diffusion. *Social Science Quarterly*, 87 (1), 190–207.

Department of Economic and Social Affairs of the United Nations. (2005). *Understanding knowledge societies: In twenty questions and answers with the Index of Knowledge Societies*, New York: United Nations.

DiMaggio, P., Hargittai, E., Neuman, W.R. and Robinson, J.P. (2001). Social implications of the Internet. *Annual Review of Sociology*, 27, 307–336.

Dobson, T.M. and Willinsky, J. (2009). Digital literacy. In, D.R. Olson and N. Torrance (eds.), *The Cambridge handbook of literacy* (286–312.). Cambridge, UK: Cambridge University Press.

Eshet, Y. (2002). Digital literacy: A new terminology framework and its application to the design of meaningful technology-based learning environments. In P. Barker and S. Rebelsky (eds.), *Proceedings of EDMEDIA, 2002 World Conference on Educational Multimedia, Hypermedia, & Telecommunication*. Norfolk, VA, US: Association for the Advancement of Computing in Education, 493–498.

Eshet, Y. and Aviram, R. (2006). Towards a theory of digital literacy: Three scenarios for the next steps. *European Journal of Open Distance E-Learning*. Available from: http://www.eurodl.org/index.php?p=archives&year=2006&hal fyear=1&article=223

Eshet-Alkalai, Y. (2004). Digital literacy: A conceptual framework for survival skills in the digital era. *Journal of Educational Multimedia and Hypermedia*, 13(1), 93–106.

Eshet-Alkalai, Y. and Chajut, E. (2009). Changes over time in digital literacy. *CyberPsychology & Behavior*, 12(6), 713–715.

Eshet-Alkali, Y. and Amichai-Hamburger, Y. (2004). Experiments in digital literacy. *Cyberpsychology & Behavior*, 7(4), 421–429.

Friemel, T.N. and Signer, S. (2010). Web 2.0 literacy: Four aspects of the second-level digital divide. *Studies in Communication Sciences*. 10(2), 147–170.

Gilster, P. (1997). *Digital Literacy*. London: John Wiley & Sons.

Gui, M. and Argentin, G. (2011). Digital skills of the Internet natives: Differences of digital literacy in a random sample of northern Italian high school students. *New Media & Society*, 2(17), 1–18.

Hargittai, E. (2002). Second level digital divide: Differences in people's online skills. *First Monday* 7(4). Available from: http://firstmonday.org/htbin/cgiwrap/bin/ojs/index.php/fm/article/view/942/864 (retrieved 5 January 2010).

Hargittai, E. (2004). The Internet access and use in Context. *New Media & Society*. 6(1), 137–143.

Hargittai, E. (2005). Survey measures of web-oriented digital literacy. *Social Science Computer Review*, 23(3), 371–379.

Hargittai, E. (2009). An update on survey measures of web-oriented digital literacy. *Social Science Computer Review*. 27(1), 130–137.

Hargittai, E. and Walejko, G. (2008). The participation divide: Content creation and sharing in the digital age. *Information, Communication & Society*, 11(2), 239–256.

Herring, C.S. (2001). *Gender and power in online communication*. Available from: https://scholarworks.iu.edu/dspace/bitstream/handle/2022/1024/WP01-05B.html (retrieved 8 August 2011).

International Telecommunication Union (ITU). (2010). *Estimated Internet users, fixed Internet subscriptions, fixed broadband subscriptions.* Available from: http://www.itu. int/ITU-D/icteye/Reporting/ShowReportFrame.aspx?ReportName=/WTI/Inf ormationTechnologyPublic&ReportFormat=HTML4.0&RP_intYear=2010&RP_ intLanguageID=1&RP_bitLiveData=False (retrieved 11 August 2011).

Internet World Stats (2011). *Middle East usage and population statistics.* Available from: http://www.the Internetworldstats.com/middle.htm (retrieved 11 august 2011).

Jenkins, H., Clinton, K., Purushotma, R., Robinson, A.J. and Weigel, M. (2006). *Confronting the challenges of participatory culture: Media education for the 21st Century, an occasional paper written for the MacArthur Foundation.* Available from: http:// www.DigitalLearning.macfound.org/site/c.enJLKQNlFiG/b.2029291/k.97E5/ Occasional_Papers.htm (retrieved 10 January 2009).

Jolls, T. and Thoman, E. (2004). Media literacy: A national priority for a changing world. *American Behavioral Scientist*, 48(1), 18–29.

Jolls, T. and Thoman, E. (2008). *Literacy for the 21st Century: An overview & orientation guide to media literacy education.* Available from: http://mcdialit.org/ medialitkit.html; (retrieved 20 November 2008).

Livingstone, S. and Helsper, E. (2007). Gradations in digital inclusion: Children, young people and the digital divide. *New Media & Society*, 9(4), 671–696.

Livingstone, S. and Helsper, E. (2010). Balancing opportunities and risks in teenagers' use of the Internet: The role of online skills and the Internet self-efficacy. *New Media & Society*, 12(2), 309–329.

New Media Consortium. (2005). *A global imperative: The report of the 21st Century Literacy Summit.* Available from: http://www.educause.edu/Resources/ AGlobalImperativeTheReportofth/153960 (retrieved 9 January 2009).

Norris P. (2001). *Digital divide: Civic engagement, information poverty, and the Internet worldwide.* Cambridge, UK: Cambridge University Press.

Perez Tornero, J.M. (2004a). *Understanding digital literacy; Promoting digital literacy,* Available from: http://ec.europa.eu/education/archive/elearning/doc/studies/ dig_lit_en.pdf (retrieved 22 December 2008).

Perez Tornero, J.M. (2004b). *A new model for promoting digital literacy.* Available from: http://ec.europa.eu/education/archive/elearning/doc/workshops/ Digital_literacy/position_papers/perez_tornero_jose.pdf (retrieved 6 July 2009).

Pinto, M. and Sales, D. (2007). A research case study for user-centred information literacy instruction: Information behaviour of translation trainees. *Journal of Information Science*. 33(5), 531–550.

Ruane, J.M. (2005). *Essentials of research methods: A guide to social science research,* Oxford, UK: Blackwell.

Sassi, S. (2005). Cultural differentiation or social segregation? Four approaches to the digital divide. *New Media & Society*, 7(5), 684–700.

Selwyn, N. (2004). Reconsidering political and popular understandings of the digital divide. *New Media Society*, 6(3), 341–362.

Semati, M. (2008). Living with globalization and the Islamic State: An introduction to media, culture and society in Iran. In M. Semati (ed.) *Media, culture and society in Iran: Living with globalization and the Islamic State*. London: Routledge, 1–13.

Tsatsou, P. (2011). Digital divides revisited: What is new about divides and their research? *Media, Culture & Society*, 33(2), 317–331.

Tyner, K. (1998). *Literacy in a digital world: Teaching and learning in the age of information*, Mahwah, NJ, US: Lawrence Erlbaum.

van Deursen, A.J.A.M. and van Dijk, J.A.G.M. (2010). The Internet skills and the digital divide. *New Media & Society*, 11(11), 1–19.

van Dijk, J.A.G.M. and Hacker, K. (2003). The digital divide as a complex and dynamic phenomenon. *Information Society*. 19, 315–326.

van Dijk, J.A.G.M. (2005). *The deepening divide: Inequality in the information society*. Thousand Oaks, US: Sage.

van Dijk, J.A.G.M. (2006a). *The network society* (2nd edn). London: Sage.

van Dijk, J.A.G.M. (2006b). Digital divide research achievements and shortcomings. *Poetics*, 34, 221–235.

Warnick, B. (2002). *Critical literacy in a digital era: Technology, rhetoric, and the public interest*. Mahwah, NJ: Lawrence Erlbaum.

Wilson, K.R., Walin, J.S. and Reiser, C. (2003). Social stratification and the digital divide. *Social Science Computer Review*, 21(2). 133–143.

Yu, L. (2006). Understanding information inequality: Making sense of the literature of the information and digital divides. *Journal of Librarianship and Information Science*, 38(4), 229–252.

Notes

1 See Department of Economic and Social Affairs of the United Nations (2005).
2 According to the International Communication Union (ITU), however, the latest statistics (2010) indicate that only a small percentage of the Iranian users (0.68%) have access to broadband connections. This gap is something that worries scholars of the field, as in the long term it could slow down Internet use, causing issues in development projects in Iran.
3 In our questionnaire we put two bogus items (Proxypod and JFV) following Hargittai's model of inquiry (Hargittai, 2009). Although these two terms are very similar to ICT terms, they express no meaning. Our findings indicate that the mean of the bogus item JFV among 43 items was the lowest one, and the mean of Proxypod was only higher than RSS, feed, XML, mirror websites, podcast and JFV. That is probably because this item is similar to other ICT terms. These results indicate that it is likely that the respondents did not answer our questions in a haphazard way. That means they did not claim they are familiar with items that do not exist. In order to evaluate the reliability of the measures used in the questionnaire we conducted the Cronbach's Alpha test. The test result for 41 variables (items) minus the 2 bogus items amounted to 0.97, which confirms we used a highly reliable set of measures in the questionnaire.
4 For arguments on self-efficacy see: Bandura (1977, 1994); Bandura and Locke (2003); Bandura *et al.*, (2001). And, for arguments on digital literacy self-efficacy see: Hargittai (2005, 2009); Livingstone and Helsper (2010).
5 The data was collected to assess the digital literacy of students. Here we tried to apply a new theoretical framework to an existing set of data.

Section 6

Under-studied countries and regions

16 The digital divide in the Latin American context[1]

Daniela Trucco
United Nations Economic
Commission for Latin America and the Caribbean

Introduction

Durkheim's sociological theory was developed a century ago, when the modernization process of industrial society was perceived to be generating a set of disintegrating processes; class conflicts, recurrent economic crisis, increased suicide rates, lack of social values, etc. (Usátegui, 2003). This social unrest had to be addressed through social regulating processes and the generation of social integration; where the state and the education system played a key role.

The main purpose of this chapter is to analyze from Durkheim's viewpoint, the contribution that educational public policy in Latin America (LA) is making to society in the digital era. In one of the most unequal regions of the world, the main risk is that the mass dissemination of information and communication technologies (ICT) could be generating new and rapidly growing differences. The approach views ICT as instruments for addressing the development needs of the region through the socialization process of children and adolescents of different social sectors of society, contributing to the formation of human capital assets in the more disadvantaged social sectors of LA's society. However, there are different types or levels of digital divides that operate simultaneously. The access gap, which is still substantial, is compounded by a second breach of use and appropriation. The analysis uses empirical data collected through countries' household surveys and through international educational assessment tests like the OECD Programme for International Student Assessment (PISA) (OECD, 2009).

The discussion focuses on the role that public policy can take on in order to counter the consequences of market-driven mass dissemination of ICT in terms of social integration (à la Durkheim). His perspective on the role of the state, as representing society's interest and education being a key tool in this process is used to follow these developments in the region. A strategic area is the public school system that can not only promote more equitable access to technology but also its meaningful use and skill development for generations to come.

**The inevitable process of Internet dissemination:
Risks and prospects**

Countries of the LA region have not been exempt from the rapid dissemination and incorporation of digital technologies – such as computers and the Internet – in everyday life. Differential access through the Internet to inconceivable amounts of information, with global reach and no time barriers, should explain important changes in social structures. Access to the Internet and to ICT devices also carries meanings linked to their use, created and disseminated especially by advertising. The most prominent of these is the promise of individual success through a lifestyle involving their use in all daily activities. Whereas whoever lacks access to these technologies appears doomed to stagnate and be marginalized (UNDP, 2006).

The process of dissemination and use of these technologies has also been the subject of public policies, as tools for development and effective government service. Such public policies have further sought to offset inequities of access by promoting a variety of initiatives to foster widespread use (UNDP, 2006). The promotion of access to these technologies through the education system has been one of the privileged public policy strategies in this region.

Durkheim would have agreed with the importance given to the education system as a strategic factor for social integration. Education was conceived by the author as crucial for socialization, where society needs to oversee that individuals acquire the common moral values and skills that allow them to maintain collective life. Society cannot survive if there is not enough homogeneity among its members; education perpetuates and reinforces that homogeneity, fixing in advance the essential similarities required by collective life in the child's soul (Durkheim, 1975, as cited in: Usátegui, 2003). Although not an opponent of private education, Durkheim saw an important regulatory and supervising role of the state in the education system. The state's intervention is required if the goal is a more equal society (Usátegui, 2003).

The education system has been conceived as a strategic port of entry into the information and knowledge society. The first school-oriented ICT policies and programs in LA emerged in the late 1980s and early 1990s, under the assumption that they were tools that would address the major challenges that countries faced in this field. Those challenges included ensuring a high quality education, improving the efficiency of education systems and guaranteeing equity in the different dimensions of those systems (Sunkel and Trucco, 2010).

At the same time, ICT mass dissemination through market-driven forces has been very rapid in recent years, especially in the richer countries of the LA region, and the youngest generations are the ones that have incorporated them to the greatest extent in their daily lives. However, as expected in one of the most unequal regions of the world, it is a process that has reproduced and even exacerbated the pre-existing social inequities. As the data analysis will show in the following section, there are different types or levels of digital divides operating simultaneously.

While access to the Internet presents a very equalizing potential, in terms of information access around the world for all its users, it also has the risk of reproducing social cleavages. The concept of a second digital divide acquires relevance in this sense, which is related to the opportunity of taking real advantage of the Internet's potential in the development of individual capabilities valuable in the current postindustrial society. This type of digital divide has been identified between those who have the necessary competences and skills to benefit from computer use and those who do not. These competences and skills are closely linked to the persons' economic, cultural and social capital (Pedró, 2009). That means that not all types of Internet use and appropriation will empower young people and help them build the capabilities required for their future development and secure their position in the economy.

Even though the process of Internet dissemination has produced an important generational gap, meaning that young people in general have integrated this technology much more rapidly than older generations, the next section's data analysis will demonstrate how class advantage still plays an important role here. Children and youngsters inherit their class position also in terms of a differential access to equipment, contacts and competences available for them, which marks a difference in their approach to digital technology. This gap carries a risk of social polarization and disintegration.

As mentioned above, countries of the LA region have put their hopes in the public promotion of Internet access and use, using the public school system as the strategic point of entry, in order to counterbalance the inequalities produced by technology dissemination. These efforts can be understood from Durkheim's perspective on the role he assigned to the state. According to his vision, the state was the great architect, constructor and producer of society and its development, through the design of rational and dynamic policies (Caputo, 1996). The state has a regulatory function for the collective interests: fixing individuals' rights (García Raggio, 1998) and generating the adequate conditions for their observance. The education system is the privileged tool the state has to pursue equal opportunities for society's new generations.

In this new globalized era the concern for social exclusion is not only connected to the categories of economic exploitation and dominance, but can also be analyzed from a cultural and subjective angle. The Internet has helped to integrate the economy from a global perspective, expanding the market's needs and logic, but leaving a portion of the population with a high risk of social exclusion (García Raggio, 1998). Durkheim's concern for social integration is, then, still very relevant.

Society, through its organized secondary institutions, with an overseeing role of the state, regulates individual interests and contributes to the encouragement of a moral existence that promotes social integration. From Durkheim's perspective, the state's function, especially through the education system, is the construction of social values, organizing society in a way that ensures fairness, that is, allowing each member to be treated as he or she deserves, inhibiting unjust or humiliating dependency, in the understanding that each person also maintains obligations to the other members of society (Richter, 1960). "The main purpose of state intervention is to free the individual from whatever environmental disabilities may keep them from realizing their potentialities" (Richter, 1960: p. 202). This view is consistent with the efforts that LA states have been promoting through their public education policies, to guarantee that no portion of the new generations will be excluded from the acquisition of these critical digital skills, and the key capital and cultural assets that are generated through ICT use. The presentation of data about the digital divide in LA, in the third section of this chapter, will analyze how successful they have been in reducing digital inequalities and promoting social integration.

The process of Internet integration in the Latin American context

Although still at a large distance from the more developed regions of the world, LA countries have shown significant progress in the home availability of digital technological equipment. Particularly in the last few years, the increase in the acquisition of home computers has been dramatic and it probably relates to technological progress and the consequent reduction of costs (see Table 16.1). The progress in Internet connection at the household level has been slower and it is probably associated with the high connectivity costs that still persist in the region. In any case, the growth in ICT penetration is significant: while at the beginning of the decade the access to the Internet was practically nil, by the end of the decade countries such as Brazil, Uruguay and Chile show connectivity levels that reach almost a third of their population.

The digital gap between richer and poorer countries is however patent. Plus, the digital gap between different socioeconomic groups within each country is significant. While on average 65 percent of households that belong to the richest income quintile have access to the Internet at home, only 2 percent of the poorest households (first income quintile) do. In general, studies show that despite this segmented access to technology, children and young people are entering the world of technology in greater numbers. In households with 12-to-19-year-olds, connectivity is rising at a faster rate than in households that do not have members within this age range (ECLAC, 2011). Figure 16.1 shows that in most countries

Table 16.1 Latin America and the Caribbean (selected countries): Percentage of households with computer and Internet access (years 2000–2009)

Country		2000	2001	2002	2003	2004	2005	2006	2007	2008	2009
Argentina	Computer	—	22	—	—	—	—	—	—	—	—
	Internet	—	9	—	—	—	—	—	—	—	—
Bolivia (Plurination State of)	Computer	—	7	7	—	—	12	—	17	—	—
	Internet	—	—	—	—	—	4	—	3	—	—
Brazil	Computer	—	13	14	15	16	19	22	27	31	35
	Internet	—	9	10	11	12	14	17	20	24	27
Chile	Computer	18	—	—	25	—	—	33	—	—	42
	Internet	8	—	—	13	—	—	19	—	—	29
Colombia	Computer	—	—	—	11	12	15	16	15	23	23
	Internet	—	—	—	5	6	6	7	7	13	15
Costa Rica	Computer	14	17	20	—	24	27	28	31	34	37
	Internet	4	5	7	—	—	10	10	12	15	18
Ecuador	Computer	—	—	—	18	—	—	18	—	23	23
	Internet	—	—	—	4	—	—	2	—	7	8
El Salvador	Computer	3	5	5	5	6	7	8	9	11	12
	Internet	1	2	2	2	2	2	2	3	4	6
Guatemala	Computer	4	—	—	—	—	—	11	—	—	—
	Internet	1	—	—	—	—	—	2	—	—	—
Honduras	Computer	—	—	—	5	5	6	8	10	—	—
	Internet	—	—	—	—	1	2	1	2	4	—
Mexico	Computer	—	12	15	—	18	19	21	22	26	27
	Internet	—	6	7	—	9	9	10	12	14	18
Nicaragua	Computer	—	2	—	—	—	4	6	—	—	7
	Internet	—	—	—	—	—	0	0	—	—	2
Panama	Computer	—	—	—	—	—	—	16	17	—	—
	Internet	—	—	—	—	—	—	8	9	12	—
Paraguay	Computer	5	—	5	6	6	9	9	11	15	19
	Internet	1	—	1	2	1	2	3	3	6	11
Peru	Computer	—	5	6	7	7	8	9	14	16	19
	Internet	—	0	1	1	1	2	3	6	7	10
Dominican Republic	Computer	—	—	—	—	—	—	—	—	—	17
	Internet	—	—	—	—	—	3	—	5	—	—
Uruguay	Computer	—	18	18	19	21	22	24	28	39	48
	Internet	—	13	14	14	13	13	13	16	23	28
Venezuela (Bolivarian Republic of)	Computer	—	—	—	10	10	10	—	15	17	—
	Internet	—	—	—	2	2	2	—	6	9	—

Source: Author's preparation based on ECLAC special tabulations of household surveys data, harmonized by OSILAC ICT Statistical Information System.

(particularly those with more advanced levels of access), the access to the Internet is higher in households with a presence of school aged youth, which is the generation that supposedly represents the window of opportunity for these countries to enter the information society well prepared. The younger generation might be pushing the acquisition of this type of equipment at home, accelerating market penetration.

However promising the progress of Internet access within the younger generations might seem, a less optimistic approach is reached once these advances are analyzed by class position. Younger generations from privileged social classes are the social group that has advanced most rapidly in the home acquisition of Internet connectivity. The burgeoning, market-driven penetration of ICT in the region is creating substantial gaps in access to equipment by social class (ECLAC, 2011). While approximately 7 percent of 12 to 19-year-olds that have access to the Internet at home belong to the highest income quintile, only 1 percent of this population belong to the poorest income quintile (Figure 16.2). The regional average however, hides the heterogeneity among LA countries and their respective living standards. Less affluent countries such as Honduras and Bolivia have fewer class differences in access to ICT, because households of the higher income quintiles have much lower living standards than those of more affluent countries, such as Brazil, Chile or Uruguay, which show a clearer class divide in household ICT access.

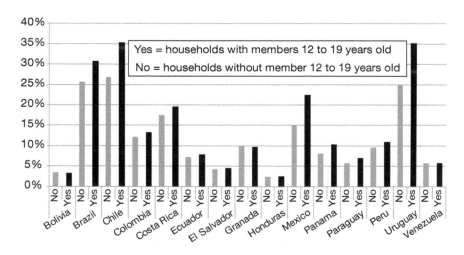

Figure 16.1 Latin America and Caribbean (LAC) (15 countries): Percentage of households with Internet access, with or without members between 12 and 19 years old (around 2009)

Source: Author's preparation based on ECLAC special tabulations of data from household surveys.

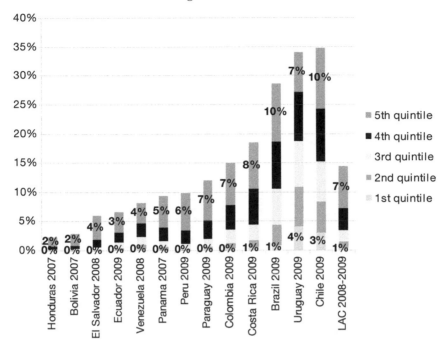

Figure 16.2 Latin America (13 countries): Percentage of people 12 to 19 years old that have Internet at home, according to country and household income (around 2009)

Source: Author's preparation based on ECLAC special tabulations of data from household surveys.

Identifying different connectivity access rates by generation leads to an examination of how much this weakens or reinforces class-based gaps (Kaztman, 2010). A look at the figures shows that in the countries where technology is more market-driven (such as Brazil, Chile and Uruguay) the class gaps for younger-generation users are not narrowing (ECLAC, 2011). They are widening (see Figure 16.3). In households without young people the gap is less than 40 percentage points, while in households with young members in the more connected countries, the gap has grown to over 50 percent.

The digital divide in LA is, in part, rooted in unequal access stemming from enormous differences in the availability of equipment. But it also has to do with the way students use and can benefit from such equipment. At this other level, inequality is evidenced in different levels of ability to use ICT productively and take advantage of their potential for developing the competencies and skills necessary for integration in the globalized world (Sunkel and Trucco, 2010).

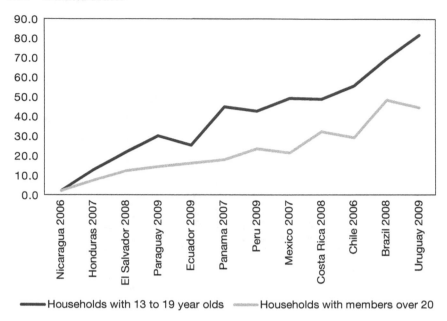

──Households with 13 to 19 year olds   ──Households with members over 20

Figure 16.3 LA (11 countries): Difference in the proportion of households with Internet connection in the highest and lowest income quintiles by presence or absence of household members aged 13–19, around 2008[a] (percentages)

Source: ECLAC (2011), on the basis of special processing of household surveys reconciled by OSILAC; and Kaztman (2010).

[a] Countries shown in order of the percentage of households with Internet connection in each country.

Data collected through international educational assessment tests like the OECD PISA (OECD, 2009) show the class differences between secondary students in terms of Internet and computer use. An optional student questionnaire is offered in the PISA measurement that allows a deeper analysis in relation to student use of ICT at school. Only four countries of the Latin America and Caribbean (LAC) region chose to participate in this additional component: Chile, Panama, Trinidad and Tobago, and Uruguay.

The main uses that young people make of computers involve the Internet, primarily as a means of communication and, to a lesser degree, to download music and games. But in these four countries, homework use of the computer and the Internet at home is the most relevant use in terms of frequency, even higher than the OECD countries' average.

Considering the high frequency users for these different areas and the students' class position, the second type of digital gap discussed before becomes evident. Class advantage in terms of taking full advantage of the Internet's potential in a broad sense is clear, which means that youngsters that are born in a more advantageous socioeconomic situation also acquire better skills and competences to participate as adults in society. OECD PISA 2009 reveals that approximately 20 to 25 percent of 15-year-old students are frequent users for schoolwork related activities (see Figure 16.4).

A striking difference between the LAC countries and the OECD countries is the distribution of these frequent scholar ICT users. While in OECD countries they are distributed almost in equal portions according to the students' economic and sociocultural quartiles,[2] LA countries show a clear digital gap according to class position. Most frequent users belong to the third and fourth superior quartiles, while very few belong to the first one. The same tendencies can be observed from the data related to communicational and recreational Internet use. These are the most

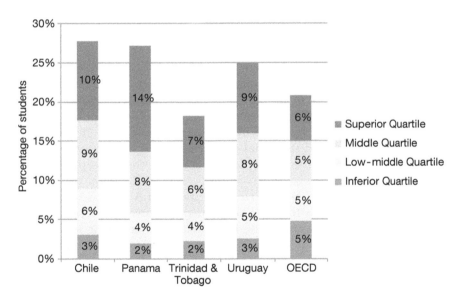

Figure 16.4 Percentage of 15 year old students that are high frequency users of ICT for school work at home, according to their economic and socio-cultural status, year 2009

Source: Author's preparation, based on ECLAC's special tabulations of PISA 2009 ICT Questionnaire data.

Note: OECD represents the weighted average of OECD countries. High frequency users were defined through a summation index of students who declare to use ICT at least once a week for the following activities: Doing homework on the computer; browse the Internet for schoolwork; use e-mail for communication with other students about schoolwork; use e-mail for communication with teachers and submission of homework or other schoolwork; download, upload or browse material from your school's website; and check the school's website for announcements.

common and natural ways for young people to approach these technologies, but class position which already generates a gap in access to the equipment, also generates a gap in terms of the use and skill development associated with it.

In general, the digital divide in LA has been understood only in terms of access to technology. Yet, as the discussion of user profiles has shown, a more profound digital gap has also emerged between those who have the social, cultural and economic position needed to take advantage of computers, and, in addition, have access to the Internet at home, and those who occupy a less favorable position in society. As happened with educational attainment differentials, there is a risk that strongly market-based advantages for families will continue to be the prime determinant of digital divides (ECLAC, 2011, p. 108).

The role of the state in the regulation of the market's divergent tendencies

Many countries in the region have made significant progress in recent years in integrating ICT into the education sector. Most of the schools in this region are part of a public education system. As part of that process, many countries have implemented policies involving the creation of institutions and the allocation of significant resources. As mentioned above, a central thrust of the efforts in the region to deploy public policies in the area of ICT for education has been to contribute to social integration and to avoid the social polarization that would result if broad segments of the population were denied access to the new opportunities offered by ICT (Sunkel and Trucco, 2010).

As Durkheim would have asserted, the state in LA countries should be playing a regulating role to diminish the market's divergent tendencies, in order to protect and include those individuals who are being left behind. Schools have been seen as strategic playing fields for reducing inequalities of access. However, if these programs in the schools are to contribute to equity, then merely reducing inequalities of access is not enough. What is needed is to ensure that ICT for education can prevent the gap in skills and behaviors among Internet users from exacerbating existing differences. The discussion that follows uses the data provided by the PISA studies to analyze how effective the state has been in achieving both objectives through its education policies in LA countries.

As Table 16.2 shows, the percentage of 15-year-old students with school access to computers has increased significantly in the LA countries that have participated in the PISA assessments. Computer coverage at schools has reached high levels, closer than household computer access to the average coverage reached in more developed regions of the world, such as the OECD countries. Moreover, contrary to the tendencies followed by household ICT access, schools' computer access shows a more equitable growth in coverage, reducing by half the social gap between students of different social backgrounds in the last decade (from 19 to 8 percentage points) (Claro *et al.*, 2011).

Table 16.2 Latin America (7 countries) and OECD average: Percentage of 15-year-old students with computer access in school, according to ESCS quartiles (years 2000 to 2009)

		Inferior Quartile (%)	Superior Quartile (%)	Class Gap (%)
Argentina	2000	48	67	20
	2006	83	95	13
	2009	80	95	15
Brazil	2000	50	70	20
	2003	37	78	41
	2006	67	89	23
	2009	89	95	6
Chile	2000	97	100	3
	2006	92	98	6
	2009	100	100	0
Colombia	2006	89	94	5
	2009	98	99	1
Mexico	2000	56	83	27
	2003	61	87	27
	2006	89	96	7
	2009	90	98	8
Peru	2000	38	66	29
	2009	71	95	25
Uruguay	2003	75	86	10
	2006	88	91	3
	2009	100	100	0
LA	2000	54	73	19
	2003	47	81	34
	2006	79	93	14
	2009	88	96	8
OECD	2000	82	85	3
	2003	75	85	10
	2006	90	90	0
	2009	98	100	2

Source: Author's preparation, based on ECLAC's special tabulations of PISA 2000, 2003, 2006 and 2009 data.

Note: LA and OECD represent the weighted average of each regions participating countries.

Internet school access has followed a similar tendency but at a lower rate, both in terms of reaching a lower percentage of schools and in terms of reducing social gaps at a lower rate (Claro *et al.*, 2011). Nevertheless, equitable growth coverage has been an important policy contribution that is also reflected in the real opportunity to use a computer at school, when looking at the student computer ratio data (see Table 16.3).

Table 16.3 shows that the gap between student to computer ratio in school for students of different social background has decreased significantly in most LA countries over the last few years. The distance between the two extreme economic and sociocultural quartiles has declined from a difference of 39 students in the year 2000 to a difference of 7 students per computer available in school in the year 2009.

The sum of these ICT access indicators in the school system shows that education policy has had significant results in terms of promoting broad

Table 16.3 Latin America (9 countries) and OECD average: Student to computer ratio at school, according to ESCS quartiles (years 2000 to 2009)

		Inferior Quartile (%)	*Superior Quartile* (%)	*Class Gap* (%)
Argentina	2000	58	32	26
	2009	34	18	17
Brazil	2000	218	42	177
	2009	45	28	18
Chile	2000	46	37	9
	2009	20	22	−2
Colombia	2009	38	26	13
Mexico	2000	37	16	21
	2009	13	10	3
Panama	2009	20	21	−1
Peru	2000	86	38	48
	2009	24	13	11
Trinidad & Tobago	2009	15	16	−1
Uruguay	2000	31	27	3
	2009	25	21	4
LA	2000	72	33	39
	2009	24	17	7
OECD	2000	11	10	1
	2009	8	7	1

Source: Claro *et al.* (2011), based on ECLAC's special tabulations of PISA 2000–2009 data.

Note: LA and OECD represent the weighted average of each region's participating countries. Uruguay's 2000 data is from the 2003 PISA.

access to ICT infrastructure and equipment. Moreover, these efforts have benefited the least favored socioeconomic sectors, reducing the distance that separated them from the more privileged sectors. However, these indicators show that there is still a long path to advance in terms of having access that allows real quality and regular use of ICT for students in school.

The data obtained through the PISA ICT special questionnaire (only applied in four countries of the LA region) demonstrate that the percentage of students that are high frequency users of computers and the Internet at school is generally lower than the percentage of high frequency users at home for the same type of activities. For example, on average 69 percent of students from these four LA countries use the computer at home at least once a week for homework, compared to 42 percent that do so at school. Another example is chatting online, one of the most widespread activities: while on average 65 percent of LA students chat at least once a week from a home computer, only 10 percent do so from a school computer.

The problem with access opportunities at schools or other places such as commercial establishments is the low intensity at which individuals can make use of the technology. Because of the cost, or due to access conditions at educational institutions, those who use these locations normally do so for shorter periods of time and thus have fewer possibilities for developing digital competencies for social and productive integration than do young people who can access the Internet at home (ECLAC, 2011).

However low this percentage of high frequency school ICT users might be, it is worthwhile analyzing what user profiles have been developed in this context and the role of the school system in generating or reducing social gaps at this level. Despite ICT access differences between LA countries and OECD countries, when analyzing user profiles, you find similar patterns of use. Moreover, LA countries show a higher percentage of ICT high frequency users at school (see Figure 16.5).

Moreover, what appears as a relevant difference in the regional user profiles is the prominent place that schoolwork ICT use has in LA countries, as compared to the OECD average. For example (see Figure 16.5), in Chile 45 percent of students are high frequency users of school Internet for schoolwork, compared to only 31 percent in OECD countries. On the other hand, both Chile and Panama have more than 30 percent of their students using school computers at least once a week for their individual homework, while in OECD countries this rate drops to 14 percent. These results are important, because they might be revealing a certain pedagogical orientation from teachers or even parents, to promote the use of ICT in support of schoolwork. This would constitute a base for what could be an interesting projection of the development of relevant and more complex skills related to ICT (Claro *et al.*, 2011), reinforcing Durkheim's perspective.

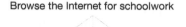

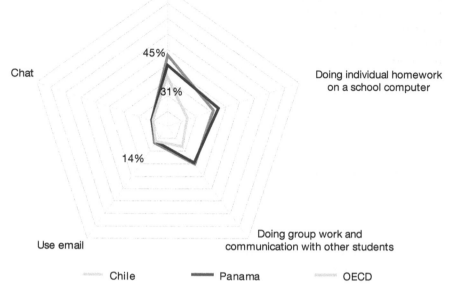

Figure 16.5 Chile, Panama & OECD average: percentage of 15 year old students who declare using school computers at least once a week, according to type of activity (year 2009)

Source: Claro, *et al.* (2011), based on ECLAC's special tabulations of PISA 2009 data – ICT questionnaire.

Note: OECD represents the weighted average of the region's participating countries.

Now, in terms of socioeconomic gaps, despite the lower possibilities of having high frequency ICT users at school, the difference in the percentage of students following this pattern of use is slightly more favorable to students that belong to less benefited social backgrounds. Figure 16.6 shows the patterns of school use for students of the four LA countries, distinguishing between those students that belong to the superior and inferior economic and sociocultural status quartiles. That means that schools have been able to provide equal opportunities of meaningful educational uses of technology at school, independent of the students' social background.

In today's increasingly global economy, the Internet and the skills developed through and with them are more and more relevant for Durkheim's concern for social integration. The analysis has shown that LA states have used education policy as one of their main strategies in promoting this integration process, and this approach has been relatively successful in terms of both providing access and promoting meaningful

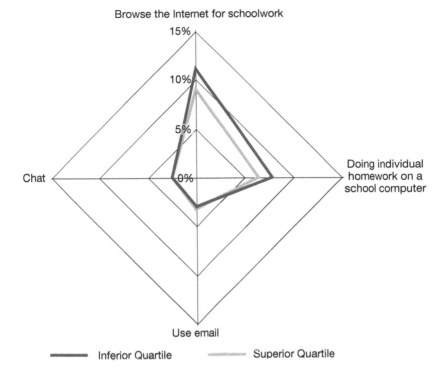

Browse the Internet for schoolwork

Figure 16.6 Latin America (4 countries): percentage of 15 year old students that use ICT at least once a week in school, by type of activity and the student's economic and socio-cultural status (year 2009)

Source: Claro, *et al.* (2011), based on ECLAC's special tabulations of PISA 2009 data – ICT questionnaire.

Note: LAC represents the weighted average of Chile, Panama, Trinidad & Tobago and Uruguay.

use to the new generations. However, the efforts must be greater in order to compensate for the huge differences generated through social class and household opportunities.

Summary and conclusions

The ongoing technological revolution advances and redefines the world's opportunities for development, for individuals and society in general. ICT dissemination is fast and moves almost in an automatic way pushed by market forces. LA has not been excluded from this process. However, the market-driven forces tend to leave some social sectors behind and to reproduce pre-existing social inequities (with the risk of exacerbating some of them) between and within nations. The great risk is an increase in social polarization, leaving social groups completely excluded from the possibility of integrating with the knowledge society. Social disintegration was one of Durkheim's main apprehensions in relation to the modernization process of his time.

That also seems to be the case up until now with regards to household acquisition of ICT equipment and the opportunities provided of use and competence development for younger generations. Greater intensity and productivity in use requires more time in front of monitors and quality programs for developing the required skills set. Here, the difference between those who access these technologies at home and those who do not currently determines the depth of the digital divide and reinforces underlying socioeconomic and capital gaps (ECLAC, 2011: p. 109).

As Durkheim would have seen it, the risks of social disintegration compel the state to play a role in counteracting these inequalities by offering more and better access to technology to those who have none at home, deepening penetration in order to increase usage time. ICT for education constitutes, following Durkheim's conception, one of the essential intellectual assets that the state should guarantee for all society's members. It has become a basic skill required to participate in today's economy, social networks and political arena both at the national and international levels.

Education policy and the school system have been a positive point of entry in the LA region. Especially in terms of providing more equitable access to technology but also in terms of offering pedagogical guidance that motivates students to use the technology autonomously both for research and homework. However, there still is much to be done in terms of promoting an equitable formation of knowledge and cultural assets. The school system is still far from providing a similar opportunity for ICT utilization to the one obtained through home access. School systems in LA countries have great challenges in terms of effectively integrating digital skills in the curriculum and promoting frequent and significant uses that will provide new generations with the required skills to compete and participate in the opportunities offered by society. This analysis shows how Durkheim's theoretical perspective, developed a century ago to understand Europe's modernization process, still has strength and analytical value. His reinterpretation enlightens the comprehension of the social consequences brought by technological changes. The velocity of these urgently demand the need for sociological reflection for which a new reading of Durkheim's papers can prove valuable.

References

Caputo, L. (1996). Durkheim, algunos elementos para la comprensión de las organizaciones sociales y los cambios en América Latina. Asunción, Paraguay: BASE Investigaciones Sociales.

Claro, M., Espejo, A., Jara, I. and Trucco, D. (2011). *Aporte del Sistema Educativo a la Reducción de las Brechas Digitales. Una mirada desde las mediciones PISA*. Santiago, Chile: ECLAC, forthcoming.

ECLAC (Economic Commission for Latin America and the Caribbean) (2011). *Social panorama of Latin America, 2010* (LC/G.2481-P). Santiago, Chile: United Nations publication.

García Raggio, A. (1998). *Transitando por los márgenes: las transformaciones del trabajo y el debilitamiento de la ciudadanía*. In E. De Ipola, (ed.) *La Crisis del Lazo Social. Durkheim, cien años después*. Buenos Aires, Argentina: Editorial Universitaria.

Kaztman, R. (2010). *Impacto social de la incorporación de las TIC en el sistema educativo*, (LC/L.3254-P), Santiago, Chile: Serie de Políticas Sociales 166, ECLAC.

OECD. (2009). *Pisa 2009 – Organisation for Economic Co-operation and Development*. Retrieved from http://www.oecd.org/pisa/pisaproducts/pisa2009

Pedró, F. (2009). *Are the New Millennium learners making their grades? Technology use and educational performance in PISA*. Paris: OECD Centre for Educational Research and Innovation (CERI).

Richter, M. (1960). *Durkheim's politics and political theory*. In K. Wolff (ed.) *Essays on sociology and philosophy by Emile Durkheim et al. with appraisals of his life and thought*. Columbus, OH, US: Ohio State University Press.

Sunkel, G. and Trucco, D. (2010). *New information and communication technologies for education in Latin America: Risks and opportunities*. (LC/L.3266-P). Santiago, Chile: Serie de Políticas Sociales 167, ECLAC.

UNDP (United Nations Development Programme). (2006). *Desarrollo humano en Chile. Las nuevas tecnologías: ¿Un salto al futuro?* Santiago, Chile: United Nations.

Usátegui, E. (2003). *La educación en Durkheim: ¿Socialización versus conflicto?* Revista *Complutense de Educación*, 14(1), 175–194.

Notes

1 Most of the information and data analysis included in this chapter was developed in the context of a project carried out by the United Nations ECLAC – Alliance for the Information Society, phase 2 – which is financed by the European Union. The author is grateful for the valuable statistical support provided by Andrés Espejo.

2 As measured by the ESCS which refers to the Economic, Social and Cultural Status. This index is elaborated based on the following variables: International Socio-Economic Index of Occupational Status (ISEI); parents' highest level of education converted into school years; PISA's family richness index; PISA's educational resources index; and PISA's index related to classic cultural possessions at home (http://stats.oecd.org/glossary/detail.asp?ID=5401).

17 The Central Asian digital divide

Barney Warf
University of Kansas

The digital divide, or social and spatial differentials in Internet access, has been the subject of a growing body of literature (Norris, 2001; Korupp and Szydlik, 2005; Warf, 2001), revealing how digital communications are enfolded in relations of wealth and power in ways that reproduce real world inequalities in virtual space. A significant literature has illustrated how the Internet is entwined with social inequalities (e.g., Witte and Mannon, 2010), and, by enforcing the information asymmetry advantage of those with access, may enhance social and spatial differences within societies. An enormous body of classical and more contemporary social theory has sketched the drivers and manifestations of social and spatial inequality, and need not be recapitulated here; suffice it to say that the literature on the digital divide has both been inspired by such theorizations and in turn traced how inequalities are manifested in terms of class, gender, and ethnic differences in Internet access (Compaine, 2001; Cooper and Compaine, 2001; Crang, Crosbie and Graham, 2006; Stevens, 2006). "Access" and "use" are vague terms, but are generally taken to mean deployment of the Internet at home or at work; rather than a simple access/non-access dichotomy, it is more useful to think of a gradation of levels of access, although data of this subtlety do not exist. For Marxists, the digital divide is yet another dimension of class inequality; for feminists, it is evidence of patriarchal limitations on women's opportunities; and for theorists who take ethnicity as their point of departure, the "racial ravine" constitutes another means by which minorities suffer from discrimination.

Despite its historical status as the crossroads of Asia, Central Asia has been peripheralized in studies of the Internet (but see Warf, 2010). This oversight may be attributable largely due to the region's marginal geopolitical status during the Cold War, the crippling legacy of Soviet political and economic policies, its relatively small population size and low Internet penetration rates, and its persistent poverty and endemic government corruption.

The Internet in Central Asia affords the opportunity to study international technology diffusion and adoption, including the incentives, policies, and barriers that shape the uneven growth of users over time and space (Caselli and Coleman, 2001; Clarke, 2004; Comin and Hobijn, 2004; Keller, 2004). The view that the diffusion of the Internet is a relatively straightforward matter of removing economic obstacles and encouraging adoption hints at technical solutions for complex social and political problems. This approach to overcoming the digital divide is redolent of older modernizationist approaches to development that portray technology adoption as a simple, linear path. Yet the digital divide in Central Asia reveals a far more complex situation, one in which political dynamics play a fundamental role in shaping who has Internet access and who does not, including frequently corrupt and oppressive governments. Indeed, Central Asia reflects mounting inequalities characteristic of neoliberalized societies worldwide, with a small, wealthy, globalized elite and large numbers of impoverished and marginalized residents (Anderson and Pomfret, 2004; Falkingham, 2005). In this light, as it emerged from the relative inequality of the Soviet era into the globalized, privatized world of neoliberalism, the region began to offer a unique laboratory in which to examine how social and spatial discrepancies are reproduced and sustained, a topic that falls squarely within conventional theorizations of inequality. This chapter examines several dimensions of the Central Asian digital divide. It begins with an overview of the broad contours that shape social and spatial inequalities in the region, including incomes and poverty, the incipient fiber optic network, satellite services, government policies, and the slow arrival of broadband. Second, it focuses on the number and distribution of Central Asian netizens, the rapid growth of the Internet in the region, and the role played by cybercafés; it also points to the urban biases in Internet use, male dominance, and touches on some of the cultural obstacles to participation online. The third part reviews Internet censorship in the region in light of many states' attempts to restrict cyber-activism, a point raised to emphasize the politics of the digital divide. The conclusion highlights the chapter's principal analytical findings.

The architecture of the Central Asian digital divide: Infrastructures and policies

Central Asian countries vary widely in terms of incomes and standards of living (Table 17.1), ranging from miserably poor Afghanistan ($US 900 GDP per capita annually) to $12,700 in Kazakhstan. With the exception of Afghanistan, where a little more than one-quarter of the population can read or write, these countries have achieved almost universal literacy, in part due to the legacy of the Soviet Union. However, most have significant pools of people living below the poverty line, including more than half the population of Tajikistan. Because digital divides the world over are closely correlated with incomes, the existence of millions of impoverished people is a significant obstacle to the implementation of equal access to cyberspace. In many countries, landline telephone systems, which are critical for dial-up access, are antiquated and in disrepair, leading to slow upload and download speeds. Such communications networks still rely heavily on copper cable wires, when most of the world's telecommunications traffic has moved decisively into fiber optic cable. Mobile or cell phone penetration rates are much higher, but vary widely, from 22.5 percent in Turkmenistan to 96 percent in Kazakhstan.

Other than the telephone network, fiber optics and satellites remain the dominant technologies facilitating Internet access, especially for the increasingly important broadband applications. In Central Asia, the principal fiber optic line is the 27,000 km-long Trans-Asia-Europe (TAE) cable, the world's longest overland route, which began operations in 1998. It begins in Frankfurt, extends to Turkey, crosses Iran, has trunk lines northward to Georgia, Armenia, and Ukraine, and follows the ancient Silk Road route into western China and hence to Shanghai (Figure 17.1). Built by a consortium of international telecommunications companies, it constitutes the major high-capacity line within the region. However, while much of the world has witnessed a glut in fiber capacity, in Central Asia fiber connections remain relatively scarce and thus expensive. Some countries, such as Uzbekistan, have a reasonably well developed fiber infrastructure, complemented with microwave radio relay links, while others, such as Kyrgyzstan, are almost bereft of fiber and must utilize other modalities.

Satellite Internet provides another opportunity for providing access where terrestrial connections are not viable or are prohibitively expensive, and many Central Asian Internet service providers (ISPs) rely on satellite

Table 17.1 Central Asian economic, literacy, and ITC statistics, 2011

	GDP per capita (PPP) ($US)	% below poverty line	Adult literacy rate	Telephone landlines per 1000 people	Mobile phone penetration
Afghanistan	900	36.0	28.1	0.4	29.0
Kazakhstan	12,700	8.2	99.5	24.0	96.0
Kyrgyzstan	2,200	40.0	98.7	9.1	62.7
Mongolia	3,600	36.1	97.8	7.0	66.8
Tajikistan	2,000	53.0	99.5	4.2	53.7
Turkmenistan	7,500	30.0	98.8	0.3	22.5
Uzbekistan	3,100	26.0	99.3	6.8	44.5

Source: CIA World Factbook; International Telecommunications Union.

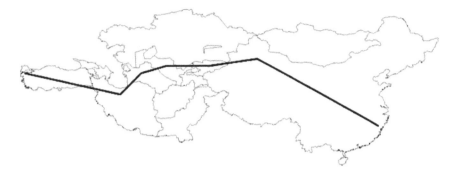

Figure 17.1 The Trans-Asia-Europe (TAE) fiber optics cable.

Source: redrawn from http://www.science-arts.org/Internet/node37.html

services. International satellite services such as Intelsat, Eutelsat, and AsiaSat offer services to Central Asian ISPs. Some governments in the region have taken steps in this direction. For example, in 2006, Kazakhstan launched its own satellite, KazSat, followed by a second in 2009, which lowered the costs of satellite telecommunication services. Private satellite ISPs also serve various Central Asian countries. Such providers include Bentley Walker, with three satellites hovering over the central Eurasian landmass, and GT&T's SkyOne, which offers broadband connections. Other trans-national satellite ISPs include IDM International, Satcom, Skyvision, BusinessCom, and the French firm e-Quai.

In addition to the Internet's infrastructure, government tele-communications policies are important in shaping the contours of Internet access in Central Asia. The neoliberal logic that celebrates markets held that deregulation and privatization would encourage competition, innovation, and risk-taking, lower prices, and improve service quality. Empirically, countries that deregulated their telecommunications markets have tended to have more competition, higher penetration rates, and lower user prices than those that did not. In Central Asia, privatization and deregulation have occurred much more slowly than in most of the world, and are often handicapped by governments fearful of losing control over a vital means of information control. In 2007, the Kazakh operator Kazakhtelecom was the region's first state-owned company to actually offer its shares for sale, but only 4.1 percent have been sold. The Kyrgyz government has gradually liberalized its telecommunications sector, which improved the affordability of Internet access there and made use of cyberspace more attractive and profitable; however, as OpenNet Initiative (2010a) points out, "Kyrgyzstan is an effectively cyber-locked country dependent on purchasing bandwidth from Kazakhstan and Russia." The privatization of the Tajik operator Tochiktelecom began in 2003, but has not advanced much since then. Mongolia has partially privatized Mongol Telecom. Some governments cling to the older model of state-owned telecommunications, such as Afghanistan and Uzbekistan, in which UzbekTelecom retains a legal monopoly status even as it is being privatized. In 2001, following a brief window of privatization that opened with independence in 1991, Turkmenistan granted a monopoly over data services to TurkmenTelecom, driving several smaller ISPs out of business. In such cases, service tends to be poor and prices for dial-up and ISPs are relatively high and certainly out of reach for low income residents.

The number of ISPs varies among Central Asian countries (Table 17.2), ranging in 2008 from 1 in Turkmenistan to 859 in Uzbekistan. These numbers reflect not only varying levels of demand for Internet services and penetration rates, but also the degree to which governments encourage, tolerate, or facilitate competition in this sector. Many ISPs in the region lack international connections and must purchase bandwidth from top-tier national providers. Some ISPs have introduced Internet cards, which have become very popular in cybercafés.

Most Central Asian netizens must rely on dial-up connections, which can be frustratingly slow in an era in which graphical material has become common on the Internet. Broadband, the latest frontier of the digital divide the world over, remains poorly developed in Central Asia. There are enormous variations among Central Asian countries in the availability and cost of broadband services (Table 17.3). The ratio of broadband subscribers per 1,000 people ranged from essentially zero in Tajikistan and Turkmenistan to almost 76 percent in Kazakhstan. These discrepancies can be explained in part by varying national levels of investment in fiber cables. Kazakhtelecom, for example, has invested in a national data transfer system that has reduced transmission prices significantly (ESCAP, 2009). Moreover, the region's telecommunications providers charge vastly different prices for domestic broadband service, ranging from relatively

Table 17.2 Number of Internet service providers in Central Asian countries, 2008

Afghanistan	46
Kazakhstan	105
Kyrgyzstan	38
Mongolia	14
Tajikistan	10
Turkmenistan	1
Uzbekistan	859

Source: OpenNet Initiative.

Table 17.3 Central Asian domestic broadband subscriptions and costs, 2009

	Broadband subscribers per 1,000 people	*Broadband subscription tariff ($US/month)*
Kazakhstan	75.9	17.2
Kyrgyzstan	0.9	48.1
Mongolia	1.8	8.5
Tajikistan	0	363.6
Turkmenistan	—	—
Uzbekistan	9.9	199.5

Source: World Bank, 2011.

low costs in Mongolia and Kazakhstan to Tajikistan's exorbitant fee of $US 363/month, which effectively, and not surprisingly, puts broadband financially out of reach for almost all of the country's residents.

The enormous popularity of mobile or cellular phones is often heralded as a means to overcome the digital divide, especially in developing countries. In Kyrgyzstan, 21 percent of netizens access the Internet using mobile devices (OpenNet Initiative, 2010a). The region also exemplifies the potential of "leap-frogging" old technologies: the Kyrgyz ISP AsiaInfo recently initiated Central Asia's first wireless broadband service in Bishkek. The Afghani government recently contracted with two Chinese firms to build a national wireless network. In Kazakhstan and Mongolia, wireless technologies now allow for the rise of yurt-based Internet access (Davison *et al.*, 2003). However, because most Internet users who access the web via wireless means are already connected, it is unlikely that increasing use of mobile phones and the mobile Internet access they provide will have significant impacts on the Central Asian digital divide.

Central Asian netizens

Data on Internet users for March 2011 were drawn from Internet World Users Statistics (www.Internetworldstats.com); unfortunately, they do not include information on the socio-demographic characteristics of users or their location within countries. As Table 17.4 reveals, the distribution of Internet users among the seven countries included in this analysis varies widely. In total, there were more than 17.7 million Central Asian netizens in December 2011; by far the largest populations of users were found in Uzbekistan (7.5 million) and Kazakhstan (5.5 million). However, like many developing regions in the world, Central Asia has witnessed astronomical rates of growth in Internet access: between 2000 and the end of 2011, the

Table 17.4 Central Asian Internet users and penetration rates

	Total users (000s)		% Growth	Internet Penetration Rate 12/2011	Facebook Subscibers (000s)
	2000	12/2011			
Afghanistan	1.0	1,256	125,500	4.2	198.0
Kazakhstan	70.0	5,449	7,471	35.1	293.0
Kyrgyzstan	51.6	2,194	4,152	39.3	49.8
Mongolia	30.0	355	1,067	11.3	182.6
Tajikistan	2.0	795	34,900	10.4	20.3
Turkmenistan	2.0	80	3,900	2.0	13.0
Uzbekistan	7.5	7,550	100,567	26.8	82.9

Source: http://www.internetworldstats.com

number of users in the region jumped by almost 10,700 percent, more than 50 percent annually. Indeed, the Internet is arguably the fastest diffusing technology in world history. Penetration rates in the region varied widely: some, such as Kyrgyzstan (39.3 percent) and Kazakhstan (35.1 percent) are above the world average of 30.0 percent, whereas in others, such as Afghanistan (4.2 percent), the Internet is a marginal presence at best, or in the case of Turkmenistan (2.0 percent), almost completely absent. Finally, the popularity of Facebook in the region should be noted, with 839,600 people using this popular social networking site (4.7 percent of the region's Internet users).

In a part of the world that does not enjoy particularly high incomes or standards of living, Internet access can be prohibitively expensive. Kapitsa (2008, p. 45), for example, notes that:

> in Kazakhstan, the unlimited dial-up Internet connection package offered by Kazakhtelecom cost about €86 per month, the unlimited ADSL connection – from €102.45 (at 64 Kbps) to €3278.57 (at 2048 Kbps) per month, and the unlimited cable Internet connection – from €9,163.09 (at 3 Mbps) to €24,432 (at 10 Mbps) per month. Taking into consideration that the average monthly salary in Kazakhstan was 292 euros (as of January 2007), it is not surprising that most of Internet users have been accessing the Internet at their workplaces.

Personal computer ownership rates are relatively low in Central Asia (e.g., two per 100 people in Kyrgyzstan in 2009, one in Tajikistan and Uzbekistan).

Because of low rates of computer ownership, and because ISP access charges are often high, many users rely upon privately-owned Internet cafés for access rather than individual accounts. Cafés are particularly important for those who lack dial-up access at home or at work or who simply cannot afford personal computers of their own. In Kyrgyzstan, for example, the majority of Internet users depend on cafés (Privacy International, 2003; Srinivasan and Fish, 2009). In Uzbekistan, roughly 40 percent of users do so from their homes, 40 percent use their place of work, but 30 percent use cybercafés (OpenNet Initiative, 2010c). In Kazakhstan, half of users have Internet access from their homes. In Afghanistan, cybercafés are essentially confined to the airport in Kabul and a few luxury hotels. In Tajikistan, there is a network of 400 cafés which are the dominant points of entry into cyberspace; the average café charges $US 0.73 per hour, compared to the national minimum salary of $US 7.00 per month. However, strict licensing requirements have reduced the number of Tajik cybercafés. In Turkmenistan, private Internet cafés are illegal, although the government monopoly TurkmenTelecom operates 15 cafés in the country (OpenNet Initiative, 2010b). Prices in these cafés in 2007 averaged $US 4/hour (compared to an average income of $US 100/month), although after President Berdymukhamedov reprimanded the Minister of Communications for such high charges they dropped to $US 2/hour. (In 2008 TurkmenTelecom began to offer dial-up home access, but at such high prices that it is unaffordable to most residents). Some assert that high fees are an implicit form of censorship designed to limit Internet access (Lambroschini, 2011). Clark and Gomez (2011, p. 8), however, argue that rather than fees, it is the technical skills of staff that make cybercafés accessible to unskilled users: "In Kazakhstan, while most staff in cybercafés are information technology students and trained in ICT, most public library and telecentre staff have almost no ICT training."

Throughout Central Asia, Internet cafés tend to be clustered in commercial districts frequented by tourists, particularly business districts, hotels, and airports. Cybercafés are also major points of government control over the Internet: those in which customers attempt to access banned websites are routinely closed, and customers who access pornography typically face steep fines. However, as Internet penetration rates climb, including more access at home, the importance of cybercafés is likely to diminish.

Some governments in the region have also promoted the public counterpart to private cybercafés. In Kazakhstan there are 460 public Internet access points, which began in 2006 (Bhuiyan, 2010), and the government has begun to provide free dial-up access in public schools. The Kyrgyz government has established 150 public access Internet centers (OpenNet Initiative, 2010a) and promoted free Internet access through schools, libraries, and even hospitals and prisons. Even Afghanistan has provided a few public tele-kiosks.

As in most of the world, the most active Central Asian netizens tend to be young and well educated, including students, government employees, and those working for large corporations. In Kyrgyzstan, one-half of users are students and 75 percent are under age 30. Ninety percent of Uzbek users have a post-secondary education (Wei and Kolko, 2005). Not surprisingly, it is often elites situated in urban areas who tend to exhibit the highest rates of connectivity. In Uzbekistan, for example, 85 percent of netizens live in urban areas (Wei and Kolko, 2005), 70 percent of whom are concentrated in Tashkent (Privacy International, 2003; OpenNet Initiative, 2010c). In Kyrgyzstan, 77 percent of Internet users are located in Bishkek. In Turkmenistan, 95 percent of users are in the capital, Ashgabat (OpenNet Initiative, 2010b). The minuscule population of Afghani netizens is concentrated in Kabul, Jalalabad, and Khost.

Because Internet penetration rates are low, and users tend to be well educated, often employed by foreign firms, or in touch with Central Asian diasporas elsewhere, the domestic share of Internet traffic in the region tends to be low. In Uzbekistan, for example, 90 percent of the country's Internet flows are international in scope (ESCAP, 2009, p. 7), indicating that the web's use to create or solidify ties among Uzbeks is limited.

In addition to economic, technical, and political obstacles, Central Asian Internet users often face cultural impediments. The widespread deployment of English on the web narrows the participation of those unfamiliar with the language, and English language websites are uncommonly used in Central Asia. As another testimony to the legacy of the Soviet era, Russian often remains the most popular language on the Central Asian Internet, although Russians are a minority people there. Numerous Russian language websites and search engines exist, sometimes comprising the vast majority, which gives a significant advantage to the Russian minority and limits Internet access to non-Russian speakers. Freedom House (2011), for example, found that 94 percent of Kazakh websites were in Russian. Because local language websites are underdeveloped, many users see the Internet as a means of accessing foreign material but as being of limited use in obtaining information about local events. In some countries, i.e., Afghanistan, low literacy rates and restrictive gender roles play a role; Afghani women have the lowest female literacy rates (9 percent) in the world. Even in countries with high literacy, a significant gender gap remains: in Uzbekistan, for example, two-thirds of netizens are male (Wei and Kolko, 2005), and in Tajikistan, more than 77 percent are men.

Censorship and the Central Asian digital divide

Repressive governments often fear the emancipatory potential of cyberspace, which allows individuals to circumvent tightly state-controlled media. Central Asia – whose governments have long been known for authoritarian rule, corruption, political systems that center upon patronage, censorship, and human rights abuses – not surprisingly exhibits numerous attempts to restrict access to the Internet as well as govern its contents. A wide variety of methods are used to restrict and/or regulate Internet access, including applying laws and licenses, content filtering, tapping and surveillance, discriminatory pricing and taxation policies, harassment of bloggers (e.g., via libel laws or invoking national security), hardware and software manipulation, and pervasive self-censorship.

Reporters Without Borders (RWB), an NGO that is the world's leading judge of censorship, ranks the world's governments in terms of the severity of their Internet censorship. Central Asian countries did not fare well by this standard (Table 17.5), with the lowest scores (least censorship) found in Mongolia (23.3) and Tajikistan (32), while Uzbekistan (67.7) and Turkmenistan (107) – one of the most closed countries in the world – ranked as two of RWB's "Internet enemies." Similarly, the OpenNet Initiative regularly conducts tests of filtering of websites in Central Asia and finds frequent, but uneven and often irregular, attempts to hinder access.

McGlinchey and Johnson (2007) studied the divergent censorship paths found in the region and concluded that in Central Asian countries where international aid groups and NGOs provide assistance with the Internet (e.g., infrastructure funding), governments tend to be more permissive and less restrictive about Internet access. They argue (p. 275) that:

> where international NGOs and bilateral and multilateral donors provide capital and assistance in drafting legislation, such as in Kyrgyzstan, Tajikistan, and to a lesser extent Uzbekistan, the formal regulatory framework is more open, clearly articulated, and permissive of electronic media. ....ICT development demands ongoing negotiations with and aid from willing foreign partners. And it is the iterative nature of this relationship that provides Western donors the ability to ensure conditionality—that is substantive reform—in return for ICT aid.

Table 17.5 Reporters Without Borders scores for Central Asian countries, 2009

Afghanistan	54.2
Kazakhstan	49.7
Kyrgyzstan	40.0
Mongolia	23.3
Tajikistan	32.0
Turkmenistan	107.0
Uzbekistan	67.7

Source: Reporters Without Borders, http://www.rsf.org/en-classement1003-2009.html

The Nazarbaev regime in Kazakhstan, for example, which can use its oil and gas revenues to purchase ICT equipment, has received less assistance from foreign organizations and has thus been relatively free to curtail Internet access. Nonetheless, since 2009 Kazakhstan has enacted draconian censorship laws for the Internet and traditional media alike (Lambroschini, 2011) under the Kazakh Agency for Information Technology and Communications. ISPs in the country must retain electronic records of the Internet activities of clients. A Kazakh journalist from the news website kub.kz, Kazis Toguzbayev, was given a two-year prison sentence in 2008 for posting an article accusing the regime of protecting the killers of opposition leader Altynbek Sarsenbayev.

Central Asian Internet censorship takes a variety of forms, and is typically justified through the excuses of protecting public morality from decadent or anti-Islamic ideas or combating terrorism and Islamist extremism. In Afghanistan, Internet usage only began in 2001 following the ouster of the Taliban, which held that the web allowed foreign and anti-Islamic obscenities to enter the country. During the 2005 parliamentary elections, the government of Kyrgyzstan launched "just-in-time" denial of service cyber-attacks against opposition party websites, and the government closed Internet connections to neighboring countries (Schwartz, 2005). The Kyrgyz government's botnet used to launch the attacks also affected servers in the US, whose protests then forced the attacks to cease. Despite its severe control over non-digital media, Kyrgyz cyberspace is relatively deregulated and the government has relatively straightforward rules governing Internet access, which may reflect its reliance on foreign aid organizations (McGlinchey and Johnson, 2007; Srinivasan and Fish, 2009).

Uzbekistan and Turkmenistan, two of RWB's Internet enemies, engage in widespread and systematic Internet censorship. Uzbekistan's government was relatively lenient regarding the Internet until 2004, when it imposed numerous controls in response to Islamist uprisings. In Uzbekistan ISPs must operate under government control, the government's web filter, Uzpak, enjoys a monopoly over international connections, monitors all Internet traffic in the country, and the state often shuts down uzbekistanerk.org and birlik.net, the websites belonging to the largest opposition parties (Privacy International, 2003; OpenNet Initiative, 2010c). Invoking an older Soviet tradition, Uzbek Internet journalists who publish criticisms of the government are occasionally forced into psychiatric hospitals. However, the regime appears to have gradually liberalized its restrictions on the use of ICT in the hopes of obtaining more foreign aid. The dictator of Turkmenistan, Saparmurat Niyazov, strove to keep that country hermetically sealed from the outside world, essentially converting the country's Internet into an intranet, although his successor, Gurbanguly Berdymukhamedov, vowed to open it up to the global Internet. This promise was belied, however, by the presence of government soldiers at the doors of Internet cafés (Eurasianet.org, 2007) and government surveillance of all ISPs using deep packet inspection techniques. As RWB (n.d.) notes, "Opposition websites such as XpoHo.tm and Gundogar, and regional news sites covering Central Asia such as ferghana.ru and eurasianet, are blocked."

A growing community of Central Asian cyber-activists resists these attempts (see EurasiaNet.org). Across Central Asia, netizens have struggled to protect Internet freedoms, including in Uzbekistan (Machleder, 2002), where the Uzbek "For a Free Internet!" campaign has monitored bills in the lower house of parliament, the Mazhlis, which attempted to extend the government's censorship. In Kyrgyzstan, the Internet and other media played an instrumental role in the Tulip Revolution of 2005 that led to the ousting of President Askar Akayev. The Tajik government's attempts to criminalize some forms of cyber-speech as libel against the state were met with heated opposition led by Nuriddin Qarshiboev, head of the National Association for Independent Media in Tajikistan. Moreover, Tajik cyber-journalists petitioned the government to abolish the requirement that the president be called "worthy" and "reliable" every time he was mentioned. More recently, those seeking to avoid government censorship can download software designed to help them do so, such as the Canadian "censorship circumvention" program Psiphon.

The blogosphere has also become an important part of the Internet in Central Asia, giving rise to new forms of participatory journalism and enlarging the sphere of public debate. Kyrgyz bloggers, for example, often see themselves as actively creating a new sphere of civil society through online forums such as Diesel and AkiPress (Srinivasan and Fish, 2009). The Kazakh government has encouraged government officials to create their own personal blogs, but has not been above arresting Internet activists such as Zhanna Baytelova and Irina Mednikova, who protested Kazakhtelecom's blocking of the opposition websites LiveJournal and Respublika (Freedom House, 2011).

Concluding thoughts

Still hampered by the crippling legacy of Soviet rule, Central Asia has been relatively slow to be enfolded into the world's telecommunications networks. Although fiber optic cables and satellite services have become more common, usage in this part of the world remains relatively low, albeit uneven among its constituent countries. Some governments have initiated the necessary steps to rectify this situation, including investments in national data networks, fiber links to schools, and deregulation of state telecommunications monopolies, but progress on this front remains glacial. Broadband technologies, key to using the contemporary Internet effectively, remain in their infancy, in part due to exorbitant charges. As a result, the Central Asian digital divide is changing largely despite the region's governments, not because of them. International diplomatic pressure and foreign NGOs have played a key role in encouraging change.

In total, more than 17 million Central Asians used the Internet in 2011. Penetration rates varied considerably, from 2.0 percent (Turkmenistan) to almost 40 percent (Kyrgyzstan). Particularly notable is the explosive growth in the number of users, however: between 2000 and 2011 the population of Central Asian netizens jumped by 10,300 percent, or roughly 52 percent per year. Because domestic ownership of personal computers is very low, many people – often the majority – rely on cybercafés to access the Internet, although some governments are promoting Internet use in schools and public tele-kiosks. Users in these countries are usually young, almost always well educated, overwhelmingly urban, and predominantly male. While most of Central Asia has achieved universal literacy, low incomes and restrictive gender roles still play a key role in shaping the digital divide. The Russian language is disproportionately reflected in the region's websites while webpages in local languages are underrepresented, adding another obstacle to Internet utilization.

Fearful of democracy and of the Internet's potential to disrupt the power of established elites, most Central Asian governments have actively sought to curtail their residents' ability to log on and to control the contents of the webpages they can access. While none of the governments have refused to interfere, Uzbekistan and Turkmenistan have engaged in the most egregious Internet censorship. Despite these political barriers, in addition to economic ones, the region's Internet users have struggled against censorship, including a small but active blogosphere of cyber-dissidents.

As the Internet gains traction in Central Asia – a process that is occurring with remarkable speed – it is likely to have a wide variety of unanticipated consequences, including the creation of new forms of civil society and new geographies of centrality and peripherality (e.g., virtual Silk Roads). Fears that cyberspace may lead to a cultural homogenization, for example, appear to be unfounded: Wei and Kolko (2005) concluded that far from simply homogenizing cultures, the Internet in Uzbekistan facilitated the expression of local languages and literature. The introduction of e-government to the region may lead to greater transparency and efficiency in the provision of public services. In short, the digital divide in Central Asia, while undergoing rapid change, simultaneously reflects the region's power relations and becomes a vital part in their transformation.

References

Anderson, K. and Pomfret, R. (2004). Spatial inequality and development in Central Asia. Research Paper No. 2004/36: United Nations University World Institute for Development Economics Research.

Bhuiyan, S. (2010). E-government in Kazakhstan: Challenges and its role to development. *Public Organization Review* 10(1), 31–47.

Caselli, F., and Coleman II, W. (2001). Cross-country technology diffusion: The case of computers. *American Economic Review* 91(2), 328–335.

Clark, M. and Gomez, R. (2011). The negligible role of fees as a barrier to public access computing in developing countries. *Electronic Journal of Information Systems in Developing Countries* 46(1), 1–14.

Clarke, G. (2004). The effect of enterprise ownership and foreign competition on Internet diffusion in the transition economies. *Comparative Economic Studies* 46(2), 341–370.

Comin, D. and Hobijn, B. (2004). Cross-country technology adoption: Making the theories face the facts. *Journal of Monetary Economics* 51(1), 39–83.

Compaine, B. (ed.). (2001). *The digital divide: Facing a crisis or creating a myth?* Cambridge, UK: Cambridge University Press.

Cooper, M. and Compaine, B. (eds). (2001). *The digital divide.* Cambridge, MA, US: MIT Press.

Crang, M., Crosbie, T. and Graham, S. (2006). Variable geometries of connection: Urban digital divides and the uses of information technology. *Urban Studies* 43(13), 2551–2570.

Davison, R., Vogel, D., Harris, R., Gricar, J. and Sorrentino, M. (2003). Electronic commerce on the new Silk Road: A cornucopia of research opportunities. http://is2.lse.ac.uk/asp/aspecis/20030040.pdf

ESCAP. (2009). Economic development through improved regional broadband networks: Macro-level study of 4 selected broadband markets in Central Asia. http://www.unescap.org/idd/working%20papers/IDD_TP_09_05_of_WP_7_2_909.pdf

Eurasianet.org. (2007). In Turkmenistan, Internet access comes with soldiers. http://www.eurasianet.org/departments/insight/articles/eav030807.shtml

Falkingham, J. (2005). *The end of the rollercoaster? Growth, inequality and poverty in Central Asia and the Caucasus.* Social Policy and Administration 39(40), *340–360.*

Freedom House (2011). Kazakhstan. http://www.freedomhouse.org/images/File/FotN/Kazakhstan2011.pdf

Kapitsa, L. (2008). Towards a knowledge-based economy – Europe and Central Asia: Internet development and governance. United Nations Economic Commission for Europe Discussion Paper 2008.1. Geneva: UNECE Information Unit. http://mgimo.ru/files/33016/ECE_DP_2008-1.pdf

Keller, W. (2004). International technology diffusion. *Journal of Economic Literature* 42(3), 752–782.

Korupp, S. and Szydlik, M. (2005). Causes and trends of the digital divide. *European Sociological Review* 21, 409–422.

Lambroschini, A. (2011). No Twitter revolt for Central Asia's closed regimes. Physorg.com (Feb. 24). http://www.physorg.com/news/2011-02-twitter-revolt-central-asia-regimes.html

Machleder, J. (2002). Struggle over Internet access developing in Uzbekistan. *Eurasia Insight* March 12, http://www.eurasianet.org/departments/rights/articles/eav031202.shtml

McGlinchey, E. and Johnson, E. (2007). Aiding the Internet in Central Asia. *Democratization* 14(2), 277–288.

Norris, P. (2001). *Digital divide: Civic engagement, information poverty, and the Internet worldwide*. Cambridge, UK: Cambridge University Press.

OpenNet Initiative. (2010a). Kyrgyzstan. http://opennet.net/sites/opennet.net/files/ONI_Kyrgyzstan_2010.pdf

OpenNet Initiative. (2010b). Turkmenistan. http://opennet.net/research/profiles/turkmenistan

OpenNet Initiative. (2010c). Uzbekistan. http://opennet.net/sites/opennet.net/files/ONI_Uzbekistan_2010.pdf

Privacy International. (2003). Uzbekistan. http://www.privacyinternational.org/article.shtml?cmd[347]=x-347-103794

Reporters Without Borders. (n.d.). Turkmenistan. http://en.rsf.org/Internet-enemie-turkmenistan,39772.html

Schwartz, S. (2005). The Kyrgyz take their stand: A democratic revolution in Central Asia? *The Weekly Standard,* April 11, 10(28), 12.

Srinivasan, R. and Fish, A. (2009). Internet authorship: Social and political implications within Kyrgyzstan. *Journal of Computer-Mediated Communication* 14(3), 559–580.

Stevens, D. (2006). *Inequality.com: Money, power and the digital divide*. Oxford, UK: Oneworld Publications.

Warf, B. (2001). Segueways into cyberspace: Multiple geographies of the digital divide. *Environment and Planning B: Planning and Design* 2, 3–19.

Warf, B. (2009). The rapidly evolving geographies of the Eurasian Internet. *Eurasian Geography and Economics* 50(5), 564–580.

Warf, B. (2010). Islam meets cyberspace: Geographies of the Muslim Internet. *Arab World Geographer* 13(3–4), 217–233.

Wei, C. and Kolko, B. (2005). Resistance to globalization: Language and Internet diffusion patterns in Uzbekistan. *New Review of Hypermedia and Multimedia* 11(2), 205–220.

Witte, J. and Mannon, S. (2010). *The Internet and social inequalities*. London: Routledge.

World Bank. (2011). *The little data book on information and communication technology*. http://siteresources.worldbank.org/INFORMATIONANDCOMMUNICATIONANDTECHNOLOGIES/Resources/ICT_Little_Data2011.pdf

18 The double digital divide and social inequality in Asia

Comparative research on Internet cafes in Taiwan, Singapore, Thailand, and the Philippines[1]

Tomohisa Hirata
Kyoto University

Introduction: The double digital divide in Asia

According to statistical data, the proportion of households with the Internet in Asian countries and some other countries in 2008 can be shown as follows.

The percentages of households with the Internet in some "technologically advanced countries" in Asia are higher than or equal to those in technologically advanced countries in other areas. For example, the percentage in the United States in 2008 was 62.5 percent and the average percentage in the five Nordic countries was 82.9 percent. At the same time, household Internet usage in most "technologically developing countries" in Asia is equivalent to that in the rest of the world. In fact, these percentages are similar to those in African countries.

Previous studies on the above situation focused on either the digital divide in each Asian country (Tarohmaru, 2004; Kagami *et al.*, 2004; Kumar, 2006) or that across the whole of Asia (Choi, 2000; Quibria *et al.*, 2002; Evers and Gerke, 2004). Some of them found relationships between the digital divide and social stratification. On the other hand, others revealed no relationship between them. However, there have been no studies that bridge these approaches and their contradictory conclusions.

The purpose of this chapter is to accomplish this task. The term "double digital divide in Asia" in the title of this chapter indicates both the digital divide within each Asian country and that across the whole of Asia.[2]

Methodology: Understanding Asia through the Internet cafe

To fulfill this purpose, I will consider Internet cafes (ICs) in the metropolitan areas of Taiwan, Singapore, Thailand, and the Philippines.

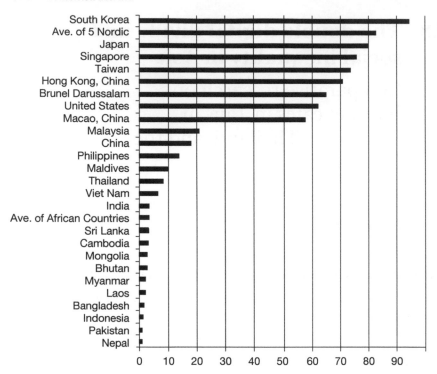

Figure 18.1 The Proportions of Households with the Internet

Note: The median of the proportion of households with the internet in African Countries is 1.5%.

Source: This figure was created by the author from data provided by ITU (2010), Taiwan Network Information Center (2008), and the National Statistical Bureau (2011).

The IC can be defined as a store which offers personal computers (PCs) and Internet access at a relatively low cost to anyone. I will treat the IC as a place where technological "have-nots" who want to use PCs and the Internet can easily become technological "haves," although only temporarily. According to my research on ICs in the above countries, they are used by not only young people, but also international/domestic migrants[3] who are a quintessential example of technological have-nots and are living in the global labor market and international/domestic stratification. Moreover, their uses of ICs are quite limited by their economic, cultural, racial, and political (legal) situations.

By focusing on ICs and their users, I will unravel the relationship between social stratification and the double digital divide in Asia. In my consideration, I will briefly refer to Weberian socio-economic theory of social stratification and some statistical data in each area. However, for the sake of precise description of ICs and their users, I will use an ethnographic approach in most of this chapter like that of Whyte (1993) and Willis (1981). More concretely, I used three empirical approaches in this research, as follows:[4]

1) Mapping ICs: By confirming the disparities in the distribution of ICs in each area, we grasp not only the financial situations and social backgrounds of the technological have-nots but also the social functions of the ICs.

2) A field survey on the efficiency of the PCs, pre-installed software, usage fees, and additional services in the ICs: PCs can vary in efficiency and additional devices which are available in accordance with user's needs. We can presume that the level of PCs in ICs is minimized to reduce the cost of installation and maintenance, while at the same time they are customized to meet most of the main users' needs. We see all the possible uses of the PCs for technological have-nots in their local ICs from this survey.

3) Semi-structured interview research with the shop managers/assistants of the ICs and their customers: Through this research, we confirm the basic attributes of the technological have-nots who are found in surveys 1) and 2) above along with a simple understanding of their life course. We also clarify the functions of ICs and the basic attributes of their managers/assistants through concrete examples.[5]

Thailand: The great barrier of two languages

In 2008, there were at least 500 ICs in Bangkok (National Statistical Office Thailand, 2008), and its total area is approximately 1565 km^2. Almost all ICs use glass panes for their frontage because their front side must be kept transparent by law, for ease of patrolling by police officers who check whether students are skipping their classes to play online games.

In Bangkok, online gaming is a popular use of ICs and this usage relates to one aspect of the distribution of ICs. In suburban places such as On Nut and Wongwian Yai, ICs are spreading. In 2011 they were offering high-end PCs for contemporary online games. Usage fees in this kind of area are from 10 to 20 THB (1 THB = 0.03 USD[6]) per hour and most ICs offer some discount packages for customers staying longer. This tendency can be seen in the vicinity of some universities where there are many young people.

However, the most concentrated area of ICs is in the Khaosan area (one of the most famous backpacker zones in the world) and the second most concentrated area is around BTS Nana station (one of the most famous nightlife spots in Bangkok).

There were 38 ICs in approximately 0.5 km^2 of the central area of Khaosan and the 1.5 km^2 centered on BTS Nana station has 26 ICs. These ICs sometimes double as travel agencies or hostels for foreign travelers and their PCs are low-end, only for viewing webpages, e-mail or social networking services. Their fees are almost exclusively 1 THB per minute, or 10 or 15 THB as the minimum charge.

Let us focus on the common factors of ICs in Bangkok. Almost all their PCs have Microsoft Windows XP English version installed. This fact requires shop managers/assistants to have reasonable English skills to manage the shops. They need to install and modify PCs which have non-native language operating systems and understand the uses of software on offer to customers. According to my research, a fair percentage of shop assistants are university students or have university degrees.

Now, I would like to turn to customers who do not belong to the categories of gaming users and travelers. A, a junior high school student, comes to ICs to do her homework two or three times per week. Ms. B, the mother of A, is from Northern Thailand. After getting married, she had three children including A; however she is now divorced from her husband. Now she manages a Thai noodle stand to cover living expenses. Her income per month is 6,000 THB. Their house rent costs 3,000 THB per month, so it is very difficult for them to buy a second hand laptop because this costs at least 6,000 THB or more in Bangkok.[7]

In contrast, ICs in travelers' areas have another type of customer. They are called "bar girls" in Thailand. Some ICs around BTS Nana station offer extra services for them. One is to resize and upload pictures to websites. And another is to translate e-mails or letters written in the Thai language to English. In a shop, it costs 30 THB per mail or 50 to 70 THB per A4-size letter. The person who translates and uploads them is a shop assistant.

Ms. C, a shop assistant, told me that those letters are mainly "love letters."[8] She works at the IC from 7:00 pm to 4:00 am, from Monday to Friday. She said the characteristics of the customers change at 2:00 am, which is when all the bars close.

Previous studies on bar girls in Thailand have pointed out that they were usually born into very poor families in rural areas and they have often had no chance to gain higher education.[9] Ms. C also told me that almost all bar girls have only graduated from primary school and they have sufficient knowledge of neither English nor PCs.

Moreover, they can hardly go to relatively cheaper ICs in residential areas. Regarding this, one of the reasons which Ms. C explained to me is the bar girls' pride. That is, some of them feel ashamed to be able to use neither English nor PCs. We can easily suppose that it would be more difficult for them to ask shop assistants to help them in residential areas because this implicitly reveals what kind of job they do. At midnight in the Nana area, it is not out of the ordinary for customers to be unable to either use English or PCs.

In the context of the language problem, another barrier to accessing ICs should be mentioned. There are from 1.5 to 2 million[10] migrants from Myanmar in Thailand and most of them are engaged in dirty, difficult, and dangerous low-paid work (Amnesty International, 2005). However I could not find them in ICs in Bangkok and the shop managers/assistants never referred to them as customers of their shops.

From the above discussion it is clear that ICs in Bangkok sometimes play a role in solving social stratification which derives from economic, cultural, and racial factors but sometimes do not. As one significant factor, the language skill required to access PCs and the Internet – English and Thai language – was focused on.

The Philippines: Ubiquitous skills, class and status

Incidentally, the specificity of language as a skill is that it is not only a skill but also that the value of language as a skill is transformed in different cultural contexts. The situation of Metro Manila is an example where this can be seen. As a reference to comprehend the total number of ICs in Metro Manila, let us see the number of ICs which had business permits in 2010 in the cities of Manila, Pasay, and Quezon.

Fourteen hundred twenty-nine shops are located in 218.67 km^2, which is approximately one-third of the total area of Metro Manila (639 km^2). This means ICs are extremely numerous in comparison with Bangkok. All the PCs in ICs in Metro Manila have Windows XP English version installed. The usage fees are from 15 to 30 PHP (1 PHP = 0.02 USD) per hour and some shops offer discount packages.

Table 18.1 ICs in three municipalities in Metro Manila

Municipality (Area)	Classification of ICs by Nature of Business	Sub Total Number of ICs	Total Number of ICs	Average Density of ICs (Shops/km^2)
Manila (38.55 km^2)	Internet Cafe	198	891	23.11
	Computers for Education	203		
	Computer Games	490		
Pasay (19.00 km^2)	Internet Cafe	92	200	10.52
	Computer Rental (and Internet)	108		
Quezon (161.12 km^2)	Internet Cafe	338	338	2.09
Total (218.67 km^2)	—	—	1429	6.53

According to a summary of the 2000 Census of Population and Housing, 81.57 percent of the total household population aged five years old and over can speak English in Metro Manila (National Statistics Office, 2005). So they can use PCs in ICs easily. However, this implies that having English skills is not an advantage over others, but rather a required skill not to drop to a lower segment of society.

In fact, the wages of shop assistants in ICs in Metro Manila are almost the legal minimum wage (426 PHP per day) or lower. In contrast, the average income of IC shop assistants who I interviewed in Bangkok was 8,000 THB per month. This is considerably higher than the minimum wage (215 THB per day) per month in 2011 (Bank of Thailand, 2011, p. 2).

Let us consider the concentrated areas of ICs in Metro Manila. The most concentrated area of ICs is in 2.25 km^2 centered near the University of the East in the City of Manila. This area has 92 ICs, 5 universities and 3 colleges. So, ICs in this area can attract young customers. These areas have two types of ICs. According to Table 18.1, they are divided into "Computers for Education" and "Computer Games." The former mainly offer PCs with relatively low efficiency to students who need to write reports or collect data to get better grades but do not have their own PCs. The latter provide high efficiency PCs for anyone wanting to play online games.

The second most concentrated area is in Pasay City. There are 35 ICs in approximately 1.0 km^2 around LRT Libertad station. In an IC around this station, Ms. D, a shop assistant, told me that there are of course gaming users in this shop, however, some residents in this area do not have their own PCs, and some do not have enough money to pay for Internet access.

This situation is not a rare case in Metro Manila, and these people use ICs for two main purposes. The first one is job hunting. In the above-mentioned IC, some adults write their CVs using PCs sometimes bringing their children, and some use the Internet for job-seeking.

In Weberian theory, classes are defined as "groups of people situated similarly in relation to commodity or labor markets on account of their possession of capital or skills" (Witte and Mannon, 2010, p. 87). According to Weber, "Ownership or non-ownership of material goods or of definite skills constitutes the 'class-situation'" (Weber, 1946, p. 405).

At first this situation fits with that in ICs in Bangkok. However, as we saw, most Filipinos in Metro Manila have English skills to access the Internet and PCs easily. Additionally, ICs accelerate this tendency because they play a role in diminishing the problem of capital possession. As a result, the possession of English skills itself is relatively devalued and this increases the competition in job hunting in Metro Manila compared to some other Asian countries.[14]

Another use of ICs in residential areas is contacting relatives and friends who work in foreign countries using English skills. The total number of overseas Filipinos as of December 2009 is 8,579,378 (Commission on Filipinos Overseas, 2009) and this number is 9.29 percent of the total population (National Statistics Office, 2012) in the Philippines.

Table 18.2 The number of overseas Filipinos by country and their status

Country	Permanent (%)	Temporary (%)	Irregular (%)	Total
Singapore	47,770 (26.22)	64,320 (39.44)	56,000 (36.34)	163,090
Taiwan	8,328 (8.83)	83,070 (88.11)	2,885 (3.06)	94,283
Total	51,098 (19.85)	147,390 (57.27)	58,885 (22.88)	257,373

Source: This figure was created by the author from data provided by the Commission on Filipinos Overseas (2009).

The number of overseas Filipinos and their situation in Singapore and Taiwan are as above. Table 18.2 clearly shows that most Filipinos in both countries are temporary and irregular. But why do they go? The reason why they travel abroad for work is not only to get money in relatively stable positions but also for a chance to improve their and their families' social status in Weberian terms. According to Weber (1946, p. 405), status is "a quality of social honor or lack of it, and is in the main conditioned as well as expressed through a specific style of life."

In my survey, overseas Filipino workers (OFWs) used the term "sacrifice for my family" to describe their situation. Actually almost all of them work abroad in order to earn money to cover their children's school expenses, which are sometimes for tuition fees for private schools. These schools offer a better learning environment but their fees are very expensive for ordinary people.

Status takes shape in stratification which is "rested on honor, or prestige, rather than on economic assets" and in addition, "family background and occupational group" play "an especially important role in distinguishing one's status position and hence, one's lifestyle choices" (Witte and Mannon, 2010, pp. 87–9) in Weberian theory. In this sense, ICs play a role in demonstrating that their status is improving to OFWs and their families. That is, in the precise moment when they and their families use the ICs for communication, ICs provide them with the evidence that the quality of their lifestyle is gradually getting higher. In the following section, we will see some examples of status stratification in the manner of use of ICs in Singapore and Taiwan.

Singapore and Taiwan: Status stratification in migration and childcare

As we saw in the first section, Singapore and Taiwan belong to the group of technologically advanced countries. So, all the shop assistants interviewed in ICs in Singapore and Taipei unanimously said that ICs are decreasing in number. However, ICs do not disappear even in these places.

Or rather, there are still many ICs for migrants. The fees are also very cheap. For example, fees in Singapore are mostly from 0.6 to 2 SGD (1 SGD = 0.78 USD) per hour, and those in Taipei are from 20 to 30 TWD (1 TWD = 0.03 USD) per hour.

For now, let us confirm the places where OFWs come together in these cities.[11] Lucky Plaza is a big shopping mall in Singapore where there are many OFWs. It has eight ICs and other shops aimed at OFWs such as money transfer shops and employment agencies. On their holidays, the OFWs use PCs for communicating with their relatives and friends.

Ms. E is from the Northern part of the Philippines. She has worked as a domestic helper in Singapore from 2009. After learning how to use PCs with the help of her employer, she often comes to ICs to communicate with her relatives. However, now she wants to buy her own laptop because in ICs there are sometimes people who complain loudly about the Internet and PCs and it is disturbing.

Regarding this, Ms. F, an OFW and a shop assistant in an IC in that mall, told me that nuisances in her work are complaints from those kinds of customers. However, she also told me with a smile that this job is not too stressful because she does not need to be polite to customers, most of whom are OFWs.

Similarly, there are four ICs in a small building in Taipei City, near which many OFWs come together. Mr. G, an OFW and a shop assistant in an IC in this building, told me that the shop is only for OFWs and therefore it makes money only in their holidays. In fact, its PCs have Windows XP English version installed and an advertisement saying "We Assist Visa to Canada" is shown on the wall. He also said that no customers annoy him because they are all Filipinos.

The above situations can be understood through the relation between class and status in Weberian theory. Weber (1946, p. 405) said that status membership "influences the class-situation in that the style of life required by status groups makes them prefer special kinds of property or gainful pursuits and reject others." Ms. E and Ms. F's thoughts about nuisances are based on their image of the ideal skilled IC user whom every IC user should aim to become. They also apply this ideal to OFWs' use of the IC. However, Ms. F and Mr. G both felt relaxed in their ICs. It is clear that this feeling is derived from the fact that these ICs become places in which mainly OFWs, who belong to the same class when in foreign countries, come together.

In contrast, a few ICs for gaming use are in middle-sized shopping malls in residential areas in Singapore. According to regulations stated by the Singapore government, ICs for gaming use are not allowed "to be set up in HDB residential zones" (Ministry of Home Affairs, 2007). The Housing and Development Board offers public housing (HDB flats) for Singaporean citizens and permanent residents at low cost. I found a few ICs on the first floors of HDB flats for migrants, however one of them had the warning "Online Gaming is strictly not allowed" on the wall.

In Chinatown in Singapore, some young children were playing games in an IC in the late evening. Mr. K, the manager of this shop, told me that almost all their parents are divorced and live in old and cheap HDB flats nearby. These single-parents who need to work a lot at night have neither enough time to care for their children nor enough money to employ housemaids. They do not buy PCs because they think there is no need. All they can do for their children is to give them 10 SGD per day as an allowance. As a result, the children have no choice but to go to ICs because they are all alone in their home and no shops except ICs are open until evening. The regulations only require ICs "not to admit persons below 16 years of age before 6.30 pm on a school day" (Ministry of Home Affairs, 2007).

In Taipei City, the most concentrated area of ICs is around Taipei Railway station and Ximen station, there are 13 ICs in 0.66 km². However, many ICs are in New Taipei City, a suburb of Taipei City. In fact, half of the total number of ICs which had business permits in 2011 (256 shops) in New Taipei City are in five districts near to Taipei City, although the total area of the five districts is only 6.05 percent of the New Taipei City area. These ICs are mostly for gaming use.[12]

In this situation, recently some parents have been using ICs as substitutes for An-qin-bans (Liu and Huang, 2011),[13] a kind of childcare facility for elementary school children. They have also played the role of private tutoring schools and have supported Taiwanese women who work after childbirth. However, their costs are very expensive, from at least 4,000 TWD to, at maximum, 10,000 TWD per month (Fukaya, 2008, p. 196).

So, if parents do not have enough money to pay for An-qin-bans, but they want to give their children a relatively safe space where someone watches over them, it is possible that they let their children go to ICs as a substitute for An-qin-bans. However, from a legal viewpoint, parents cannot use ICs for this purpose in Taiwan. Taking an ordinance enacted in Taipei City as an example, IC managers/assistants "shall not admit people less than fifteen years of age, unless accompanied by parent(s) or guardian(s), into business sites" (Law Regulation Database in Taipei City, 2002).

These two cases show us that some children whose families belong to lower economic groups in Singapore and Taipei City sometimes have no choice but to use PCs and the Internet in ICs. Their parents are trying to keep their status in their own way for example by providing a safe space or a minimum allowance for their children. They seek what is called "good" but this is sometimes incompatible with another "good."

So, we can treat these families as a case of class and status stratification in Weberian theory. Because, especially for the children, their family background imposes IC use on them as a lifestyle as in class. From this viewpoint, we can see Ms. D's situation as a similar case because now she uses PCs only for communicating with her relatives although she has the PC skills to use it for other purposes. Investigating these ICs plays a role in distinguishing those people who can use PCs and the Internet without ICs, from others who have no choice but to use ICs to access these lifestyles.

Conclusions: Rethinking the digital divide in Asia

From the above discussion, we revealed that capital for an educational environment that offers the opportunity to learn something, including the IT skills and the required language skill, is a crucial factor for the digital divide in every case. In this sense, it is true to some degree that, as some previous studies have pointed out, the capital for an educational environment (including private and public environments) is a key factor in solving the problem of the digital divide in Asia.

However, it is also true to some degree that other previous studies have found that the gap of the digital divide in Asia is decreasing (or is expected to in the near future) especially from the viewpoint of capital such as GDP, some of which is used for educational purposes. In fact, ICs in Bangkok and Metro Manila play an important role in diminishing this gap, and it is highly likely that the global labor market accelerates this tendency. As a result, there is a possibility for the migrants and children we saw in the above section to be ignored in these two approaches because they can be treated as having the skills to access PCs and the Internet, and their situation can be regarded as a transition to a "more equal" society.

So our task is to focus on the diversity of choices which is the final goal of education and IT. More concretely, further subjects for research in terms of the double digital divide in Asia will be: 1) to seek ways of broadening peoples' choices for their lives through their current uses of PCs and the Internet, and 2) to consider ways of realizing a society which is open to a diversity of peoples' choices.

References

Amnesty International. (2005). *Thailand: The plight of Burmese migrant workers.* Retrieved May 30, 2012 from http://www.amnesty.org/en/library/asset/ASA39/001/2005/en/7003d6fd-d4e2-11dd-8a23-d58a49c0d652/asa390012005en.pdf

Aoyama, K. (2009). *Thai migrant sex workers: From modernisation to globalisation.* New York: Palgrave Macmillan

Bank of Thailand. (2011). *Inflation report July 2011.* Retrieved May 30, 2012 from http://www.bot.or.th/Thai/PressAndSpeeches/Press/News2554/n2654e.pdf

Burrell, J. and Anderson, K. (2008). "I have great desires to look beyond my world:" Trajectories of information and communication technology use among Ghanaians living abroad/ *New Media & Society* 10(2), 203–224.

Chen, W. and Wellman, B. (2004). The global digital divide – within and between countries. *IT & Society,* 1(7), 39–45.

Choi, B. (2000). *Digital divide in the APEC: Myth, realities and a way forward.* Seoul: Korea Institute for International Economic Policy.

Commission on Filipinos Overseas. (2009). *Stock estimate of overseas Filipinos as of Dec. 2009.* Retrieved May 30, 2012 from http://www.cfo.gov.ph/pdf/statistics/Stock%202009.pdf

Ehrich, R.S. and Walker, D. (2000). *Hello my big big honey!* San Francisco, CA, U.S.: Last Gasp.

Evers, H-D. and Gerke, S. (2004). *Closing the digital divide: Southeast Asia's path towards a knowledge society,* (Working Papers on Contemporary Asian Studies No. 5). Scania, Sweden: Center for East and South-East Asian Studies, Lund University.

Fukaya, M. (ed.). (2008). *Cross-national survey on child-care anxiety.* Tokyo: Gakubunsha. (in Japanese).

Hongladarom, S. and Entz, A. (2003). *Turning digital divide into digital dividend: Anticipating Thailand's demographic dividend.* Retrieved May 30, 2012 from http://homepage.mac.com/soraj/web/DemDividend.pdf#search='turning digital divide into digital dividend'

International Telecommunication Union, (ITU). (2010). *Measuring the information society.* Geneva: Place des Nations.

Kagami, M., Tsuji, M. and Giovanni, E. (eds.). (2004). *Information technology policy and the digital divide: Lessons for developing countries.* Northampton, MA, U.S.: Edward Elgar.

Kumar, D. (2006). *Information technology and social change: A study of the digital divide in India.* Jaipur, India: Rawat Publications.

Law Regulation Database in Taipei City. (2002). *Taipei Municipal Self-Government Ordinance for Management of Information Leisure Service Providers.* Retrieved May 30, 2012 from http://163.29.36.23/taipei/eng/showmaster.jsp?LawID=E040001-20020425

Liu, Y.Q. and Huang, B.C. (2011, August 18). Internet cafe=An-qin-ban? With meals and games, staff become housemaids. *Ctitv.com.* Retrieved May 30, 2012 from http://www.ctitv.com.tw/news_video_c14v51499.html (in Traditional Chinese).

Ministry of Home Affairs. (2007). *Home team speeches in 12 November 2007.* Retrieved May 30, 2012 from http://www.mha.gov.sg/news_details.aspx?nid=MTE0Mg%3D%3D-Q%2FQO32vXIO4%3D.

National Statistics Bureau. (2011). *Population and housing yearly statistics.* Retrieved May 30, 2012, from http://eng.stat.gov.tw/public/data/dgbas03/bs2/yearbook_eng/y008.pdf

National Statistics Office. (2012). *2010 census and housing population.* Retrieved May 30, 2012 from http://www.census.gov.ph/data/census2010/index.html

National Statistics Office Thailand. (2008). *Results of surveys on Internet services in 2008.* Retrieved May 30, 2012 from http://service.nso.go.th/nso/nsopublish/service/survey/interCafeRep_51.pdf (in Thai language)

National Statistics Office. (2005). Special release No. 153: *Educational characteristics of the Filipinos.* Retrieved May 30, 2012 from http://www.census.gov.ph/data/sectordata/sr05153tx.html.

Quibria, M. G., Ahmed, S. N., Tschang, T. and Reyes-Macasaquit, M-L. (2002) *Digital divide: Determinants and policies with special reference to Asia* (ERD Working Paper Series No. 27). Manila: Asian Development Bank.

Taiwan Network Information Center. (2008). *Network statistics database online search system.* Retrieved May 30, 2012, from http://statistics.twnic.net.tw/item04.htm (in Traditional Chinese).

Tarohmaru, H. (2004). Social stratification and Internet use: Critique of digital divide studies. *Soshioroji*, Vol. 48 (3), 53–66, (in Japanese).

Warf, B. and Vincent, P. (2007). Multiple geographies of the Arab Internet. *Area*, 39(1), 83–96.

Weber, M. (1946). *From Max Weber: Essay in sociology*, Translated by H.H. Gerth and C.W. Mills. New York: Oxford University Press.

Whyte, W.F. (1993). *Street corner society*, 4th Edition, Chicago, U.S.: University of Chicago Press.

Willis, P.E. (1981). *Learning to labor: How working class kids get working class jobs*. New York: Columbia University Press.

Witte, J.C. and Mannon, S.E. (2010). *The Internet and social inequalities*. New York: Routledge.

Notes

1 This work was supported by a JSPS Grant-in-Aid for Research Activity Start-up (21830052) and The Kyoto Erasmus Program: A Program for the Overseas Development of Future Research Project Leadership on Sustainable Social Development in Asia.
2 From the same perspective, Chen and Wellman (2004) discuss the global digital divide in and between the U.S., the U.K., South Korea, Japan, Germany, Italy, China, and Mexico.
3 Regarding international migrants' uses of ICs in Europe and Middle East, see also Burrell and Anderson (2008) and Warf and Vincent (2007).
4 The following surveys have been conducted two or three times in each area by the author. The periods were as follows:
    Taipei: February 13–16, 2010; September 12–27, 2011.
    Singapore: June 1–7, 2010; August 15–19, 2010; August 8–16, 2011.
    Bangkok: February 23–March 1, 2010; July 23–August 8, 2011.
    Metro Manila: March 1–10, 2010; August 16–31, 2011.
5 The number of informants in each city is approximately 20. When conducting daytime interview surveys in each city, I did so with the aid of interpreters.
6 All exchange rates in this chapter are as of May 30, 2011.
7 Regarding the problem of access to computers for children, political moves and plans for solving it repeatedly came to naught because of their insufficient investigation into the socio-economic situation in rural areas in Thailand (Hongladarom and Entz, 2003, pp. 13–6).
8 A similar phenomenon occurred in the previous medium, handwritten letters (Ehrich and Walker, 2000, p. 7).
9 For example, see Aoyama (2009).
10 This number includes temporary and illegal migrants.
11 Especially in Singapore, there are some other concentrated areas of ICs where migrants come together such as Little India (Indian migrants) or Geylang (Chinese migrants).
12 Additionally, some commuters who work at night in Taipei City use ICs for taking a rest.
13 The case to which I refer here is in Takao City, but there are similar cases in Taipei.
14 Regarding this, many informants evaluated the IC as both a good and bad place for children from the viewpoint of ease of access to information. In fact, all ordinances relating to ICs enacted by the above three cities referred to protection from pornography as their purpose.)

19 Dimensions of the mobile divide in Niger

Gado Alzouma
American University of Nigeria

Introduction

The rapid appropriation of information and communication technologies in Africa has sparked an abundant literature centered on the "transformative" character of computers and mobile phone technologies. For many authors (Davison *et al.*, 2000; Steinmueller, 2001; Fleming, 2003; Waverman *et al.*, 2005) ICTs use will enable Africa to achieve leapfrogging development. That is why a number of international organizations and agencies have now placed ICTs at the heart of their development strategies through programs and projects centered on education, health, trade, governance, gender, etc. In recent decades these initiatives have been particularly concerned with the way computers and the Internet can be used to promote and foster both the economic and the social well-being of African communities. However, with the advent of the mobile phone, it is around the possible leveling effect of this technology, that much developmentalist discourse tends now to focus (Hyde-Clarke and van Tonder, 2011). It is argued that the mobile phone, unlike the computer, is ubiquitous, cheap, offers innovative functions (such as the ability to access the Internet), and presents few barriers to adoption by all social strata and classes, including the poorest. More and more scholars and development actors now believe that it will be the use of the mobile phone that will finally reduce, if not eliminate, the digital divide. Authors like Geser note, for example, that "by being adopted, irrespective of education and family background, the cell phone bridges at least some gaps between different social classes" (Geser, 2004, p. 6). For his part Boyera writes: "One of the most promising directions to bridge the Digital Divide is to provide eServices on mobile phones" (2007, p. 1). In those arguments, the underlying assumption is that having or not having the technical object is the main barrier or inequality between users.

In contrast to these statements, this article takes a more cautious approach and argues that the digital divide, as recently emphasized by Witte and Mannon (2010), has many dimensions and should not just be viewed as the sole difference or inequality in terms of physical availability or access to ICTs, particularly the mobile phone. The mere possession of a technical object, including access related to the Internet using that technology, e.g., a mobile phone, does not eliminate inequalities between those who possess it. Multiple levels of access do exist that are closely linked to the position that agents occupy in the social space and that will vary, depending on the degree of economic, social, and cultural resources these agents are endowed with. Using a Bourdieusian framework, this paper identifies some of these inequalities as they exist in Niger. It also explains how differences and inequalities are manifested in both intensity of use and opportunities for use. The paper is partially based on statistics from some international organizations – the International Monetary Fund (IMF), the International Telecommunication Union (ITU), and the United Nations Procurement Division (UNPD) – concerning access to ICTs in Niger. These sources are complemented by a few groups of data collected using semi-structured interviews during the summer of 2011 from rural Nigerien mobile phone users who seasonally migrate to Niamey, the capital city of Niger.

The paper has three main parts. The first presents the sociology of Bourdieu in its relation to the sociology of Weber, in its relation to the concepts of inequality and social class, and the way the "Webero-Bourdieusian" theoretical heritage can be used to explore and explain the digital divide. The paper then presents Niger in the context of the global digital divide with a particular focus on its (the digital divide's) economic dimensions and how the inequalities in terms of access to ICTs and the Internet are manifested at the Nigerien national level. The last part examines the cultural, symbolic, and social dimensions of the digital divide and emphasizes certain aspects that are often not addressed in the literature.

Theoretical framework: From Weber to Bourdieu

The sociology of Bourdieu borrows from Marx, Durkheim, and Weber. However, the Weberian theoretical heritage in Bourdieu's work is more explicit in certain of his texts than in others (Bourdieu, 1971). The Weberian legacy is most evident in Bourdieu on issues of inequality, social class, domination, and the concepts of field and habitus. Bourdieu particularly took up, from Weber, the idea that inequality has an economic dimension (resulting in the existence of social classes), a social dimension (status, in the hierarchical sense of that word, depends on the positions occupied by agents), and a political dimension. These three dimensions are three orders of phenomena or three hierarchies that do not always overlap. For Bourdieu, one can understand them as forms of unevenly distributed resources for the possession of which the members of a society (structured as various fields) are engaged in a permanent struggle. The resources that are available to individuals and groups, the resources they can mobilize, constitute their capital, an economic concept borrowed from Marx that Bourdieu extended to cultural, symbolic, and social aspects, following, in so doing, Weber. The capital presents itself in three forms:

> as *economic capital,* which is immediately and directly convertible into money and may be institutionalized in the forms of property rights; as *cultural capital,* which is convertible, on certain conditions, into economic capital and may be institutionalized in the forms of educational qualifications; and as *social capital,* made up of social obligations ("connections"), which are convertible, in certain conditions, into economic capital and may be institutionalized in the form of a title of nobility (Bourdieu, 1986, p. 242).

The capital, in all its forms, can be accumulated and transmitted from one generation to another just as it can be won or lost over time. This capital inheritance explains the constant reproduction of inequalities over time, and their expansion and reconfiguration, which when combined, give its structure to the society. Thus, Bourdieu states that:

> the structure of the distribution of the different types and subtypes of capital at a given moment in time represents the immanent structure of the social world, i.e., the set of constraints, inscribed in the very reality of that world, which governs its functioning in a durable way, determining the chances of success in practices (1986, p. 241).

What Bourdieu means is that, in all spheres of social activity, agents act under structural constraints and within the limits of the capital they are endowed with, based on the possibilities offered by the position they occupy.

From this perspective, analyzing the digital divide would be tantamount to examining how the differential distribution of capital (under its various forms) is manifested in and governs the access to the Internet in Niger. Therefore, the differences, or more precisely the inequalities which will be discussed in the following text, are not only those existing between the users who have access to the Internet and those who do not have access ("haves" and "have-nots"), namely, those inequalities that exist between countries and between individuals and groups based on the level of their wealth or their income. These inequalities are important, and it is they that will be presented and analyzed in the first instance. However, this paper also focused on differences in position or the inequalities that exist between those users that do have access to the Internet or the mobile phone. Unlike the first (the economic forms of inequality), the latter are understood as being the result of an uneven distribution of both the cultural and the social capital.

Access to the Internet in Niger

With the notable exception of the mobile phone penetration rate of 24.5 mobile phone subscriptions for 100 inhabitants, ICT indicators are very low in Niger. The International Telecommunication Union's 2011 report on ICT development ranks Niger among the two last countries in the world with an ICT Development Index (IDI) of 0.92 in 2010 (ITU, 2011, p.13). That same year (2010), only 1.2 percent of Nigerien households had a computer and only 0.2 percent had access to the Internet.

Because of their high cost, computer ownership, Internet subscriptions as well as traditional forms of access to the Internet (including cybercafés) are out of reach for the vast majority of the Niger population. Indeed, access to the Internet is far more expensive in Niger than it is in most developed countries: "Experts say that this cost is 500 times fold the actual rate in Europe" (Ibrahim, 2007, p. 121). However, it has also been suggested that the effect of the difference on access between countries like Niger and developed countries is mitigated by the multiple means or "locations" of use such as defined and listed by the ITU: "home, work place, place of education, another person's home, community Internet access facility, commercial Internet access facility, any place via a mobile cellular telephone, [and] any place via other mobile access devices" (ITU, 2010, p. 19). Users who use other means or locations are much more numerous than those who access the Internet through a computer they own or those who subscribe to the Internet "by a factor of 2–3 in developed countries and more in developing countries" (World Bank, 2009, p. 159). That is why certain authors (Kwaku and Lemaire, 2006; Boyera, 2007) argue that the nature of the global digital divide could be changed with a wider access to the Internet through mobile phones because access to mobile phones is far higher than access to computers, particularly in developing countries.

Therefore, the inequality between Niger and other countries is far less important when it comes to mobile phone subscriptions (24.53 for 100 inhabitants in 2010) than it is when it comes to Internet access. This difference in the access to the Internet and the access to mobile phones is principally explained by the lower cost of mobile phones compared to computers. Even in a country like Niger, many people who are defined as "poor" have a mobile phone albeit to a lesser extent than those defined as having high income. However, only a tiny minority of the population owns computers, principally because of their cost. Therefore in Niger, like elsewhere in the world, the economic capital is the determinant factor in Internet access and use.

However, as will be seen below, the crude figures that help capture the inequalities in economic capital and thus access to the Internet also hide other important disparities between users. Some of those disparities are for example location (rural/urban) or education, which are often correlated with income but also with the types of technical objects used, the patterns of use. Those disparities are better understood in terms of other elements of Bourdieu's theory, namely social capital and cultural capital.

Dimensions of the digital divide at the national level

The rural-urban divide

In Niger, the first difference between users is the difference that exists between urban users and rural users. Because most telecommunication infrastructure, services, and opportunities to access the Internet are concentrated in the cities, urban residents have a higher opportunity for access to the Internet than rural residents:

> Niger has witnessed a huge telecommunications penetration, particularly as a result of mobile telephony with subscriptions increasing from 57,541 in 2002 to 546,094 in 2006... However, despite this significant increase, 79% of the rural councils (169 councils out of 213) are not covered by fixed telephone or GSM telephony. 84% of the rural councils (178 councils out of 213) are not covered by GSM (IMF, 2008, p. 61).

The rural-urban disparity is, therefore, very high in Niger.

In addition, in Niger, rurality is correlated with poverty, illiteracy, and the general deprivation of populations with respect to the possession of technical objects. For example, if one defines poverty as "a state of individual or collective destitution which places man in a situation of shortage or lack of essential needs" (IMF, 2008, p. 17), the need to communicate could be understood as one of those basic needs. So while general poverty is very high in Niger (affecting 63 percent of the population according to the IMF), it is even higher in the rural areas: 65.7 percent in rural areas and 55.5 percent in urban areas (IMF, 2008, p. 19). It should also be noted that the urban poor live in peripheral areas of the cities "on under-developed plots or lands" (IMF, 2008, p. 20), which lack adequate basic infrastructures and facilities of all sorts, including communication facilities.

Finally, even among those who do have access to ICTs, opportunities to use them, the degree of use and the intensity of use will vary depending on whether one is a rural or urban user. The INS-PNUD survey (2009) shows for example that rural people, unemployed workers, and people with a low level of education use mobile phone less often than do urban dwellers or those with a high/higher level of education. This second group of users also spends much more on their mobile phone than does the other group. The average expenditure in mobile telephony is higher in urban areas than in rural areas. However, while rural people spend less on their mobile phones than do city dwellers, these expenses also account for a larger share of the rural household budgets than for urban household budgets. Among rural people and the poor (in both rural and urban environments), expenditures on mobile phones, although low, weigh more on other expenditures that are essential, such as clothing and food. Therefore, the desire to join the technical universe often produces indebtedness among the members of this group. These differences in expenditures and the effect of expenditures on mobile telephony can further reflect class inequalities that constitute, according to Witte and Mannon, the main dimension of the digital divide: "The most consistent and striking sources of variation were found along the traditional markers of class, namely education and income" (2010, p. 113). Education in general, or what Bourdieu calls cultural capital, is an important dimension of the digital divide in Niger as well.

Mobile phones and illiteracy

According to Bourdieu, "any given cultural competence (e.g., being able to read in a world of illiterates) derives a scarcity value from its position in the distribution of cultural capital and yields profits of distinction for its owner" (1986, p. 243). In the same way that the economic capital is unequally distributed between agents and, therefore, yields different profits and successes (such as differential access to ICTs), literacy, which is a dimension of the cultural capital is also unevenly allocated and yields specific forms of profit. Therefore, the cultural capital (such as higher education), because it can be converted into economic capital, is one means of "appropriating the accumulated and objectively available resources" (Bourdieu, 1986, p. 243), among which are technical objects (cars, televisions, computers, mobile phones, etc.). We should also understand "appropriation" in the sense of "domestication," namely the possibility and opportunity given to different users to master technical objects and use them for their own benefit. Indeed, ICTs are probably the best example of the cultural capital in its "objectified state," in other words the cultural capital as "objectified in material objects and media," or the immaterial (knowledge) made material, tangible. Although the cultural capital is "transmissible in its materiality" (Bourdieu, 1986, p. 243), the possibility to own, appropriate or master advanced technical objects, such as computers (and even, to some extent, own and use mobile phones) still depends on cultural competencies (technical, literacy or educational skills for example) of social agents. Nowhere else is this more obvious or important than in Africa where illiteracy still prevails in large sections of society.

For example in Niger over 60.1 percent of adults cannot read or write (at least in languages used in Western-style or modern education; i.e. French in the case of Niger). These rates are even more important when it comes to gender literacy since 80 percent of women can neither write or read (Macro International, 2007). Illiteracy is thus the biggest barrier to Internet access. It (illiteracy) is an obstacle that cannot be surmounted either by the implementation of cybercafés in rural areas or by free access to multipurpose community tele-centers. As Parkinson says:

> People using computer-related services (in telecentres) tend to have higher levels of education (secondary or above) and often have had some prior exposure to computers through school, work, or are introduced through a friend or family member... telecentres, have not proven a robust method of overcoming the multiple barriers to access that many people face (2005, p. XVII).

It could be added that the possession of new generation mobile phones that certain authors hail as a panacea for Internet access does not remove the illiteracy barrier. It can be seen in the relatively higher degree of access to other information and communication technologies among Nigerien households irrespective of income. For example, neither the cost of radio, nor the cost of television, let alone the cost of a mobile phone, has become a barrier to their possession to the same extent that illiteracy has for overall Internet access. Thus, in 2006, 73.1 percent of urban households and 56.6 percent of rural households in Niger did own a radio; 34.1 percent of urban households and 6.2 percent of rural households had a television, and 6 percent of urban households and 0.7 percent of rural households had a fixed line telephone (Macro International, 2007). Then, it can be said that the main reason for possessing radios, televisions, and telephones is that their users do not need to know how to read and write to use them. However, these same individuals cannot access the Internet if they are illiterate, no matter their economic capital; people may well have the material means to appropriate cultural goods (namely the economic capital) at least relatively as in the case of radios, televisions, and mobile phones, and yet lack the symbolic means (the cultural capital) to access technical goods (computers and the Internet). As Bourdieu says:

> To possess the machines, he (the social agent) only needs economic capital; to appropriate them and use them in accordance with their specific purpose (defined by the cultural capital, of scientific or technical type, incorporated in them), he must have access to embodied cultural capital, either in person or by proxy (1986, p. 243).

By "appropriate," Bourdieu means the capacity, for a social agent endowed with the required skills or technical competencies, to master and use a technical object in accordance with his/her intended goals. These skills and competencies are part of his/her habitus, i.e., the dispositions cultivated in him/her, the know-how (*savoir-faire*).

They (the skills and competencies) have obvious consequences for patterns of mobile phone use. In Africa, most users use the mobile phone only to call and receive calls. While the use of SMS is especially popular among young educated people (Vold Lexander, 2011), it is not so for all users. Those who do not know how to read and write do not use SMS or only rarely use it, often in a limited way. For example, Z, who usually uses intermediaries to read SMS or save names of callers, says:

> I sometimes receive messages but most of the time I receive phone numbers that I have asked for. I know which buttons to press to see the number and save it. Although I am illiterate I know how to read numbers one after the other.

Finally, illiterate people mainly use a mobile phone to maintain contact with family members and for business. These limited uses of the mobile phone principally characterize those users who are weakly endowed with cultural capital (literacy and digital literacy). The lower the cultural capital, the more limited the number of uses. More importantly, in countries like Niger and most African countries, social agents lack, to a certain degree, both economic capital and cultural capital; therefore, the overwhelming majority use mobile phones under that double constraint.

The mobile divide: Poverty, lifestyle, and phone use

"*You have to try, to try, to try...*" In terms of cultural capital, it could be argued that mobile phone ownership and use is part of the lifestyle, which for Bourdieu manifests a set of tastes, beliefs, and practices that characterize a specific social class or a fraction of a social class. The lifestyle is the product of the living conditions which in turn generate a different class habitus:

> Because different conditions of existence produce different habitus... the practices engendered by the different habitus appear as systematic configurations or properties expressing the differences objectively inscribed in conditions of existence in the form of systems of differential deviations which... function as life-style (Bourdieu, 1984, p. 190).

The habitus operates under structural constraints (the capital owned by agents and their position in the field; for example the field of technology consumption) that restrict both possible choices and direct actions. In this respect, it is well known that the mobile phone, at least in its beginning, was a sign of distinction (a status symbol for Katz and Sugiyama, 2006) for some classes and the manifestation of conspicuous consumption in the same way that the ringtone, the mobile phone color, its brand and its functionalities express today personal choices that are widely associated with a certain lifestyle. As a sign of conspicuous consumption, the mobile phone reflects the possession of a certain degree of economic capital and as a sign of social distinction denotes the possession of a particular social and cultural capital.

It is especially evident in societies, such as the Nigerien society, where class differences espouse extreme configurations, with wide gaps (in income) between groups of unequal economic status that the weight of the habitus regarding consumption choices becomes the greatest. This is particularly salient in terms of the ownership of mobile phones whose apparent "democratization" and apparent "levelling effect" (Geser, 2004) conceal in fact deep inequalities.

One of those inequalities (which also marks the ownership of computers) is the kind of device that users own, its level of performance, its condition, and the functionalities it offers. As noted earlier, the new mobile devices (Smartphones) have more advanced features than the ordinary mobile phones do: One can browse the web, as well as access social media and send mail (using SMS). Audio and video functionalities (camera, radio, television and photography) are also available; but these phones are generally more expensive (in Niger they cost a minimum of US$ 50 or one-fifth of the annual income of the average citizen) and only a tiny minority of people can afford them. Indeed, even the cost of the cheapest mobile phone seems prohibitive in terms of the average Nigerien's income: "The price of the cheapest mobile phone... in Niger is equivalent to 12.5 kilograms of millet, enough to feed a household of five for five days" (Aker and Mbiti, 2010, p. 5). This is a first level of inequality since the majority of mobile phone users buy inexpensive and less efficient devices. In addition, 37.6 percent of users say they acquired their phones as a gift (INS-PNUD, 2009), which is some indication of the group's extremely low purchasing power. The devices they own cannot perform most of the functions people in developed countries take for granted:

> Many of the low-end handsets found in the markets and shops in developing countries [have] no browser of any kind and [do not] support GPRS (General Packet Radio Service) or any other form of data transmission... But this is not the only problem. Network coverage in many rural areas lacks data support even if the phones did have it, although this is admittedly changing (Banks, 2008).

Even when the region is covered, rural users are often confronted with a weak signal or absence of signal altogether, depending on where they are located in their villages. One of my interviewees told me that they have to walk outside of their village to be able to make calls or hear calls. Therefore, calls cannot be received or made on a regular basis or at will. They are often "planned ahead of time" or made through individuals in the village who are located near where calls can be received. Calls are also often missed or "cut" (dropped) during conversations and users have to resume the process. As another of my interviewees told me: "You have to try, to try, to try..." thereby underlining the tedious, time-consuming and frustrating aspect of a phone call in some Nigerien rural areas. Along with the cost, this situation has consequences in terms of the quality of the conservations and their length because conversations are most often shorter or halted (Alzouma, 2006, 2008).

For the same reasons, what people use their phones for (call choices) is restricted: "I reduce my calls to the minimum. I only call when it is necessary," says O, a peasant. As for S, he adds: "I am more often called than I make calls myself. In fact I rarely call and when I do so, it is almost always to ring and hang out and have the person I am calling to call me back." Calls are not made on a regular basis: "It could go for days before I call," S says. The INS-PNUD survey notes that "The distribution of the population of phone users by degree of use shows that 63% of them use weakly that communication device, while only 37% report using it frequently in their daily lives" (INS-PNUD 2009, p. 26). Therefore, having a mobile phone does not mean that it is actually used or that it is used as often as one would like. Those who are endowed with low economic capital make calls less often, and when they do so, almost always they have to wait to be called (being at the mercy of their interlocutors) (Alzouma, 2006, 2008; Donner, 2007). In rural areas, they are faced with a lack of electricity and are obliged to resort to various "tricks," such as the use of batteries to recharge their phones (Alzouma, 2008). Their devices remain unused for long hours or even for days. On average, poor households also have a lower number of mobile phones per household than do high income households. Consequently, more individuals in the same household must depend on fewer phones.

Conclusion

As seen in this discussion, the digital divide cannot be solely reduced to unequal access to computers or mobile phones. Even when most people do have a mobile phone, social inequalities (including those inequalities related to the use of that technology) are not suddenly erased by having possession of the technical device. The physical availability of mobile phones is just one dimension of the digital divide. Among many others are also literacy, income, or even level of access and certain structural constraints (location, availability of electricity, affording the calls) within which the use of the technology takes place. Those structural constraints do not affect all users the same way and to the same degree. Depending on how they (the users) are economically, culturally or socially equipped (the volume, structure and distribution of the capital they are endowed with under its diverse forms) to face these constraints, their potential to benefit from the use of technology may be different. Finally, it should be noted that there is interplay between the economic capital, the cultural capital and the social capital. Also, the factors associated with these different forms of capital, namely the rural/urban divide, the differential access to the Internet, and the disparity in cultural/technological competence, play in ways that are so intricate that no statistical analysis or theoretical rendition would be sound enough to capture all the complexity of their interrelations.

References

Alzouma, G. (2006). Social aspects of cell use in Africa. Presentation of the Global Media Research Center, 23 January 2006. Carbondale, US: Southern Illinois University. Retrieved 22 October 2011 from http://mcma.siu.edu/podcasts/GMRC_Alzouma_jan_16_06_PDF.pdf

Alzouma, G. (2008). Everyday use of mobile phones in Niger. *Africa Media Review*, 16, 49–69.

Aker, J. and Mbiti, I.M. (2010). Mobile phones and economic development in Africa. *Journal of Economic Perspectives*, 24, 207–232.

Banks, K. (2008). Mobile phones and the digital divide. *IDG News Service*, 29 July 2008. Retrieved 22 October 2011 from http://www.cio.com/article/439927/Mobile_Phones_and_the_Digital_Divide

Bourdieu, P. (1971). Genèse et structure du champ religieux (*Genesis and structure of the religious field*). *Revue Française de Sociologie*, XII, 295–334.

Bourdieu, P. (1984). *Distinction: A social critique of the judgment of taste*. New York: Routledge.

Bourdieu, P. (1986). The forms of capital. In *Handbook of theory and research for the sociology of education*. New York: Greenwood, 241–258.

Boyera, S. (2007). The mobile web to bridge the digital divide? Paper presented at the IST-Africa Conference 2007, Maputo, Mozambique. Retrieved 4 March 2012 from www.w3.org/2006/12/digital_divide/IST-africa-final.pdf

Davison, R., Vogel, D., Harris, R. and Jones, N. (2000). Technology leapfrogging in developing countries – An inevitable luxury? *The Electronic Journal of Information Systems in Developing Countries*, 1, 1–10.

Donner, J. (2007). The rules of beeping. Exchanging messages via intentional "missed calls" on mobile phones. *Journal of Computer-mediated Communication*, 13, 1–19.

Fleming, S. (2003). The leapfrog effect: Information needs for developing nations. In *Managing globally with information technology*. Hershey, PA, US: Idea Group Publishing, 127–139.

Geser, H. (2004). *Towards a sociological theory of the mobile phone*. University of Zurich. Retrieved 21 October 2011 from http://socio.ch/mobile/t_geser1.pdf

Hyde-Clarke, N. and van Tonder, T. (2011). Revisiting the "leapfrog" debate in light of current trends of mobile phone Internet usage in the Greater Johannesburg area, South Africa. *Journal of African Media Studies*, 3(2), 263–276.

Ibrahim, A.A. (2007). Niger in global information policy. In *Global information policy*. A. Kamal (ed.). Teaneck, NJ, US: Fairleigh Dickinson University, 117–138.

Institut National de la Statistique and Programme des Nations Unies pour le Développement (INS-PNUD). (2009). *Impact de la téléphonie mobile sur les conditions de vie des utilisateurs et des intervenants du marché. Rapport Final*. Niamey, Niger: INS.

International Telecommunication Union (ITU). (2010). *Core ICT indicators 2010*. Geneva, Switzerland: ITU.

International Telecommunication Union (ITU). (2011). *Measuring the information society*. Geneva, Switzerland: ITU.

International Monetary Fund (IMF). (2008). *Niger: Poverty reduction strategy paper*. IMF Country Report No 08/149. Washington DC: IMF.

Katz, J.E. and Sugiyama, S. (2006). Mobile phones as fashion statement: Evidence from student surveys in the US and Japan. *New Media and Society*, 8, 321–337.

Kwaku Kyem, Peter A. and Lemaire, P.K. (2006). Transforming recent gains in the digital divide into digital opportunities: Africa and the boom in mobile phone subscription. *Electronic Journal of Information Systems in Developing Countries*, 28, 1–16.

Macro International. (2007). *Niger: Enquête démographique et de santé et à indicateurs multiples 2006. Rapport de* synthèse. (Demographic and Health Survey – Multiple Cluster Indicators: Synthesized Report). Claverton, Maryland, US: Macro International Inc.

Parkinson, S. (2005). *Telecentres, access and development. Experiences and lessons from Uganda and South Africa*. Bourton-on-Dunsmore, UK: ITDG Publishing; Kampala: Fountain Publishers.

Steinmueller, E. (2001). ICTs and the possibilities for leapfrogging by developing countries. *International Labour Review*, 140, 193–210.

Vold Lexander, K. (2011). *Names U ma puce: Multilingual texting in Senegal*. Working paper presented to the Media Anthropology e-seminar, European Association of Social Anthropologists, 17–31 May 2011. Retrieved 21 October 2011 from http://www.media-anthropology.net/file/lexander_multilingtext.pdf

Waverman, L., Meschi, M. and Fuss, M. (2005). The impact of telecoms on economic growth in developing countries. *Vodafone Policy Paper Series*, No. 2, March 2005. Retrieved 29 October 2011 from http://www.gsmworld.com/documents/L_Waverman_Telecoms_Growth_in_Dev_Countries.pdf

Witte, J.C. and Mannon, S.E. (2010). *The Internet and social inequalities*. New York: Routledge.

World Bank. (2009). *Information and communication technologies for development 2009: Extending reach and increasing impact*. Washington DC: World Bank.

Afterword

Internet freedom, nuanced digital divides, and the Internet craftsman[1]

Sascha D. Meinrath
James Losey
Benjamin Lennett
New America Foundation, Open Technology Institute

The international consensus that communications is a fundamental human right is emerging as we begin to understand the key role that the Internet plays in numerous spheres of social life. In 2010, United Nations Secretary-General, Ban Ki-moon, stressed the importance of access to the Internet and information in his remarks to the General Assembly (United Nations, 2010), and Spain and Finland have elevated broadband access to a legal right (BBC, 2010; Morris, 2009). The economic and democratic potential of Internet connectivity has driven 20 European Union nations and the United States to set goals for universal broadband access (see European Union, n.d.).

However, while most commentators and policy makers have focused on the benefits of broadband and Internet connectivity, two significant dilemmas receive less attention. First, the challenges faced by the unconnected (the "Dark Side of Metcalfe's Law" – see Tongia and Wilson, 2011) remain less explored. While the evolution of communications technologies opens the door for greater equality (making information and knowledge increasingly available to many), history demonstrates that availability alone is insufficient. As telecommunications experts Rahul Tongia and Ernest Wilson (2010) posit, "The more people included within and enjoying the benefits of a network, the more the costs of exclusion grow exponentially to the excluded." A second oft-overlooked fact is that all connectivity is not created equal; in the Internet age, which technologies and devices you use to connect increasingly determine your online opportunities. This differentiation is rapidly creating a more nuanced digital divide that manifests itself, not just in terms of who has access to broadband and who does not, but what users can actually do with their connectivity.

These twenty-first century divides are driven by a worsening trend among communication providers to increasingly lock down networks and devices. The Internet, though predicated on an open, decentralized architecture, is becoming increasingly subject to command-and-control that limits how we communicate. In the coming years, how these new divides are addressed will have far reaching implications that will either fulfill the promise of the Internet as a universal and equal communications medium, or serve to re-enforce existing societal inequities. By highlighting the nuanced nature of today's digital exclusion, this book has drawn attention to new forms of discrimination and dis-empowerment that are becoming hallmarks of the next generation of broadband networking. These problems are surmountable, but only if we understand the nuances and how to address them.

The digital divide has traditionally been defined as a "gap between people with and without Internet access," but DiMaggio *et al.* (2004) stress the importance of the point that "understanding of digital inequality requires placing Internet access in a broader theoretical context." For example, although the U.S. government claims that 95 percent of the population has access to broadband, only 68 percent of all Americans, and less than 50 percent of African-Americans and Hispanics actually use broadband at home (Economics and Statistics Administration and National Telecommunications and Information Administration, 2011). The rural/urban divide is also quite pronounced, with home broadband use at 60 percent in rural communities compared to 70 percent among urban constituencies (ibid.).

Broadband adoption differentials around the globe parallel these findings. The Organization for Economic Cooperation and Development's (OECD) broadband penetration rates (i.e., subscribers per 100 inhabitants) show Denmark leading OECD nations with a penetration rate of 38 percent, followed closely by the Netherlands, Switzerland and Norway (OECD, 2010). The U.S. is ranked fourteenth with a penetration rate of 27 percent (before Finland but lagging behind Germany, the U.K., Canada, Sweden, France, and South Korea, among others) while the broadband penetration in some OECD countries such as Mexico, Chile, and Turkey is as low as 10 subscribers per 100 inhabitants (OECD, 2010). Globally, the International Telecommunication Union estimates that home broadband penetration rates range from 23 percent in the developed world versus 4 percent in developing countries (see Chart 1.4 in International Telecommunications Union, 2010).

The stark difference between *access* and *adoption* is only part of a considerably more complex digital divide ecosystem. A study by the Investigative Reporting Workshop at American University found that the best *values* for broadband were in the affluent areas while poorer areas may pay slightly less, on average, for *significantly* slower broadband speeds (Dunbar, 2011). This divide is even more pronounced when you factor in the fact that actual broadband speeds may be only half of advertised speeds (OfCom, 2011; Federal Communications Commission, 2010).

In addition, the network management practices used by many providers can also inhibit digital freedoms for already disadvantaged communities.

In 2012 a joint study between the Body of European Regulators for Electronic Communications and the Europe Commission (2012) found widespread restrictions on wire-line and wireless broadband connections including slowing speeds and setting data caps. Additionally, restrictions on VoIP and peer-to-peer protocols impact one out of every five subscribers.

These restrictive trends are enabled by several key technological advances. For example, the IP Multimedia Subsystem (IMS), a still-evolving technology primarily used on mobile networks (Waclawsky, 2005) allows a provider to break the open Internet into a closed, small set of differentiated services (e.g., email or voice traffic) and then charge for them on an individual basis. Likewise, Deep Packet Inspection (DPI) technologies allow a network operator to identify, monitor, and restrict access to specific kinds of Internet applications and content. Providers are also interested in using these same DPI technologies to track users and exploit user data for targeted advertising (see Federal Trade Commission [2010, 2011] regarding the "Matter of protecting consumer privacy in an era of rapid change: A proposed framework for businesses and policy makers").

Thus far, only the Dutch government has passed a network neutrality law that would ban restrictive practices on both mobile and wire-line networks (van Beijnum, 2012). Legal scholar, Tim Wu in a review of information technologies of the past hundred years, finds that technology has an unfortunate history of moving from open to closed (2010, p. 6). This devolution poses significant dilemmas for closing the digital divide by creating an unequal hierarchy of digital opportunities and new divides. DiMaggio *et al.* stress that understanding the digital divide requires that we fully understand the benefits a user is able glean though their connectivity (2004). The closed mobile computing space foreshadowed by Harvard Law Professor Jonathan Zittrain in 2008 is now a widespread reality: from restrictions on tablets like the iPad to devices that resist user modification or even render themselves inoperable if legal, though unauthorized, software is detected on them (Lee, 2012; Meredith *et al.*, 2010).

Given current trends, those who can afford to access the Internet through a higher speed or a more open wire-line connection will have considerable advantages over users that can only afford more limited and restricted wire-line or mobile connectivity. As providers further limit user freedom, the promise of the Internet and broadband as a resource for economic and societal empowerment, especially for society's least advantaged, will go unfulfilled.

New York University professor, Richard Sennett, posits that craftsmanship, whether of a new cabinet or a new media, is a "basic human impulse, the desire to do a job well for its own sake" (2008, p. 9). The ability to localize, improve, question, and explore the tools we use is an important facet of being human. Early Internet adopters, in addition to possessing certain technical skills, were empowered to fundamentally shape the medium, acting as *Internet craftsmen* to build, improve, and innovate the technology.

As this volume documents, Internet service providers (ISPs) are moving away from open and participatory architecture and systematically erasing these freedoms and opportunities. Today, ISPs are focusing on locking down every facet of their networks, designing systems that prioritize consumption not creation, and creating barriers to user-driven communications, adaptations, and innovations. Metcalfe's law assumes that a new network participant gains the benefits gleaned from the other members of the network. As we are seeing today, however, companies are garnering enormous profits by commoditizing every form of communications possible and the inefficiencies caused by these practices (in terms of lowered information flow, network congestion at centralized monitoring points, greatly decreased innovation at the edges of the network, etc.) are coming at the literal expense of edge users.

However, technologies exist today that would dramatically lower the cost of communications, increase adoption rates, fuel the development of new services and applications, and are synergistic with pre-existing infrastructure. Digital justice advocates should be aware of these emerging technologies and actively support their development and adoption.

Using off-the-shelf Wi-Fi routers with upgraded software, mesh networking facilitates local-to-local communications, allowing individuals to stream video, share local media, and use VoIP for free telephone calls (Meinrath and Pickard, 2009). Current implementations range from covering a few blocks in Detroit, Michigan (Breitbart and Chodoroff, 2010) to covering hundreds of square kilometers in Vienna, Austria (Forlano *et al.*, 2011). The impacts from these networks can be quite extraordinary: "[In] Berlin, a city that has struggled with depopulation, high unemployment and budget deficits since the fall of the Berlin Wall, the community wireless network Freifunk has provided free Internet access to residents who cannot afford commercial services since 2002" (Forlano *et al.*, 2011).

Peer-to-peer networking on mobile handsets creates additional opportunities for edge-user empowerment. In Australia, the Serval Project (see http://www.servalproject.org) has developed mesh networking for cell phones running the Android operating system. Their system allows users to make free voice calls through a local network or, by adding Asterisk or another VoIP gateway, to almost anywhere in the world (Johnston, 2011).

Gnu Radio and the OpenBTS projects are developing alternatives to local mobile networks. OpenBTS created an open-source GSM air interface, enabling users to build their own cell phone networks and provide low-cost or free services (Burgess, 2010). Gnu Radio, a software development toolkit that performs signal processing and permits users to develop software radios using cheap hardware, could put these adaptive networking technologies into the hands of the masses (see http://gnuradio.org/redmine/wiki/gnuradio). Many of these projects are currently collaborating on the development of the Commotion Wireless Project, a free "open-source communication tool that uses mobile phones, computers, and other wireless devices to create decentralized mesh networks" (Commotion Wireless, n.d.).

Yet the trajectory of regulation prevents the implementation of these innovations. For example, spectrum reforms to allow widespread use of cognitive radio technologies (especially shared and opportunistic spectrum access) have been met with hostility by regulators and incumbent telecommunications companies worldwide. Instead, the overarching focus has been on maintaining artificial scarcity through an almost singular focus on spectrum auctions and granting exclusive licenses to a small group of providers. However, as smart radio technologies mature, the gap between technological capabilities and permissible use will increase – a process that will eventually lead to the rise of a generation of "electromagnetic jaywalkers."

Bridging today's digital divides means reforming policies and regulations, but also understanding that Internet craftsmen are digital literacy crusaders that bring new thinking and innovative technologies to the fore. Bridging the digital divide means getting rid of antiquated barriers that prevent the Internet craftsmen and local communities from implementing outside-the-box thinking, but it also means making it illegal to develop new barriers that prevent tinkering and innovations at the edge of the network. Eliminating twenty-first century digital divides means providing the resources and opportunity necessary for anyone to develop innovative infrastructure, new services and applications, and improvements to communications that better meet their own needs and those of their communities. This is the challenge that the next generations of digital justice advocates face and must overcome.

References

BBC. (2010, July 1). Finland makes broadband a "legal right." BBC, Online at: www.bbc.co.uk/news/10461048.

Body of European Regulators for Electronic Communications. (2012, May 29). A view of traffic management and other practices resulting in restrictions to the open Internet in Europe. Online at: https://ec.europa.eu/digital-agenda/sites/digital-agenda/files/Traffic%20Management%20Investigation%20BEREC_2.pdf

Breitbart, J. and Chodoroff, B. (2010, August) Community wireless mesh prototype in Detroit, MI, U.S. Online at: http://www.newamerica.net/node/34925

Burgess, D.A. (2010, September 25). The man burns in 341 days. *The OpenBTS Chronicles.* Online at: http://openbts.blogspot.com/2010/09/man-burns-in-341-days.html

Commotion Wireless (n.d.). Home. Accessed 2012, October 31. Online at: https://commotionwireless.net/

Dunbar, J. (2011, February 28). Wealthy suburbs get best broadband deals: D.C., rural areas lag behind. Washington, DC: Investigative Reporting Workshop. Online at: http://investigativereportingworkshop.org/connected/story/washington-dc-broadband-speed/

DiMaggio, P., Hargittai, E., Celeste, C. and Shafer, S. (2004). From unequal access to differentiated use: A literature review and agenda for research on the digital divide. In K. Neckerman (ed.). *Social Inequality.* New York: Russell Sage Foundation, 355–400.

Economics and Statistics Administration and National Telecommunications and Information Administration. (2011). Exploring the digital nation. Washington, DC: NTIA. Online at: http://www.ntia.doc.gov/files/ntia/publications/exploring_the_digital_nation_computer_and_internet_use_at_home_11092011.pdf

European Union. (n.d.). Annex 2 – Key targets of national member states broadband strategies. Online at: https://ec.europa.eu/information_society/activities/broadband/docs/annex_2.pdf

Federal Communications Commission. (2010, August). FCC broadband performance OBI technical paper, no. 4. Online at: www.fcc.gov/Daily_Releases/Daily_Business/2010/db0813/DOC-300902A1.pdf

Federal Trade Commission. (2010, February 28). Comments of AT&T Inc. Online at: www.ftc.gov/os/comments/privacyreportframework/00420-58059.pdf

Federal Trade Commission. (2011, February 18). Comments of Verizon and Verizon Wireless. Online at: www.ftc.gov/os/comments/privacyreportframework/00428-58044.pdf

Forlano, L., Powell, A., Shaffer, G. and Lennett, B. (2011, February). From the digital divide to digital excellence: Global best practices to aid development of municipal and community wireless networks in the United States. Online at: http://www.newamerica.net/publications/policy/from_the_digital_divide_to_digital_excellence

International Telecommunications Union. (2010). Measuring the information society 2010. Geneva: International Telecommunications Union. Online at: http://www.itu.int/ITU-D/ict/publications/idi/material/2010/MIS_2010_without_annex_4-e.pdf

Johnston, C. (2011, January 31). Researchers enable mesh WiFi networking for Android smartphones. *Ars Technica.* Online at: http://arstechnica.com/gadgets/news/2011/01/researchers-enable-mesh-wifi-networking-for-android-smartphones.ars

Lee, T.B. (2012, October 26). Jailbreaking now legal under DMCA for smartphones, but not tablets. Online at: http://arstechnica.com/tech-policy/2012/10/jailbreaking-now-legal-under-dmca-for-smartphones-but-not-tablets/

Meinrath, S. and Pickard, V. (2009). The rise of the Intranet Era: Media, research and policy in an age of communications revolution. In K. Howley (ed.). *Globalization and communicative democracy: Community media in the 21st century.* London: Sage Publications. Online at: http://www.newamerica.net/publications/policy/rise_intranet_era

Meredith, D., King, J., Meinrath, S. and Losey, J. (2010, October 13). Mobile devices are increasingly locked down and controlled by the carriers. Washington, DC: New America Foundation, Open Technology Initiative.

Online at: http://oti.newamerica.net/blogposts/2010/mobile_devices_are_increasingly_locked_down_and_controlled_by_the_carriers-38418

Morris, S. (2009, November 17). Spain govt to guarantee legal right to broadband. Online at: http://www.reuters.com/article/2009/11/17/spain-telecoms-idUSLH61554320091117

OECD. (2010, June). Broadband statistics, 1d(3), fixed broadband subscriptions per 100 inhabitants, by technology. Online at: http://www.oecd.org/dataoecd/21/35/39574709.xls

OfCom. (2011, March 2). Average speed is still less than half advertised speed. Press release. Online at: www.media.ofcom.org.uk/2011/03/02/average-broadband-speed-is-still-less-than-half-advertised-speed/

Sennett, R. (2008). *The craftsman.* New Haven, CT, U.S.: Yale University Press.

Tongia, R. and Wilson III, E.J. (2010, March). The dark side of Metcalfe's Law: Multiple and growing costs of network exclusion. Presented at Beyond Broadband Access Workshop, Washington, DC. Online at: http://www.cstep.in/docs/Network%20Exclusion%209-22-09.pdf

Tongia, R. and Wilson, E.J. III. (2011). The flip side of Metcalfe's Law: Multiple and growing costs of network exclusion. *International Journal of Communication* 5, 665–681.

United Nations. (2010, May). Governments must stand up for press freedom. Press release. Online at: http://www.un.org/News/Press/docs/2010/obv875.doc.htm

van Beijnum, I. (2012, May 10). Netherlands becomes world's second "net neutrality" country. Online at: www.arstechnica.com/tech-policy/2012/05/netherlands-becomes-worlds-second-net-neutrality-country/

Waclawsky, J.G. (2005). IMS: A critique of the grand plan. *Business Communications Review,* 35(Oct.), 54–55.

Wu, T. (2010). *The master switch.* New York: Random House.

Note

1 Adapted from *A growing digital divide* by Meinrath, Losey, and Lennett. *IEEE Internet Computing.* July/August 2011.

Index

Locators in **bold** refer to figures/tables

abilities 241; *see also* skill sets (digital)
academic community: *see* higher
  education
access, computer/internet 18, 24,
  110–11, 115; Asia 150–4, **161–2**,
  271–8, **272–5**, 285–94, **286**; benefits
  of 62–4, 113; Central and Eastern
  Europe 189; Egypt 211–12; Estonia
  196–8; global distribution 147;
  importance of 45–7, **46–7**; Israel
  223–4; Japan 88–90, **89–90**; mobile
  89; physical and material 37–40, **39**;
  research questions 57–8, 62–4; role
  in Arab Spring 214–16, **216**; Russia
  119, **120**, **122–3**, 124–8, **125**, **127**;
  South Eastern Europe 170–2; *see also*
  first order digital divide;
  motivation; usage, computer/
  internet
accessing ability 241
activism, online: *see* cyber activism
activities, online: *see* entertainment
  applications; serious applications
adolescents 179–90
adoption (new technology) 58, 91;
  attitudes 226–7; broadband 85–91,
  101–2, 310; China/Taiwan/Hong
  Kong 151–4; European Union (EU)
  64; resources and appropriation
  theory 32–40; S-curve 38–40
advancement, technological: *see*
  development, technological
Afghanistan **274**, **276**, 278
Africa: *see* Niger
age 42, 44–5; Central and Eastern
  Europe **184**, **186–7**; China/Taiwan/
  Hong Kong 155–7, **161–2**; Estonia
  195, **200–1**; Iran 245; Middle

Eastern populations 215; Russia
  126–8, **129**; Taiwan 155; United
  States **81**
agency 201–3
agreeableness 37
alienation 3, 20, 124
alternatives to the internet 45
America, North: *see* United States
American Life Project 43, 71–82
analytical models **184**
analyzing ability 241
anxiety 37, 226–7
appropriation (theoretical
  frameworks) **32**, 32–5, **34**, 112
Arab Spring 8, 209–19, **216**
Arabia 8
arithmetic 238
articulation, double 17
Asia 150–4, 271–8, **272–5**, 285–94,
  286; *see also* Central Asia; China;
  Hong Kong; India; Taiwan
attitudes 55, **184**, 226–7, **231**
auction services **95–8**
Australia **88**, **90**
Austria **88**, **90**
authoritarian regimes 212; *see also*
  censorship, internet

Bahrain 216–17
Balkans 167–77
Bangkok (Thailand) 287–9
BCG e-Intensity Index 119
Belgium **88**, **90**
Big Five (personality dimensions) 37
Blogger 217
Bourdieu, Pierre 55, 194, 298–9, 302
Brahmins 140
Brazil 6, 107–15; *see also* Latin America

BRIC (Brazil, Russia, India and China) 6; *see also* individual countries respectively

broadband: adoption 85–91, 101–2, 310; applications **95–6**, 96–9; definition 91

Bulgaria 7, 179–90, 188

Cairo 209–11, 213, 217

Canada **88, 90**

capital: economic 134, 299; social 17–19, 22–3, 70–1, 79–82, **80–1**, 115

capital, cultural: *see* cultural capital

capitalism 17, 21–6, 147–8, 194

caste system 136–9

Castells, M. 18, 68–9

categorical inequality 29–35, **32**

causality 184

cell phones 300, 302–6, 312–13

censorship, internet 159–60, 311; Central Asia 278–81, **279**; China 217–18; Egypt 216–17; Middle East 216–18; *see also* liberalization

Central and Eastern Europe 179–90

Central Asia 270–1, 281–2; censorship 278–81, **279**; infrastructure and policies 271–5, **272–5**; netizens 275–8, **276**

chances, life: *see* life chances

change, socio-cultural 19–20

childcare 291–4

Chile **88, 90**

China 7, 147–50, 159–60; first order digital divide **153**; internet censorship 217–18; trends in digital access 152, **161–2**

class 3, 20; Brazil 108; caste system (India) 136–9; Estonia 194–5; Max Weber 168–9; Russia 118; United States 68, 224–5

coherence, social 4

Coleman, J. 70

collaboration, online 167–8, 172–7; *see also* cyber activism

communal action: *see* Gemeinschaft

communication skills **41**

Communism 7–8, 193–5, 223; Central Asia 270–1, 281–2; *see also* Estonia

competencies 241; *see also* skill sets (digital)

computer science 172; *see also* science and engineering

confidence 183–90

configuration 17–26

conflict perspectives 134–5, 182, 184, 224–5, 229

connection speed (internet) 60, **272–5**, 276, 310–11; *see also* broadband

conscientiousness 37

consumerism 21, 195

consumption 21, 68, 92–3, **95, 121, 129**; conspicuous 305; Estonia 195; habitus 226; India 137, 142–3; prioritization of 312

content-creation skills **41**

content-related skills 40–1, **41**

craftsmanship 311–12

creating ability 241

cultural capital 18; Brazil 134–5; broadband use 90–1, 93–4, 96, 99, 101–2; Israel 225–6; Niger 299, 302–6

cultural perspectives 137, 196–7, 225–7, 229–34

cultural transition: *see* transition, socio-cultural

cyber activism: Arab Spring 209–19; Central Asia 278–81, **279**

cyber cafés 277, 285–94, **286**

cycle, product 110

Czech Republic **88, 90**

daily internet usage 242–3, **243**, 245–6

data sources 6–10; Brazil 110–11; reliability 43; South Eastern Europe 170–2

democratization 85, 114–15; Middle East 212; Niger 305

demographics: Arab Spring 214; Central Asia 275–8, **276**; theoretical frameworks 29

Denmark **88, 90**

dependency 22

development, technological 18–19, 22–3, 148, 267–8; Africa 297–300, 312; e-social development 115; Far East **161–2**; modernizationism 271; NGOs 279; scholarship 237; subjective poverty 113; United States 67, 224

diachronicity 110

differentiation 309; Central and Eastern Europe 180–4, 188–90; emerging digital differentiation 179–84; Estonia 194–5, 204; theoretical frameworks 19–20, 26, 31 diffusion of technology 35, **39**, 55–6, 110; Central Asia 270–1; Latin America 254–6; normalization vs. stratification models of 38, 148–50

digibetism 196

digital divide: first order 150–4, **153** *see also* access; second order 154–7, **156**, 179–90 *see also* usage; three-tiered model 238

digital era: *see* information age

digital inequality: *see* inequality

digital literacy: *see* media literacy; skill sets

digital natives 180

digital skills: *see* skill sets

digital stratification: *see* stratification

digital technology: *see* information technology

digital usage: *see* usage, computer/ internet

disintegration: *see* integration

dissemination of internet technology: *see* access; diffusion of technology

distance, social 114–15

division of labor 130–1; Durkheim, Emile 4, 108, 118; functionalism 92, 210; Weber, Max 20

The Division of Labor in Society (Durkheim) 118

domestic use of ICT: *see* home use of ICT

double articulation 17

doxa 226

drop-outs: college 141; internet users 36

Durable Inequality 30–1

Durkheim, Emile 1, 4, 20; cyber activism 210, 218; Latin America 108, 253–6, 267–8; Niger 298–9; Russia 130

early adopters 30

Eastern Europe 7–8; Central and Eastern Europe 179–90; South Eastern Europe/Balkans 167–77

economic capital 134, 299

economic transition: *see* transition, socio-cultural

education 42, 44–5, **47**, 172; broadband use 99; Central and Eastern Europe **184**, **186–7**, 189; China/Taiwan/ Hong Kong **161–2**; e-learning **96**, 171; higher **72–4**, 172–6, 237–47;

India 141; Iran (University of Tehran) 237–47; Israel 229; Middle East 215; social policies 113–14; South Eastern Europe 172–6; United States 72–5, **76**, **81**; *see also* students

e-economy 21, 45

effects focus, internet research 62–4

Egypt 8, 211–14, **216**, 216–17

e-learning **96**, 171

elite, information 5, **48**

e-literacy: *see* skill sets (digital)

e-mail 36, 45, 120, **121**, 232, **233**, 288

emerging digital differentiation 179–84

emerging economies 6–7

employee referral programs 142

enablement 119

engagement 119

Engels, Friedrich 20

engineering: *see* science and engineering

entertainment applications 44, 92–9, **121**, 182, 199, 260–1

entrance exams 141–2

environment, information 199–204

equality: definition (internet access) 118–19; relationship to national prosperity 216; *see also* inequality

e-social development 115

Estonia 7–8, **88**, **90**, 193–204

ethnicity 31, **76**, **81**, 270; Estonia 195–7, **198**; Israel 222–34, 229–30; United States 224–5

EU Kids Online 180

EU27 **59**

Eurobarometer surveys **59**, 59–60

European Union (EU) 6, 38, 55–64, **57**, **59**, **61**; *see also* Eastern Europe

evaluating ability 241

exclusion: *see* inclusion/exclusion

extraversion 37

Far East: *see* China; Hong Kong; Taiwan

feminism 270

fiction **95–6**

Finland **88**, **90**

first order digital divide 149–50, 150–4, **153**; *see also* access, computer/internet

flows, information 17–18, 312

formal skills **41**

France **88, 90**
free will 201–3
frequency (internet use) 128–30,
    198–204, 265–8, 301
FSU (former Soviet Union) 7–8, 193–5,
    223
functionalism 92, 118, 210–11, 218–19

gaming 44, 155; Singapore and Taiwan
    292–3; Thailand 287
gaps: knowledge 44, 64, 91, 172–7; sex/
    gender 90, 126; usage 43–5, 154, 157;
    see also digital divide; sex/gender
Geiger, Theodor 55
Gemeinschaft 169, 173
gender: *see* sex/gender
gender gap: *see under* gaps
gender regime 199–200
generalizations 130
Germany 6, 56, **88, 90**, 312
gerontocracy 195
ghettos 24
Gini coefficient **216**
global informational capitalism 17,
    21–6, 147–8, 194
Greece **88, 90**

habitus 55, 194, 226, 312; *see also*
    attitudes
Hargittai, Eszter 42, 61–2, 128, 173–4
health services 63, **95–6**
higher education **72–4**; South Eastern
    Europe 172–6; University of Tehran
    237–47
highly developed countries 6
Hinduism 140
Holland 35–7, 42–7, 182, 311
home use of ICT 310; Brazil 110–11;
    Central and Eastern Europe 182,
    186–7; Central Asia 277; European
    Union 58–60; Israel 225, **229–30**;
    Latin America 256, **258–61**, 265,
    268; Russia **123**
Hong Kong 7, 147–50, 158–9; first
    order digital divide **153**; second
    order digital divide **156**; trends in
    digital access 151–2, **161–2**
Household Download Index 119
household income: *see* income
Hungary 7, **88, 90**, 179–90, 188–9

Iceland **88, 90**
ICT industry (India) 138–9

illegal immigrants 109
illiteracy 109
immigrants 222–3, 228–34, **229–31,
    233**
inclusion/exclusion 23, 26, 47–9, **48**;
    BRIC (Brazil, Russia, India and
    China) 6, 115; China/Taiwan/Hong
    Kong 159; India 140–2; United
    States 69
income 72–5, **76, 81**, 99; China/
    Taiwan/Hong Kong **161–2**;
    diffusion of technology 110; Russia
    124–6
India 7, 134–43
individualism 20–3, 25–6, 29, 124
inequality 17–26, **34**; categorical
    29–35, **32**; durable 30–1; Middle
    East 213–14; network society 47–9,
    48; opportunities and outcomes
    118–21; relational 29–32;
    relationship to national prosperity
    216; *see also* positional inequalities
information age 17, 21–3, 26
information elite 5, **48**
information environment 199–204
information flows 17–18, 312
information skills **41**
information society 21–3; continuum
    vs. two-tiered model 31–2;
    Eurobarometer surveys **59**, 59–60;
    privilege/disadvantage 159–60
information technology 17–22, 35;
    alternatives to the internet 45;
    industry in India 138–9; integration
    in Latin America 256–62, **257–61**;
    mobile phones 300, 302–6, 312–13;
    social shaping of 19–20, 85
informational capitalism 17, 21–3, 26,
    148
informationalism 148
integration (social): Durkheimian
    paradigm 253–6, 266–8; Estonia
    197, 200; Latin America 262, 265
integration of internet technology:
    Central and Eastern Europe 182;
    European Union 62–3; Latin
    America 256–62, **257–61**
intensity (internet use) 128–30,
    198–204, 265–8, 301
inter-generational digital transfer
    172–6, 184, 190
International Telecommunication
    Union (ITU) 147

The Internet and Social Inequalities (Witte & Mannon) 210
internet access: *see* access, computer/internet
internet cafés (ICs) 277, 285–94, **286**
internet censorship: *see* censorship, internet
internet competence: *see* skill sets (digital)
internet content **41**
internet effects research 62–4
internet penetration: *see* access, computer/internet
internet skills: *see* skill sets (digital)
internet use: *see* usage, computer/internet
internet users/non-users 88; Central Asia 275–8, **276**; Estonia 197–8, **198**; European Union 59–63; Netherlands **46**; Russia 126–8; sex/gender of 90, 126; skilled vs non-skilled 247, 277; United States 67–8, 75–82, **76–82**
internetization 193
interpersonal relationships 17–19, 115, 174; *see also* social media
interregional differences in internet coverage (Russia) **123**
Iran 8–9, 237–47
Ireland **88, 90**
Israel 8, **88, 90**, 222–4, 232–4; conflict perspectives 224–5; cultural perspectives 225–6; data and results 228–32, **229–32**
Italy **88, 90**

Japan 6; broadband availability 88–90, **89–90**; broadband policy development **86**, 86–7; cultural capital 90–1; growth of broadband applications 86–7, **87–8**
job hunting 45, 290

Kazakhstan **272**, **274–6**, 277
knowledge gap 44, 64, 91, 172–7
Korea **88, 90**
Kyrgyzstan **272**, 272–5, **274, 276**, 278

labor, division of: *see* division of labor
language barrier 142, 287–9
Latin America 253, 268–9; dissemination of internet technology 254–6; internet

integration 256–62, **257–61**; role of the State 262–8, **263–4, 266**; *see also* Brazil
liberalization 7, 195, 212, 217; *see also* censorship, internet
Lievrouw, Leah 199
life chances 20–1, 24–6; cultural perspectives 68–9; role of the State 109–15
lifestyles 37, 75–9, 93, 134–8, 226, 304–6; *see also* doxa; habitus
literacy 109, 302–4; India 136–7; Iran 238; media 40, 239–41; Middle East 213, **216**; *see also* new literacies
literacy, digital: *see* digital literacy
Luxembourg **88, 90**

Mannon, S. E. 5, 71–2, 137, 148, 193, 202, 210, 215, 224–6, 297–8, 302
marriage 139
Marx, Karl 1–3; Brazil 107–8; Central Asia 270; China/Hong Kong/Taiwan 147–8; Niger 298–9; Russia 130
material access 40
Matthew effect 149, 154, 184, 187–9
MDCs (more developed countries) 6
media literacy 40, 239–41
medical services 63, **95–6**
medium-related skills 40–1, **41**
mentality 55, **184**, 226–7, **231**
methodology 29, 42; Central and Eastern Europe 185; Iran 240–2; Israel 228; Japan 94–6; Russia 128, 130; South Eastern Europe 170
Metro Manila (Phillipines) 289–91
Mexico **88, 90**
Middle East 8–9, 212–14, 218–19; *see also* Afghanistan
migrants 291–4; *see also* immigrants
minority groups 227; Central Asia 278; Estonia 195–7, **198**, 200; Israel 222–34; Middle East 215–16; *see also* ethnicity
mobile internet access 297–8, 312; Brazil 111; India 135; Israel 224; Japan 89; Niger 300, 305–6; Russia **120**
mobile phones 300, 302–6, 312–13
mobility, social 22–3; *see also* social capital
models: analytical **184**; normalization vs. stratification 38, 148–50; path **187**

modernization theory 210
Mongolia **272**, **274**, 275, **276**
monthly internet audience in Russia 119–20
more developed countries (MDCs) 6
Mosco, Vincent 3
motivation 35–7, 91, 101, 226–7
Mubarak, Hosni 209, 211
multicollinearity 185, 228
multi-dimensional approach 18–19, 23–5, 196–7
multimedia literacy 40, 239–41
music downloads 45, 93–9, **95–6**, 260–1

Nadwas, Tweet 209
natives, digital 180
neo-functionalism 118; *see also* functionalism
neo-liberalism 22; Egypt 209–10; Niger 273; *see also* global informational capitalism
net-evaders 36
Netherlands 35–7, 42–7, **88**, **90**, 182, 311
netizens: *see* internet users/non-users
network theory 39
networked individualism 22–3
networked society 21–3, 47–9, **48**, 69
neuroticism 37
New Left 130
new literacies 167–8, 175; *see also* skill sets (digital)
New Zealand **88**, **90**
news services 45, 77–9, **79**
Niger 297–307; internet access 300–6; theoretical frameworks 298–9
Norris, Pippa 213–14
North America: *see* United States
Norway **88**, **90**
numeracy 238

occupation **47**; Asia 291; India 134–43; Israel 229–32; Russia 126–8, **127**
occupational prestige: *see* prestige
OECD (Organization for Economic Cooperation and Development) 7, 87, **88–90**, **263–4**, **266**, 310; *see also* PISA (Programme for International Student Assessment)
OFW (overseas filipino worker) 291–2
omnivorous use 93–4
online activities: *see* entertainment applications; serious applications

online collaboration 167–8, 172–7; *see also* cyber activism
online competencies: *see* skill sets (digital)
online public sphere 8, 19, 26, 167, 173–4; *see also* social media; social networks
online skills: *see* skill sets (digital)
open category (OC) 136–7
openness 37
operational skills **41**
opportunities 118–21
Organization for Economic Cooperation and Development (OECD) 7, 87, **88–90**, **263–4**, **266**, 310; *see also* PISA (Programme for International Student Assessment)
other backward classes (OBCs) 136–7
outcomes 118–21
overseas filipino worker (OFW) 291–2

parental background/education 183–4, **184**
participating ability 241
participation: *see* inclusion/exclusion
path models **184**
patriarchy 271
patterns, consumption: *see* consumption
peer-to-peer networks 312
penetration of information technologies: *see* access, computer/internet
performance tests (digital skills) 41–3
personal inequalities 33
personality characteristics 37
perspectives: conflict 134–5, 182, 184, 224–5, 229; cultural 137, 196–7, 225–7, 229–34; functionalist 92, 118, 210–11, 218–19
Pew Internet and American Life Project 43
Philipines **289**, 289–91, **291**
physical access 37–40
PISA (Programme for International Student Assessment) 253, 260–7
Poland 7, **88**, **90**, 179–90, 189
political alleigances 108
political engagement 21, 85, 209–19, 278–81, **279**
political measures to address inequality: Brazil 112–14; European Union 56–7, **57**; India 143; Latin

America 262–8, **263–4**, **266**; South Eastern Europe 177
Portugal **88**, **90**
positional inequalities 33; European Union (EU) 62; United States 72–5
post-Fordist welfare 23–4
post-socialist transition: *see* Communism; Estonia
poverty 22, **272**, 304–6
power 3–5, 17–25, 30–2, 92, 169; Central Asia 282; conflict perspectives 224; state 219
prestige 3–4, 291; cultural perspectives 225–7; India 137; Israel 225–32; South Eastern Europe 169; *see also* social/socioeconomic status
private use of ICT **186–7**
privilege 218; Brazil 114; Central and Eastern Europe 185–8; Estonia 194–6; European Union 56, 62–4; Far East 148, 158–60; India 136–42; Latin America 258–65; Middle East 8; Russia 130; United States 215
product cycle 110
production, relations of 17–19, 24–5
professors 174–5
Programme for International Student Assessment (PISA) 253, 260–7
programming **41**, 175
The Protestant Ethic and the Spirit of Capitalism (Weber) 69
public policy: *see* political measures to address inequality
public sphere, online 8, 19, 26, 167, 173–4; *see also* social media; social networks
purposes of internet use: *see* entertainment applications; serious applications
Putnam, R. 70

Qatar **216**
questionnaires **46**, 227, 240–2

race: *see* ethnicity
referral, employee 142
regime, gender 199–200
regulation: *see* political measures to address inequality; state, role of
relational inequality 29–32
relations of production 17–19, 24–5
relationships, social 17–19, 70, 115, 174; *see also* social media

research questions **57**, 57–64, 149
residential segregation 223
resources (theoretical frameworks) **32**, 32–5, **34**
'rich get richer' 149, 154, 184, 187–9
The Rise of the Network Society: The Information Age: Economy, Society, and Culture Volume I (Castells) 68–9
Romania 7, 179–90, 188
rural areas: Brazil 110–11; Niger 301–2, 305–6; Russia **129**; Taiwan 151; United States 75, 77
Russia 6, 118–31, 193–5
Russian Federal State Statistics Service Household Budget Survey 6, 118
Russia Longitudinal Monitoring Survey (RLMS) 126

safety skills 183
satellite internet 272–3
saturation (diffusion of ICT) 38–9; European Union (EU) 56; Taiwan 149, 151
Saudi Arabia **216**, 217–18
scheduled castes (SCs) 136–42
scheduled tribes (STs) 136–42
scholarship 1–5, **57**, 130, 149, 310
schools **125**; Asia 151–2, **161**; Brazil 111–14; India 136, 142; *see also* higher education
science and engineering 141–3, 172
S-curve (adoption) 38–40
second order digital divide 149–50, 154–7, **156**, 179–90, 237–47; *see also* usage, computer/internet
second world 7–8, 193–5, 223, 270–1, 281–2
Second World War 21–2
SEE (South Eastern Europe) 167–77
segregation 223
self-confidence 183–90
self-efficacy 242–7
Serbia 7, 167–77
serious applications 44–5, 92–3, **121**, 182, 199
sex/gender 30–1, 45, 75, **81**; broadband applications **95–6**, 96–9; Central and Eastern Europe **184**, **186–7**; Central Asia 278; China/Taiwan/ Hong Kong 152–3; Estonia 195, 199; Iran 244–5; Middle East 213; Russia 126–8; Western Society 227
shopping **95–6**, 99

Singapore **291**, 291–4
skill sets (digital) 18, 60–1, **61**; content
    and medium related **41**; Iran 238–9,
    244, 245–7; performance tests 40–3;
    Philippines 289–91; safety 183;
    South Eastern Europe 171; *see also*
    literacy
skilled users 247, 277
Slovak Republic **88, 90**
Slovenia **88, 90**
SME (social media and entertainment
    related internet use) **200–3**, 200–4;
    see also entertainment applications
SNS site 200, **233**; *see also* social media
social capital 17–19, 22–3, 70–1, 79–82,
    80–1, 115
social class: *see* class
social coherence 4
social distance 114–15
social inequality: *see* inequality
social media: Arab Spring 209–19; and
    entertainment related internet use
    200–3, 200–4; South Eastern
    Europe 167–77
social mobility 22–3
social networking sites (SNS) 200, **233**
social networks 17–19, 18, 115, 174
social participation: *see* inclusion/
    exclusion
social policies: *see* political measures to
    address inequality; state, role of
social relationships 17–19, 70, 115, 174;
    see also social media
social shaping of technology 19–20, 85
social stratification: *see* stratification
sociality 168–9, 177
social/socioeconomic status 62, 92;
    Estonia 194–202; Israel 227; Max
    Weber 108, 291; *see also* prestige
socio-cultural change 19–20
sources, data: *see* data sources
South Eastern Europe (SEE) 167–77
Spain **88, 90**
Stände 168–9, 176
state, role of: Brazil 110, 112–14; Latin
    America 262–8, **263–4, 266**; state
    owned broadcasters 212; welfare
    21–5
statistics: data sources 6–10; reliability
    43
status, social: *see* social/socioeconomic
    status
Steinert, H. 23–4

strategic skills **41**
stratification 1–3, 7–11, 86, 92; Central
    and Eastern Europe 182; classical/
    Weberian theory 68, 107–9, 130,
    167–8, 172–7; diffusion of
    technology 38; Estonia 193–204;
    India 136, 140; internet effects
    research 62–4; Iran 246–7; neo-
    functionalism 118; role of the State
    112–14; social status 291–3; United
    States 67
stress 37
students: Central and Eastern Europe
    179–90; Latin America 262–7; SEE
    (South Eastern Europe) 172–6;
    University of Tehran 237–47
surveillance 24
surveys 227, 240–2
Sweden **88, 90**
Switzerland **88, 90**
symbolic capital: *see* cultural capital
Syria **216**, 217–18

Taipei (Taiwan) 291–3
Taiwan 7, 147–50, **291**, 291–4; internet
    access and activities 158, **161–2**;
    second/first order digital divide
    153, 156; trends in digital access
    151
Tajikistan **272**, 275, **276**, 277
teaching professionals 174–5
technological development: *see*
    development, technological
technology, digital/information 17–22,
    35
technophobia 37, 226–7
telematics 109
telephones, mobile 300, 302–6, 312–13
Thailand 287–9
theoretical frameworks 1–5, 17–26,
    298–9; appropriation and resources
    32–5, **34**; BRIC countries 107–15;
    conflict perspectives 134–5, 182,
    184, 224–5, 229; cultural
    perspectives 137, 196–7, 225–7,
    229–34; functionalism 92, 118,
    210–11, 218–19; generalizations 130;
    internet effects research 62–4; Iran
    239–40; modernization theory 210;
    network theory 39; relational
    inequality 29–32; Weberian 168–9
thief nets 214
3G 135

three-tiered model 238
Tilly, Charles 30–1
tipping point 38–9, **39**
training: *see* education
transition, socio-cultural 19–20, 22–3,
    167–77, 193–204, 294
tribes, scheduled (STs) 136–42
Tunisia 212, **216**, 217–18
Turkey **88, 90**
Turkmenistan **272, 274, 276**
Tweet Nadwas 209
21st century literacies: *see* skill sets
    (digital)
Twitterati 209

UCLA Internet Reports 43
unemployment rate: Estonia 195–6;
    Germany 312
United Arab Emirates **216**
United Kingdom **88, 90**
United States 38, 67–8, **88, 90**;
    community types 75–9, **76–9**;
    comparison with Estonia 204;
    cultural perspectives 68–9;
    education and income **72–4**, 72–5,
    81; internet and social capital 70–1,
    79–82, **80–1**
urban areas 77, 110–11, 135; Niger
    301–2; Russia **129**; Taiwan 151
usage, computer/internet 43–5,
    58–60, **59**, 75–82, **78, 80–1**;
    broadband 92–4; China/Taiwan/
    Hong Kong 154–7; Estonia **198**,
    198–204, **200–3**; gap 43–5, 154,
    157; at home 58–60, 110–11, **123**,
    182, **186–7**, 225, **229–30**, 256; Iran

242–3, **243**; private use **186–7**;
    Russia 119, **120**; *see also* access,
    computer/internet; home use of
    ICT; intensity (internet use);
    second order digital divide;
    versatility (internet use)
USSR 193–5; *see also* Russia
Uzbekistan **272, 276**, 277

values: *see* lifestyles
van Deursen, A. 40–4
van Dijk, J. 5, 42–4
versatility (internet use) 198–204

Weber, Max 1, 3–4, 20; Brazil 108;
    Estonia 194; India 134–5; Israel 225;
    Niger 298–9; Russia 130; South
    Eastern Europe 167–9; stratification
    theory 167–8, 172–7
welfare, state 21–5
WI (work and information related
    internet use) **200–3**, 200–4; *see also*
    serious applications
wireless 312
Witte, J. C. 5–6, 71–2, 137, 148, 193,
    202, 210, 215, 224–6, 297–8, 302
word of mouth 77
World War II 21–2

Yemen **216**
youth 195; adolescents 179–90; Latin
    America **258–61**, 258–67; Middle
    East 215; *see also* students

zero-inflated Poisson (ZIP) model
    99–100, **100**